A Traffic of Dead Bodies

A Traffic of Dead Bodies

ANATOMY AND EMBODIED SOCIAL IDENTITY IN
NINETEENTH-CENTURY AMERICA

Michael Sappol

PRINCETON UNIVERSITY PRESS

PRINCETON AND OXFORD

Copyright © 2002 by Princeton University Press
Published by Princeton University Press, 41 William Street,
Princeton, New Jersey 08540
In the United Kingdom: Princeton University Press, 3 Market Place,
Woodstock, Oxfordshire OX20 1SY

Second printing, and first paperback printing, 2004
Paperback ISBN 0-691-11875-2

The Library of Congress has cataloged the cloth edition of this book as follows

Sappol, Michael.
A traffic of dead bodies : anatomy and embodied social identity
in nineteenth-century America / Michael Sappol.
p. cm.
Includes bibliographical references and index.
ISBN 0-691-05925-X
1. Dead–Social aspects–United States–History–19th century.
2. Human anatomy–United States–History–19th century.
3. Human dissection–United States–History–19th century.
4. Body, Human–Social aspects–United States–History–19th century.
I. Title.

RA619 .S37 2001   2001021127

British Library Cataloging-in-Publication Data is available

This book has been composed in Baskerville types

Printed on acid-free paper. ∞

pup.princeton.edu

Printed in the United States of America

3   5   7   9   10   8   6   4   2

To my daughters Nell and Eve,
whose love and playfulness sustained me through the years
of research and writing,
and to the memory of Catherine Low,
who long ago encouraged me to be a historian.

AN IRISHMAN'S IDEA OF A POST-MORTEM.—
During the performance of an autopsy by us, an
Irishman who happened to witness the removal of
the heart and lungs from the body, exclaimed to a
bystander, "Bedad, that's rough. I'd die first,
before I'd let him do it to me."

FILLER ITEM, *MEDICAL RECORD* 12
(6-9-1877): 367

❧ CONTENTS ❧

ACKNOWLEDGMENTS   xi

Introduction   1

1. "The Mysteries of the Dead Body": Death, Embodiment, and
   Social Identity   13

2. "A Genuine Zeal": The Anatomical Era in American Medicine   44

3. "Anatomy Is the Charm": Dissection and Medical Identity in
   Nineteenth-Century America   74

4. "A Traffic of Dead Bodies": The Contested Bioethics of
   Anatomy in Antebellum America   98

5. "Indebted to the Dissecting Knife": Alternative Medicine and
   Anatomical Consensus in Antebellum America   136

6. "The House I Live In": Popular Anatomy and Embodied Social
   Identity in Antebellum America   168

7. "The Foul Altar of a Dissecting Table": Anatomy, Sex, and
   Sensationalist Fiction at Mid-Century   212

8. The Education of Sammy Tubbs: Anatomical Dissection, Minstrelsy,
   and the Technology of Self-Making in Postbellum America   238

9. "Anatomy Out of Gear": Popular Anatomy at the Margins
   in Late Nineteenth-Century America   274

Conclusion   313

NOTES   329

BIBLIOGRAPHY   385

INDEX   423

⋙ ACKNOWLEDGMENTS ⋘

THIS BOOK, a revision of my doctoral dissertation, "The Cultural Politics of Anatomy in Nineteenth-Century America: Death, Dissection, and Embodied Social Identity" (Columbia University, 1997), was written with the sustenance and assistance of many people and institutions. I want especially to thank Elizabeth Blackmar, my dissertation advisor and mentor. She served as an exemplary intellectual and moral presence, and provided emotional support and nurturance at every turn. Her contribution stretches far beyond the dissertation stage of the project. A full accounting of people to whom I am indebted would take up several pages; here, I can only give a partial listing (more names are credited in the endnotes): Dorothee Ahrens; Andrea Balis; Michael Berkowitz; Monique Bourque, Richard Bushman; Steve and Mary DeGenaro; Jim Edmonson; Amy Fairchild; Elizabeth Fee; Deborah Franklin; Sara Gronim; Karen Halttunen; William Helfand, Tim Hickman; Elizabeth Hovey; Jenna Johnson; Thomas LeBien; Marie I. Lovrod; Craig Lowy; Elizabeth Lunbeck; Rebecca MacLennan; Brooks McNamara; A. Deborah Malmud; Regina Morantz-Sanchez; Alice Nash; Mary Northridge; Ruth Peyser; Melissa Ragona; Charles Rosenberg; David Rosner; Nancy Leys Stepan; Anders Stephanson; Paul Theerman; Spencer Turkel; Susan Wells; Michael Zakim; and the members of the Columbia University Dissertation Seminar in American History.

Research librarians and curators played a key role in the making of this study. I want to thank Kathy Davis and the staff of Interlibrary Loan, Butler Library, Columbia University; the staff of the American Antiquarian Society, especially Joanne Chaison and Caroline Sloat, who did so much to make me feel at home; Charles Greifenstein, Jeff Anderson, Chris Stanwood, Kevin P. Crawford, and other staff members of the Library of the College of Physicians of Philadelphia; Gretchen Worden, director of the Mütter Museum, Philadelphia, who shared many wonderful finds and jokes with me; Eric Meyerhoff and Caron Capizzano of the Ehrman Medical Library, New York University Hospital; Richard Wolfe, Thomas Horrocks, and the staff of the Francis A. Countway Library of Medicine, Harvard University Medical College, Boston; the reference librarians of Butler Library and Law Library, Columbia University; Marvin Taylor, Special Collections, Health Sciences Library, Columbia University; the staff of the Massachusetts Historical Society and the Center for the Study of New England History, Boston; Ed Morman, Lois Fischer Black and the staff of the Malloch Reading Room, New York Academy of Medicine; the staff of the books and manuscripts collections of the New-York Historical Society; Steve Greenberg and the staff of the National Library of Medicine.

The research and writing of this book was supported in part by grants from the National Science Foundation, which contributed $5000 toward the cost of research; the Whiting Foundation Dissertation Writing Fellowship; a short-term research fellowship from the American Antiquarian Society, Worcester, MA; a Mellon Short-Term Research Fellowship and a full-year Scholarship-in-Residence from the Francis Clark Wood Institute for the History of Medicine, the Library of the College of Physicians of Philadelphia; a Mellon Short-Term Research Fellowship from the Institute for the Study of New England History, Massachusetts Historical Society, Boston; and a Gilder-Lehrman Fellowship for the Study of American Civilization.

A version of chapter 7 was published as "'The foul altar of a dissecting table': Anatomy, sex and sensationalist fiction in antebellum America," *Transactions & Studies of the College of Physicians of Philadelphia*, ser. 5, 20 (1998): 65–97. A version of chapter 8 was published as "Sammy Tubbs and Dr. Hubbs: anatomical dissection, minstrelsy, and the technology of selfmaking in postbellum America," *Configurations* 4.2 (1996): 131–83.

A Traffic of Dead Bodies

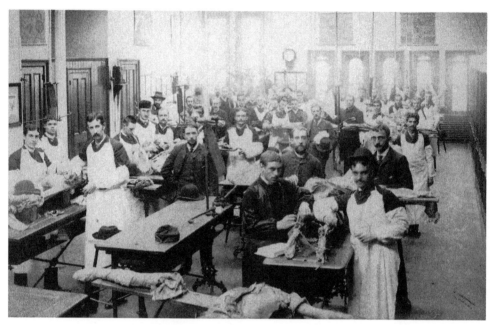

Students in the dissecting hall, Medical College, New York University, 1885. Courtesy of New York University Medical Center Archives.

INTRODUCTION

THIS IS A book about anatomy, about students and cadavers, professors and bodysnatchers, physicians and patients, politicians and the public. This is about riots against medical schools and about the teaching of anatomy in common schools, about laws forbidding medical graverobbery and about laws permitting the requisition of paupers' bodies, and about anatomy books, lectures, and museums for middle-class women, working-class men, and children of every class. This is about how people in the America of centuries past—black and white, male and female, rich and poor, healthy and diseased, living and dead—came, voluntarily and involuntarily, to be "laid bare," "fixed," and "dissected under white eyes."[1] This book is about how the anatomical body became our body.

What follows is a series of interlinked narratives and interpretations about anatomy, death, and the body in late-eighteenth- and nineteenth-century America. My subject is the anatomical acquisition, dissection, and representation of bodies—and how such activities contributed to the making of professional, classed, sexed, racial, national, and speciated selves. "Our social identities, the kind of persons we take ourselves and others to be," philosopher Rom Harré argues, "are closely bound up with the kinds of bodies we believe we have."[2] We all have bodies, *are* bodies, but our vocabulary and grammar of embodiment vary according to location in history and society. On close inspection, the biological *given* turns out to be a cultural accomplishment. Its status as "the real" is part of a historical project, or rather several overlapping, layered projects. At a phenomenological level, who you are depends on what body you are bequeathed, what aspects of that body you take up, how that body is discursively marked, dressed, posed, operated, what languages are used to describe it, what gestures it is permitted—and how such markings, dressings, poses, and gestures are coaxed, compelled, regulated, performed, and received. Like political boundaries, these are often legitimated by a material given: bodies come in different shapes, sizes, colors, and abilities. But the actual drawing of lines, the divisions inside the body, the boundaries between *inside* and *outside*, and between types of bodies—and the constitutional arrangements that govern these internal and external estates—are drawn and redrawn by polite negotiation and *force majeure*, with certain parties empowered to perform border patrol and policing duties. Here and there the lines are set down, with certain things left undecided, out of an impasse or omission or inertia.

Over the course of the nineteenth century, such boundaries were increasingly constructed and contested within the idiom of anatomy. In this cultural poetics, the *dissector*, the generator of meaning, was identified with *mind*; the *dissected*, those whose bodies were appropriated as the medium through which meanings were generated, were identified with *body*. These roles were not freely chosen or strictly assigned, but were assumed or resisted in specific places and ways, by specific actors. Internally the dissector/dissected distinction modeled a divided self. Externally it modeled and staked out divisions between bodies. The anatomist, recruited from the middle and upper echelons of society, served as an iconic representation of *spirit*. The cadaver, conscripted from the ranks of black people, criminals, prostitutes, the Irish, "freaks," manual laborers, indigents, and Indians, served as an iconic representation of *matter*.

A WEB OF PROLIFERATING ANATOMICAL NARRATIVES

Two intersecting matrices form the subject of this study: anatomy's contribution to the making of American professional medical identity; anatomy's contribution to the making of American class identity and the modern self. Medical education in America expanded rapidly in the nineteenth century, from four schools in 1800 to more than 160 in 1900. For the many young men who were seeking to acquire a secure bourgeois identity as well as a livelihood, doctoring was a popular career choice, one that had the advantage of relatively low capital requirements. But, as medicine became a well-traveled avenue of social mobility, the profession was beset by growing pains. From the 1830s onward, medical elites, and would-be elites, periodically worried about the "degradation" of the vastly expanded profession, and decried the poor social and intellectual quality of medical students and practitioners. Even worse, the "regulars" found themselves besieged by competition from alternative sects, who criticized the profession for its social pretensions and unscientific remedies, and who successfully lobbied state legislatures to withold sanctioning legislation and funding.

Under such circumstances, the identification of the profession with anatomy enabled the American profession to invest itself with the authority and prestige of the most advanced European medical science and distinguish itself from midwives, folk healers, the clergy, and other rivals. More than that, it enabled men within the profession to distinguish themselves from the pack of practitioners by virtue of their anatomical acumen and commitments. The American medical profession, following trends in Britain, France, and Germany that dated back to the mid-eighteenth century, became ever more attached to an anatomical understanding of the body and an increasing role for anatomy in the medical curriculum.

Dissection was a potent method of producing and disseminating knowledge—a powerful technology for operating upon the human body—but also a powerful metaphor. Anatomists crossed and mastered the boundary between life and death, cut into the cadaver, reduced it to constituent parts, and framed it with moral commentary. The effect of the dissector's work was to suggest that social, economic, and political practices and categories were natural; the dissector claimed the status of an epistemologically privileged cultural arbiter. "The Scalpel is the highest power to which you can appeal, . . . its revelations are beyond the reach of the cavils and the various opinions of men."[3] And anatomy circulated: anatomical terms, illustrations, instruments, protocols, and narratives served as a bountiful source of images for poets, polemicists, artists, and novelists. The organs of the body have always been laden with ascribed meanings, have always stocked speech and literature with images, but anatomy endowed the parts with elaborate boundaries, names, and topographical details, and set them within a complicated bodily "economy." More than that, the central act of anatomy, dissection, was compelling. Eighteenth- and nineteenth-century wits typically brandished the anatomical metaphor as their most menacing insult, as in John Kearsley, Jr.'s attack on Gerardus Clarkson, printed in a 1774 Philadelphia newspaper: "[I]t truly is your own sanctified Self . . . that I intend to dissect. . . . You have once undergone a muscular Dissection by me, which you have not had Sensibility enough to feel, but now to make you feel, you must undergo a Dissection of the Nervous System."[4]

Such statements suggest the intensity of the powers invested in dissection, powers acquired and experienced (in greater or lesser degree) by every formally educated physician. In dissecting the cadaver, the student penetrated, surveyed, and appropriated the interior of the body—and transformed himself. Anatomical dissection served as the ritual that inducted young men into the cult of medical knowledge; the shared anatomical experience initiated the student into the fraternity of dissectors. Dissection was dangerous and difficult. Its attributes were at once masculine and professional—not permitted to women, who were barred from entering the body (and from entering the profession, until a few breached the barrier in the late 1840s)—and not permitted to members of the public, who were required by long-established custom to respect and safeguard the dead.

Given this funerary obligation, dissectors had difficulties obtaining bodies. Most states allowed executed criminals to be dissected, but not enough people were hanged. The only remaining source of cadavers was the grave. Medical grave robbery ("body snatching" or "resurrectionism") aroused popular anger and revulsion. The unearthing and dissection of bodies was seen as an assault upon the dead and an affront to family and community honor. Between 1785 and 1855, there were at least seventeen anatomy riots in the United States, and numerous minor incidents, affecting nearly every institution of medical learning. Outraged citizens reclaimed their dead, mobbed body snatchers and anatomists, stormed medical colleges, rioted in the streets against militia and police. The distress of the public, and the threat of violence, induced state legislatures to pass laws instituting or increasing statutory penalties for grave robbery. Schools were obliged to close, relocate, or be very circumspect. Availability of anatomical "material" often decided the success of a medical college; many schools had to import bodies from distant sources at great cost.

The opposition to dissection and grave robbery, and the increasing competition for cadavers among schools, spurred anatomists to lobby for legislative relief. Starting with Massachusetts in 1831, states began passing "anatomy acts" which consigned to medical schools the bodies of the "unclaimed" (those without money for burial who died in workhouses, hospitals, and similar institutions). Such measures assured the "respectable" classes that their graves would not be plundered to provision the dissecting table, while providing anatomists with a steady supply of free cadavers, and rescuing the profession from the taint of association with unsavory lower-class body snatchers. Anatomy acts would abolish the "traffic" in bodies, and placate middle-class opponents who associated the body trade with other "skin trades"—slavery and prostitution. At the same time, the anatomy lobby assured taxpayers that dissection of indigents would reduce public expenditures for pauper burials and discourage poor people from seeking public relief. Paupers could posthumously repay their debt to society, it was argued, by acquiescing in the dissection of their bodies; the resultant improvement in medical science and the general quality of medical practice would benefit everyone. To those who charged sacrilege, anatomists replied that popular customs regarding the dead body were based on mere superstition. Neither Christian theology nor science sanctified the dead body; after death, spirit departed, leaving the material residue as the legitimate object of scientific inquiry and appropriation by medical or state authority.

Poor people and middle-class egalitarians were unconvinced. They rejected anatomy acts as ghoulish and undemocratic—a vampirical form of seigneurial privilege. The class basis of such measures was evident. The upper classes were not obligated to contribute their bodies, only the indigent. Incarceration in the almshouse and burial in potter's field already signified social death: anatomy acts added to that the penalty of dissection, hitherto associated only with heinous capital crimes. The dissected body was an effigy, mocked by body snatchers and medical students alike. The dissector was a butcher who reduced the human body to the status of thing, to the condition of "meat." Dissection was a rape of the body, body snatching a rape of the grave. The contrast with the "beautiful deaths" depicted in sentimental fiction could not be greater. The utilitarian ethic of the anatomist ("the uses of the dead to the living"), like the commercial ethic of the body snatcher, violated the sacrosanct boundary separating death from life. Dissectors and body snatchers risked the wrath of the community—a fact that antebellum politicians were keenly aware of.

Agitation for anatomy acts therefore did not at first resolve the conflict, but rather transposed it to legislative arenas where it got tangled up with party and medical politics. In most states, opposition blocked passage. Of five anatomy laws enacted before 1860, three were repealed—and New York's act was passed only in 1854, almost thirty years after it had first been proposed. Given these conditions, local and regional black markets in cadavers flourished. People of all classes tried to protect their bodies from "the surgeons": corpses were buried deeply; graveyard vigils were held; defensive coffins were devised. But the poor had fewer economic, political, and social resources with which to defend their dead: a disproportionate number of anatomical subjects were black, Indian, or Irish.[5]

From 1865 to 1890, the number of medical schools in America doubled. The growing demand for cadavers, in turn, led to a succession of new bodysnatching incidents—people were murdered so that their bodies could be sold to medical schools; the stolen body of a president's son, missing from its crypt, turned up in a college anatomy department. Beset by scandal, anatomists renewed efforts to mobilize political elites and win public support for anatomy legislation—and succeeded. The post-Civil War political climate was conducive to measures that disciplined the "dangerous classes," and that fostered the teaching of anatomy. Advances in medical knowledge and technique—the adoption of anesthesia and antisepsis, and the triumphs of Pasteur and the new microbiology—vindicated reformers' calls for scientific medical education and research, and therefore more dissection. By 1913, of states with medical schools, every state except Alabama, Louisiana, Tennessee, and North Carolina had passed a law permitting medical schools to appropriate the bodies of the indigent poor for dissection.[6] Body-snatching scandals disappeared from the front pages. Anatomical dissection, so fiercely contested for much of the eighteenth and nineteenth centuries, was made invisible, regularized. And so it remains today.

The principal elements of the above narrative—anatomy's role in the production and dissemination of knowledge, its transgressive power as a symbolic act, the corresponding prestige of anatomical authority, the public demand for anatomical healers, but also popular revulsion, resentment, and resistance to the anatomical taking of bodies—are difficult to reconcile. The story is further complicated by the wider diffusion of anatomy, a cultural domain that contemporaries termed "popular anatomy."

In the antebellum era, educators and medical authors began promoting the teaching of anatomy, physiology, and dissection. A knowledge of anatomy, they argued, was needed to educate and morally uplift the northern working class, young women, black people, savages, and American youth. Knowledge of the internal boundaries and functions of the body could be useful as a form of self-discipline—and for radical reformers, empowerment—as well as a scientific legitimation of, and adjunct to, temperance, public hygiene, and other reforms. Anatomical dissection, far from being butchery, was the quintessential epistemology of scientific, "civilized" man, a systematic and careful division and reduction of the material world, a triumph of mind over matter, reason over emotion. Anatomy, it was asserted, provided a geography of embodiment that could produce morally ordered, physiologically self-governed "individuals"—and a morally ordered, physiologically self-governing society.

In this form, anatomy circulated far beyond professional medical discourse and practice. In the late 1830s, popular alternative medical cults, the botanics and homeopaths who had originally defined themselves in opposition to anatomical medical orthodoxy, reversed field and began criticizing regular medicine for being insufficiently anatomical, and for monopolizing anatomical knowledge. Around the same time, the teaching of anatomy and physiology to children became the hobbyhorse of the movement to establish state and municipally supported public education. By 1885, most states outside the South required some teaching of anatomy and physiology in the public schools at both the primary and secondary levels. But anatomy was not merely a matter of reform from above, or even the middle: there was a large market for anatomical discourse, even anatomical spectacles—public lectures on anatomy attracted audiences in the thousands, popular anatomical books attracted readerships in the hundreds of thousands. Many cities had popular anatomical museums whose audiences ranged from respectable citizens to the working-class and immigrant poor. The care and cultivation of this anatomical public was lucrative: anatomical entrepreneurs could make comfortable livings and, in some cases, fortunes.

The political content of their teachings varied. Much of it took the form of a pietistic natural theology, but radical agendas flourished within popular anatomy. The numerous journals of "medical reform," which sprouted across America in the middle decades of the nineteenth century, proclaimed that the provision of anatomy to the public was the critical basis for the democratization of medicine and society. They regularly featured articles on anatomy for their lay readers. In the 1840s, some popular anatomists began arguing that a knowledge of anatomy was emancipatory, especially the anatomy of sexual reproduction. Scientific knowledge of the body would dispel the superstitious and irrational beliefs and customs promulgated by religion, would help to end the cruel and inequitable domination that women suffered at the hands of husbands and fathers, would help to end the enslavement of one human by another. The anatomically conscious individual was rational and self-regulating, and did not require any coercive policing by church, state, race, or family.

But other meanings attached themselves to anatomy, other possibilities. In diffusing so widely, the disciplinary or emancipatory aspects of anatomical discourse inevitably became blurred, subverted, sensationalized, and eroticized. Insofar as the anatomical body became identical with the body, the anatomical body could also stand for the desiring and pleasure-experiencing body. Anatomy could stand for the power of body *over* mind. Thus cultural critics of anatomy, on both the left and the right, recurrently equated embodied reason with calculating desire; and entrepreneurs capitalized on the anatomical body as an incitement of desire. Anatomy was up for grabs. The anatomical scenario of dissector and dissected, of the body and its geography, could be appropriated by free-thinkers and pious believers, by pornographers and social conservatives.

This study, then, seeks to complicate the cultural history of medicine in late-eighteenth- and nineteenth-century America—and the larger cultural history of nineteenth-century America—by telling it from an anatomical perspective. Such an approach has the virtue of illuminating the relation between professional ideals, class formation, and embodied social identity. It provides a novel view of the emerging boundaries of professional medicine and popular culture, one that includes patients, lecture audiences, fiction readers, anatomy rioters, religious healers, folk healers, irregular sects, and factions within the medical profession. Then we can begin to ask: What benefits (social, professional, epistemological, political) accrued to those who identified with anatomical medicine and the anatomical body? What were anatomy's cultural possibilities? What were the costs of remaining outside the anatomical circle?

A SKELETON'S KEY

A Traffic of Dead Bodies follows this sequence: Chapter 1, "'The Mysteries of the Dead Body': Death, Embodiment, and Social Identity," rummages through early modern discourses and practices of embodied personhood, of the living and dead body, to see what cultural domains anatomy arose out of, defined itself in opposition to, competed with, and assimilated. Chapter 2, "'A Genuine Zeal': The Anatomical Era in American Medicine," discusses anatomy as a productive science and an icon of science, an epistemological gold standard that successive waves of medical professionals in late-eighteenth- and nineteenth-century America enthusiastically sought affiliation with. Chapter 3, "'Anatomy Is the Charm': Anatomical Dissection and Medical Identity in Nineteenth-Century America," focuses on the anatomical rituals and performances that were important in the making of American professional medical identity. Chapter 4, "'A Traffic of Dead Bodies': The Contested Bioethics of Anatomy in Antebellum America," discusses the logistical, ethical, and political problems engendered by the anatomical demand for cadavers, and the response of anatomists, contemporary cultural commentators, state legislatures, and communities. Chapter 5, "'Indebted to the Dissecting Knife': Alternative Medicine and Anatomical Consensus in Antebellum America," takes up the case of the alternative medical sects, and shows how, after a season of opposition, they too came to affiliate themselves with anatomy. Chapter 6, "'The House I Live In': Popular Anatomy and Embodied Social Identity in Antebellum America," surveys popular anatomical entrepreneurs, books, and lectures, and analyzes the ideological uses of anatomy in bourgeois self-making discourse and radical cultural politics. Chapter 7, "'The Foul Altar of a Dissecting Table': Anatomy, Sex, and Sensationalist Fiction at Mid-Century," looks at how some mid-century novelists exploited and mocked the anatomical act of dissection, to entertain, titillate, and horrify a large popular readership, and to critique the bourgeois order. Chapter 8, "The Education of Sammy Tubbs: Anatomical Dissection, Minstrelsy, and the Technology of Self-Making in Postbellum America," continues the discussion of the politics of popular anatomy into the 1870s, focusing on Dr. Edward Bliss Foote and his extraordinary series of anatomy and physiology books for children, *Sammy Tubbs the Boy Doctor and Sponsie the Troublesome Monkey*, especially volume 5, the first anatomically explicit sex education book for preadolescent children. Chapter 9, "'Anatomy Out of Gear': Popular Anatomy at the Margins in Late-Nineteenth-Century America," examines the rise and fall of popular anatomical museums, which presented sensationalist and pornographic anatomical displays to an audience largely consisting of working-class men.

Taken together, these chapters are about how the anatomical body became a socially privileged source of the "self," became useful to the discourse and performance of professional medical identity in the era of bourgeois professionalism, and of bourgeois identity in the era of bourgeois hegemony. As staged in sickbeds, medical colleges, professional journals, morgues, public school classrooms, graveyards, legislatures, courtrooms, novels, and newspapers, anatomy was a cultural poetics crafted out of the intersections of mind, body, and spirit, science and superstition, law and desire, order and chaos, human and animal, male and female, white and black, respectability and worthlessness, health and disease, life and death. As the anatomical body, the self was encased firmly within flesh. In this idiom, it was outfitted with an extravagantly detailed interior with anterooms and workspaces and workers, or several layered interiors—corresponding to the structure of a building, or the rise of man from savagery to civilization, or the rise of Homo sapiens from primitive life forms. And, inescapably, anatomy put the body, in whole and part, in dialogue with authoritative medical discourse.

The search for vocabularies that could expressively define, mark, and regulate the bourgeois self was set within a corresponding struggle over the content of that identity, and over who would be eligible to acquire and police it. As is evident from the repeated invocation of the term "bourgeois"—"a very difficult word to use in English," according to Raymond Williams—"class" will be a privileged subject of discussion here.[7] In the past forty years or so, American historians have richly documented the premise that nineteenth-century Americans were obsessively concerned with the notion of social class, and in particular their own class identity. American egalitarianism notwithstanding, people of many different backgrounds—farmers, artisans, petty traders, merchants' clerks, emancipated slaves—were activated by a desire for improved social standing (albeit with much ambivalence) and a new identity. The claimants of this new social identity sought to identify themselves as members of a circle of "respectable," "refined," "cultivated," "modern," "genteel" persons, and were provided with the resources to make such claims by a market of proliferating cultural goods and services. "Gentility," an anonymous antebellum pamphleteer asserted, is "an abstract qualification, the importance of which will be manifest, from the fact, that it is one which Twenty Millions of persons in this country are striving to *attain* and *maintain*."[8] That is, for many Americans there was a compelling goal, to precipitate one's self and family out of the "million" and into a new class of persons, which for the purposes of this study will be denominated "bourgeois," a term of convenience that fuses middle and upper classes, while also setting that group in an ambivalent opposition to both the old-style aristocracy and "the people."

ANATOMY, CLASS, AND SOCIAL PERFORMANCE

> I . . . cohered and received / identity, through my body,
> / Of all that I had, I had / nothing except through my
> body / . . . . what identity I am, I owe / to my body
>
> WALT WHITMAN (*circa* 1855)[9]

This quest for a new social identity, it should be emphasized, was ideological, social, and material. Resources were required to assert and maintain social claims—and courts of local, regional, national, and international public opinion set standards and limits on them. In thinking about class in nineteenth-century America, we should not be led astray by the refusal of social groups to conform strictly to the language of class as it was then deployed, words like "the middle classes," "the labouring classes," "the masses," "the million," "the poor," "the aristocracy," "the best families," "Brahmins," etc. The gaps between such terms indicate not a lack of precision, but rather the ambivalence, subtlety, fluidity, not only of language but of social relations and practices, and also the various social and cultural structures in which they originated. Articulated in a number of different cultural sites, class identity took shape in the form of a *gradient* with *thresholds* and *prerequisites*, albeit variable and contested. Bourgeois identity depended on a genteel vocabulary of manners, domestic servants, fine clothes, the ownership of a carriage, a home furnished with aesthetically pleasing and comfortable furniture, the ability to make "intelligent" conversation, acceptance of one's calling card, etc. Attaining and crossing such thresholds required access to resources, in the form of ownership of the means of production or a certain amount of material wealth, cultural capital, kinship, and professional and local connections. The term "bourgeois" is useful as a shorthand term in demarcating a matrix of such gradients and tying them to a corollary ethos, social vision, and ideology. Bourgeois social identity was not necessarily equivalent to the sociological position of being in the "middle classes"—a group whose members were typically in some anxiety about their ability to sustain and improve upon their performance of gentility, and often troubled by the antidemocratic implications of the project—but also included dominant elites, at one end of the spectrum, and upwardly striving skilled manual laborers, at the other.

What makes matters confusing is that social identities were relational, negotiated, and subject in every domain—including anatomy—to the resignifying vagaries of fashions that continually demanded new costumes, new sets, new manners, new stagings, new performances, new thoughts. Social identity was a moving target. What counted as "civilized" and "respectable" in a backwoods county of Virginia would not suffice in Boston, and what counted as civilized and respectable in Boston might be seen as uppity and pretentious in backwoods Virginia. What counted as civilized and respectable in Boston in 1830 would not suffice in 1860. And, in both places and times, the very desirability of civilization and respectability as markers of social identity counted for more among some people than others, more among women than men, or more among Unitarians than Baptists.

Social identity was performed for a variety of audiences (including an internalized audience), within a large ensemble of actors, and—collectively and individually—was scripted, choreographed, staged. Such audiences were powerful and often highly critical (though some members were more powerful and critical than others). They rewarded good performances and punished bad ones, and kept the actors on their toes by continually revising the meanings of gestures (what signified gentility one year might signify vulgarity the next), continually raising the bar. The word "performance" is used here in the "performative" sense developed by Judith Butler.[10] Performances are not merely theatrical: we are handed scripts (social status, gender, national identity, religious identity, etc.) which we then perform—and revise—according to our placement in, and ability to negotiate, a highly variable constellation of social forces. Social performances always "cite" prior practice, although sometimes such practice is cited negatively (e.g., long hair on men in the 1960s cited negatively the convention that masculine identity was signified by short hair; the rejection of that convention served to establish generational and political identity, and potentially served as the entering wedge for a critique of the entire canon of performances that established masculine identity). "Discourse," then, is used here as a subset of "performance," as a particular category of "speech acts" which serve to inform and articulate the meaning of performances, and make reference to the larger ensemble of performances from which they are derived. Language intentionally and unintentionally informs, but also has material effects. Timothy Lenoir: "We can read not only what language is saying, its content, cause or philosophy . . . we can also read what language is *doing*, its material deployment, the social intervention it is accomplishing."[11]

The mid-nineteenth-century canon of bourgeois identity was meaningful only insofar as it defined itself in opposition to others: wage laborers who worked with their hands, aristocrats, slave owners, animals, savages, etc. At the same time, bourgeois discourse, by its insistence on a universal morality based on productivity and progress, invited working men and women to remake themselves in the bourgeois image. Such invitations were not always made in good faith and the responses of working-class people were varied and complicated—but some accepted the invitation and adopted (or adapted) bourgeois notions of temperance, domesticity, professionalization, etc. Some even turned bourgeois notions of universal man, improvement, confidence in human agency, against the bourgeoisie— in performances that paradoxically displayed the markers of bourgeois social identity (literacy, the dominance of reason over the passions). Once articulated, ideologies and performances cease being individual, or even class, property. No doctrine or practice is so coherent, so exclusively assigned, that it cannot be made to serve other ends. This analysis then follows from Gramsci's notion of hegemony: the most powerful group asserts and enforces foundational or cognitive categories that dominated groups and individuals stretch, twist, subvert—and, given the opportunity, appropriate or overthrow.

I began this study with the premise that the fortunes and uses of anatomy in nineteenth-century America were linked to the creation of a distinctively bourgeois social order and culture. But the course of my research led me to appreciate how various that bourgeoisie was. Certain segments championed anatomy; others opposed it; everyone modified and adapted it; and the lines of debate were far from predictable. Anatomy empowered a succession of medical elites, and provided a discursive vocabulary that helped construct, administer, and model self and society, but it had subversive as well as totallizing implications. Declassé, egalitarian, fringe types were sometimes fervent supporters of anatomy acts, while *Harper's Monthly*, the standard bearer of bourgeois ideology and culture in America, opposed them (at least for a moment). If the working class and yeomanry feared the anatomist, dime museums on the Bowery presented grotesque anatomical spectacles that fascinated, informed, shocked, and titillated a largely proletarian audience.[12] Anatomy's appeal was also ideological: In anatomy's universalist forms, as proselytized by popular anatomical lecturers and authors, every man could know his own body, could be his own anatomist. In its construction of a universal humanity as a species, the epistemology and methodology of anatomy was available as a means whereby working people, African-Americans, and the immigrant poor could be inducted into the bourgeois order, partly on terms of their own making.

I have thought that it would be helpful to inquire into the different uses and meanings of anatomy in "an age when every thing [was] remodelling, and old forms of government and ancient modes and customs [were] breaking up," a place and time when America was transformed into a fluid and fast-changing capitalist class society, a place and time in which the conspicuous performance of social identity took a dizzying profusion of forms.[13]

In this period of "remarkable change," anatomy played a vital and hotly contested part in the cultural politics of medical professionalization and bourgeois self-making. The ultimate result was the victory of the bourgeois medical profession and the instatement of the anatomical body as the bourgeois self. By the late 1880s, the cultural politics of anatomy had become institutionalized. The contest between anatomist and the working poor for rights in the body, and the contest within the bourgeoisie to define the canon of personhood, had become encrypted within social and cultural routine: in sickbeds, hospitals, classrooms, lecture halls, museums, and cemeteries. But victory is never total. A new generation of unorthodox healers and cultural dissidents emerged to appropriate and struggle against professional medical authority and the medicalized self. Ambivalent, anxious representations of the new configuration of cultural power continued to circulate in newspapers, urban folklore, medicine shows, movies, and pulp magazines, where mad doctors, body snatchers, specimens in jars, and the living dead haunted the American imagination. As everybody knows, they still do, in horror films, bestselling novels, magazine articles, TV shows, and here, in the pages that follow.

❧ 1 ❧

"The Mysteries of the Dead Body"

DEATH, EMBODIMENT, AND
SOCIAL IDENTITY

*Is there a permanent relationship between one's idea
of death and one's idea of oneself?*

PHILLIPPE ARIÈS[1]

ON A SUMMER DAY in 1818, the villagers of Ipswich, Massachusetts gathered together. As eight empty coffins were solemnly lowered into the earth, Reverend Robert Crowell preached a lengthy sermon. The previous winter, someone (later found to be Dr. Thomas Sewall, a local physician) had plundered eight graves "for anatomical purposes," a fact that was only discovered months later, and which "spread . . . unusual distress through a very extensive and respectable circle of relations and friends." The stolen, and unrecovered, bodies represented a cross-section of the village: "Mrs. Mary Millet, aged 35; Miss Sally Andrews, 26; Mr. William Burnham, 79; Mr. Elisha Story, 65; Mr. Samuel Burnham, 26; Isaac Allen, 10; Philip Harlow, 10" and "Caesar, a coloured man." The theft of the young woman's body was held to be particularly disturbing. "[T]he melancholy tidings," Crowell said, "gave such a shock to all in the place, as was never felt before."[2] Outraged, a number of villagers came together and pledged the considerable sum of $500 to catch the perpetrator and bring him to justice.[3]

From the late-eighteenth century to the late-nineteenth century, medical grave robbery was a common occurrence in America, and the fear of body snatching and consequent anatomical dissection was widespread in any area within reach of anatomists or their agents. In the winter of 1884–85, Hannah Stout, the twenty-three-year-old daughter of a prosperous Indiana farmer, succumbed to a rare degenerative disease (possibly fibrodysplasia ossificans) that turned her muscular and connective tissue to a substance resembling bone. Worried that her body would be stolen by doctors who would dissect it in an anatomical theater before an audience of colleagues and students, or perhaps exhibit it as a specimen in an anatomical museum, her family decided to bury her on their own property, "just under the window," where family members and friends could more easily mount a watch over her grave.[4]

Hannah Stout's disease made her body a sought-after commodity, but any body might be requisitioned, any graveyard quarried. The fear of that possibility forced a revision of customary death procedures. Those who could afford it buried their dead in well-crafted fortress-like coffins (sometimes sealed in lead solder), buried deep within the earth or locked behind the stout walls of a mausoleum, guarded by nightwatchmen and dogs. Those with fewer resources had to endure the depredations of professional and student graverobbers. *Freedom's Journal*, an Afro-American newspaper of the late 1820s, advised its readers of a cheap and "easy way . . . to secure dead bodies":

> As soon as the corpse is deposited in the grave, let a truss of long wheaten straw be opened and distributed in layers, as equally as may be with every layer of earth, until the whole is filled up. By this method the corpse will be effectually secured; . . . the longest night will not afford time sufficient to empty the grave, though all the common implements of digging be used for that purpose.[5]

Even as Americans took elaborate pains to defend the bodies of their dead, physicians sought to discredit the resistance. In the nineteenth century, the medical profession typically dismissed opposition to dissection as the relic of a bygone primitive age when the "prevalent opinion [was] that the touch of a dead body communicated a moral pollution."[6] Such views, anatomists agreed, still had currency in the "modern" America of the mid-1800s, especially among the lower classes. F. H. Hamilton, professor of anatomy at a small school in upstate New York, felt it his duty to inform his pupils of the "difficulties which . . . oppose the progress of the anatomical student . . . , the power of superstition." The opponents of anatomy, Hamilton contended, were people lacking "liberal and rational education," unredeemed by "the light of reason and revelation"; they were like children who believe in "nursery tales" or "superstitious old women."[7] In the same vein, Robley Dunglison, professor of "the Institutes and Practice of Medicine" at Jefferson Medical College of Philadelphia, used the occasion of his 1841 introductory lecture to lament that, although "science is proceeding with rapid strides, the belief . . . that the body bleeds on the touch of the murderer, still exists" among the poorest segment of the population: "Constantly, in my attendance on the inmates of [the Philadelphia almshouse], I see the protecting amulet placed near the heart . . . and a case has recently has come to my knowledge, in which the touch of the hand of a dead man was employed to dispel a tumour on a child's face." These "irrational practices," and "the wide extent of credulity and superstition" among the poor and laboring classes, were, in Dunglison's view, the main obstacles to public acceptance of anatomy.[8] The resistance to anatomical dissection, a chorus of physicians and enlightened sympathizers affirmed, was delusionary, ignorant, and primitive—an assessment that, up until the 1970s, was largely shared by historians of medicine.[9]

Yet that resistance was not so foreign to the beliefs of the anatomist. Anatomy disrupted the customs, lore, and discourse of death and the body—but also drew power from such customs, via disruption *and* affirmation. To focus on the belief systems of anatomical resisters is to put the cart before the horse. The ideological and cognitive system of beliefs about the body that fell under the rubric of the term "anatomy" precipitated itself out of the matrix of beliefs that were retrospectively dismissed as "superstition." Anatomy defined itself in opposition to that matrix, and yet bore some hereditary affinities to it. While anatomist and anatomy rioter differed on particulars of interpretation and practice and position, they also shared a larger cultural logic founded on three theorems.

First, while funerary practices varied according to ethnicity, social class, religion, and geographical location, and changed markedly over time, two incommensurable beliefs about the dead pervaded late-eighteenth- and nineteenth-century American culture: that the dead body was powerless, endangered, and required protection; and that the dead body was powerful and dangerous to the living, something to be guarded against. Which position received the most emphasis shifted according to historical and social location, but, in either case, the passage from life to death was fraught with risk, for both the living and the dead, an imperative that motivated Americans of all classes, religions, ethnicities, and professions.

Second, anatomists and their opponents appraised social interactions and categories through a common lens: the mind/body binary, with mind customarily privileged over body (although that could be reversed or travestied). This is not to say that there was always agreement on the assignation of the terms. The anatomist could be seen as a flesh eater or disembodied reason. The dead could serve as icons of spirit or corporeality.

Third, nineteenth-century America was convulsed by the ups and downs and pellmell growth of boom-bust capitalism; unplanned territorial expansion and urban development; a succession of technology-driven revolutions in industry, agriculture, transportation, communication, and marketing; political upheavals associated with party, class, and sectional conflict; disruptive religious revivals and innovations; the formation of a new social classes, with status performed through a fickle and proliferating set of cultural fashions and procedures that amounted to new practices and beliefs of personhood. Under such conditions, social identities were precarious and demanding, hard to maintain. If Americans in this period were especially obsessed with death and death ritual, it was because the occasion of death offered the opportunity to dramatize and fix social identity via deathbed and funerary ritual and via biographical narrative. But there was also a danger: at the moment of death one could be tagged a freak, a pauper, a sinner, a vulgarian, an animal, an entertainment, a thing, or nothing at all—and here the anatomist's intervention was found to be particularly threatening, but also valued as a claim to cultural and social authority.

"Conjurin'" versus "Buzzardism": Anatomy, Animism, and the Dead

In her exemplary social history of dissection in nineteenth-century Britain, *Death, Dissection and the Destitute*, Ruth Richardson starts from a premise similar to Dunglison's: anatomy disturbed a relict and persistent strain of death practices and beliefs among the very poor, who were excluded from participation in the bourgeois culture of conspicuous funerary consumption and who stubbornly resisted the exhortations of Protestant reformers.[10] In Richardson's view, nineteenth-century anatomy continued and expanded the Protestant attack on animism, the belief that nature (human and nonhuman) is inhabited and acted upon by spiritual entities and forces of varying degrees of power. Calvinists complained that non-Christian animistic beliefs and rituals had been assimilated into Christianity. Catholicism had coopted or tolerated practices that had been designed to appease or manipulate spirits, ghosts, gods, demigods, and demons. These included the custom of aligning the grave so that the corpse's feet were pointed toward the rising sun; the custom of burying the dead around sunset; ritual or festive eating and drinking in the presence of the dead; the placing of a dish of salt mixed with earth on the dead body; belief in the efficacy of prayer in interceding for the dead; belief in the curative or magical powers of the dead bodies (or body parts) of saints, murder victims, or murderers; belief in ghosts; the belief that the soul remains in the body for a specified period of time after death; etc. The Protestant critique of superstition, Richardson argues, was "totalizing." It interpreted long-standing death practices as travesties of Christian ceremony, willful violations of scriptural commandments, theological doctrine, and church law, or just plain sorcery. This despite the fact that funerary customs such as sin eating (where a stranger is paid to "eat" the sins of the deceased), the Irish wake, and the African-American funeral celebration, as Richardson rightly reminds us, were sometimes performed with solemnity and piety, and nearly always (despite their animist origins) woven into the fabric of Christian, even Calvinist, practice.

Certainly, in the eighteenth century, the dead body could be credited with remarkable powers. For example, a widely distributed 1767 report narrated the "curious" events surrounding the murder of Nicholas Tuer in Bergen County, New Jersey. The coroner's jury ordered a suspect, a "negro man, named Harry . . . to touch the dead man's face with his hand." When he did so, it was said that "blood immediately ran out of the nose of the dead man." Undertaken a second time, the experiment produced the same result, whereupon the suspect confessed to the murder.[11] As noted above, Dunglison and other nineteenth-century anatomists labeled such stories rank superstition, the kind of beliefs that science defined itself in opposition to, but in its eighteenth-century textual setting the story figures as a testimony to a "curiosity," a kind of scientific report. The coroner himself ventured no explanation of the matter; that was for his audience to ponder. Contemporary readers, if they credited the report as truthful, could regard it as grist for medico-philosophical inquiry, or just an entertaining conundrum—and not necessarily confirmation of the magical powers of the dead body.

Whether beliefs in the supernatural powers and qualities of the dead body were widely held by any large class or group in nineteenth-century America is an open question. But even if such beliefs were widespread (the evidence is mixed), did they motivate the opposition to anatomical dissection? Until recently, black people, the poor, criminals, prostitutes, Indians, the Irish, and members of other immigrant groups made up a greatly disproportionate number of anatomical subjects.[12] And while members of these (overlapping) subaltern or subordinate groups did hold distinctive beliefs about death and the body, they also shared many of the dominant beliefs about the dead body, in particular the belief that the period following death was a kind of "sleep" or "repose," and that dismemberment or rough treatment disturbs that sleep. The logic of funerary ritual oscillated between two poles: the living needed protection from the dead, who retained, at least for an interval, a powerful (but ineffable) ability to do grievous (magical, moral, or physiological) harm to the living; the helpless dead needed protection from the powerful (and all too effable) living. The deceased remains "human" and has to be honored for a "decent" period of time with some form of privileged "respect" that ritually affirms the humanity of the dead individual. Those people who were refused the right to participate fully in the community or polity were particularly insistent about this. They regarded the taking and dissecting of their bodies as the final and definitive annulment of their social being.[13] Over the course of the nineteenth century, the theme of the protection of the defenseless dead, always dominant in the opposition to anatomical dissection, became increasingly important in the larger funerary culture. Paradoxically, as we shall see in chapter 3, it was within the rituals of anatomical dissection and medical student life that the theme of the powerful body (which tests the courage and strength of the anatomist) was conserved and adapted.

From at least the 1840s onward, in the Philadelphia Almshouse where Robley Dunglison held the office of resident physician, bodies were regularly taken for the use of Philadelphia medical schools, a practice of dubious legality. In a letter of protest, the inmates complained of "buzzardism." To them, the resident physicians and employees were vultures circling around their bodies, eagerly anticipating their deaths so that they could feast on the remains.[14] Those who consumed human flesh in this way were "inhumane," predatory animals. They denied the persons so eaten the privileged status accorded to the human species, reduced them to the status of carrion. Reverend Robert Crowell, in his 1818 eulogy to the desecrated bodies at Ipswich, cited the Bible on this point: "of Ahab and Jezebel it was declared, by Elijah, from the mouth of the Lord, that the dogs should eat their carcasses. The judgment was even extended to their posterity: 'Him that dieth of Ahab in the city, the dogs shall eat; and him that dieth in the field, shall the fowls of the air eat.'" Crowell explained that "No one . . . can treat the body of any rational spirit with disrespect . . . , without lessening their value of the life." The appropriation of a body for any use whatsoever—"to know that they have . . . been torn from their coffins, for monied and scientific speculation, and exposed to the rude gaze of unbearded youth"—was a transgression. It was especially cruel to put the cadaver on display; the prospect of "an exposure of their bodies upon anatomical theatres," Crowell argued, caused the living much "suffering in anticipation."[15] The cutting up of a body was worse still; in reducing the body to pieces, the self suffered an attack, a violation.[16]

If so, then the cultural logic of death required a protective sequestering of the body, and a series of gestures that signaled respect for the personhood of the deceased. The deathbed vigil, the wake, the death shroud, burial in a coffin or tomb, embalming, served to set apart the dead person from the living, providing temporary protection from the predations of desecrators, curiosity seekers, and vermin. The damage inflicted by natural processes was delayed and made less visible; human attacks against the dead were warded off.[17]

Ruth Richardson conflates this repertoire of funerary customs and beliefs (in the nineteenth century, shared for the most part by the rich, middle class, and poor) with the more eccentric "reality" of popular residual death practices, depicting both "as a palpable resistance to 'scientific' medicine," and so stands the medical narrative of reason against superstition on its head. Her warm appreciation of folk customs leads her to argue that they are reasonable, just, and richly human; it is science and the professional classes that are unreasonable, unjust, and inhumane.

Michel Foucault went much further in his critique of the narrative of medical progress.[18] According to Foucault, the "moral obstacle" to anatomical medicine was a straw man, not a real obstacle at all: "experienced only when the epistemological need had emerged; scientific necessity revealed the prohibition for what it was: Knowledge invents the secret."[19] For Foucault, prior practices were irrelevant; the cult of anatomical medicine fabricated and elicited its own opposition. This line of thinking has the virtue of calling into question the self-justifying romances produced by nineteenth-century anatomists and their sympathizers, but takes us too far in the other direction: anatomy did not arise out of a void and did not create the ensemble of practices it claimed to supersede (although it frequently did caricature them to the point of unrecognizability). At the very least, prior cultural beliefs and practices supplied anatomy's opposition with a vocabulary and a compelling rationale; the fact that anatomy elicited and drew strength from its opposition does not logically require that we disregard the resistance to anatomy.

In an article on anatomy riots and anatomy law in late-eighteenth-century New York, historian Steven Wilf shows that medical graverobbery and dissection disturbed longstanding non-Christian funerary beliefs, especially among Afro-Americans and Africans, who, according to one 1786 report, threw themselves overboard and drowned rather than submit to the possibility of posthumous dissection (the ship's captain had already ordered the shipboard dissection of one dead slave).[20] But Wilf cautions that African funerary beliefs, no matter how deeply held, cannot explain the depth of opposition to anatomy; rather, bodysnatching and the prospect of dissection caused plebeian men and women of all cultural groups to react "viscerally." The intensity of their empathic fellowship with the dissected meant that they could almost "feel" the dissector's scalpel carve into their flesh, which in turn triggered a "visceral" response: rioting, fearful tremors, overwhelming grief and anger. Wilf's interpretation has the unfortunate effect of reinstating the mind/body binary: it implies that the behavior and beliefs of the upper classes are mediated, attenuated, or falsified by spirit and reason; the behavior and beliefs of the lower classes are directly produced on the body, by the body. But Wilf is on to something: the opposition to anatomical dissection was not visceral but "visceralist." That is, the anatomy rioters participated in a pervasive cultural system that identified manual laborers, petty tradesmen, the illiterate, "unwashed" poor ("the people") with "flesh," and the governmental apparatus, and church, social, and intellectual elites with disembodied "spirit." Not surprisingly, plebeian men and women saw the anatomical appropriation of their dead, and claims to authority over the body generally, as an attack; and on more than one occasion responded with "rough music" that asserted the power of the body against the mind. In eighteenth-

century terms, the medical taking, surveying, and cutting open of bodies
was an act of enclosure, much like the gentry's appropriation and enclosure of common woods, fens, and pastures in contemporary England.

"A Mass of Corruption": The Body versus the Self

> Whilst we are at home in the body, we are absent from
> the Lord.
>
> 2 Corinthians 5:6.

> Sin . . . hath marred both soul and body, and causes the
> latter to corrupt and moulder again to dust. But then it
> will be raised again, no more to die; and be reunited
> with spirit.
>
> Reverend Robert Crowell (1818)[21]

If the anatomist enclosed the cadavers of the poor, appropriating what
had never been property for exclusively private purposes, he performed
an analogous operation through anatomical discourse. The anatomist removed the dead body from its communal surroundings, opened it up and
inscribed it with internal boundaries, turning it into a representation that
had the functional purpose of showing the living body's hidden reality.
This act of representation worked to dematerialize the body, to remove it
from the realm of direct bodily experience, but also provided a new vocabulary with which to think about and experience the body. Eventually,
this paradox would come to shape how the mass of people would regard
their own bodies.

Jonathan Sawday, a literary historian, has argued that a "culture of dissection" held sway in early modern Europe.[22] But Sawday's detailed reading of canonical and obscure artifacts of high culture gives little indication of the boundaries of that culture, its relation to the less exalted
world that it sat atop. Consider, for example, another early modern meaning of the word "anatomy." In seventeenth- and eighteenth-century almanacs, a plebeian genre, "the anatomy" was a crude diagram of the astrological division of the body. It implicitly affirmed the body's metaphorical
power and connection to cosmic forces, to the universal signs of the zo-
diac. It might be used to coordinate healing practices like venesection
and purging with the phases of the moon—but made not the slightest
reference to Vesalian anatomy and the culture of dissection.[23]

"The anatomy" was but one shard of cultural flotsam that early modern
anatomy bumped up against. Before anatomical discourse pervaded think-

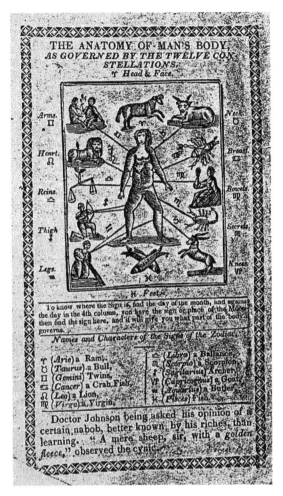

Figure 1.1. The anatomy. David Young, *The New-York
Farmer's Almanac for the Year of Our Lord 1818* (New
York, 1817). Courtesy of the National Library
of Medicine.

ing about the body, many different notions of self shared the space that
the anatomy would come to monopolize. Notwithstanding Vesalius and
Harvey, seventeenth- and eighteenth-century narratives of disease emphasized the body's permeability and susceptibility to the shaping forces of
the external environment, the decisive influence of hot weather, humid-
ity, cold, wind, diet, etc., with little visualization of the body's internal

boundaries.[24] According to Foucault, the eighteenth-century mania for taxonomy in medicine concerned itself with the classification of signs and symptoms that were evident on the surface of the body, and made little effort to correlate disease symptoms with the body's internal landmarks.[25] Eighteenth-century therapeutics tended to assume that health could be achieved by balancing a hydraulic flow of countervailing forces. These forces were not precisely mapped within the body—proper medical treatment should restore the equilibrium by drawing off excess fluid, by puking, sweating, blistering, or bleeding without identifying the precise itinerary of the body's internal fluids. Over the course of the nineteenth century this conception of the body gradually gave way to a logic that abstracted the body from its cosmological, political, and social surroundings (literally and figuratively) and stressed the taxonomic fixity of species, gender, race, diseases, and internal organs and tissues.[26]

In the seventeenth and eighteenth centuries, medical discourse described the body in anatomical, astrological, and/or humoral terms, but that body was not necessarily identical to the self. The self, prior to the triumph of anatomy, refused or exceeded the material body; the self was identified with spirit. By that reckoning, people who worked with their hands, those who were identified with body (and who provided the fodder for the dissecting tables), lacked selfhood altogether, an appraisal that they understandably found objectionable.

At the same time, the dead body exceeded discourse, even as it was mapped by Vesalius and his successors.[27] In much of seventeenth- and eighteenth-century Anglo-American culture, the Word was identified with life and spirit, the Body with death and materiality, a set of associations that was especially pronounced in Calvinism. The dead body was a thing external and opposed to the articulated self, a thing "of all uncleanness." This, more than anything, helps to explain the remarkable slippage in Puritan theology, where death liberates the essential self from its corporeal shell, frees the soul to live an ethereal eternal existence—or incarcerates (extinguishes) the self for eternity within the worm-eaten, suffering flesh (a favorite image that unites the Freudian Thanatos and Eros in the phallic figure of the worm consuming the body). For Calvinists, life was a period of temporary detention within the decomposing corpus; the final judgment was either liberation (heaven) or eternal imprisonment within the body. The death of the body is life, the life of the body is death.

Under the doctrine of original sin, the body was identified with carnality, which connoted the erotic sensuality of "fleshy" embodiment, alongside a propensity for disease and corruption, which was associated with the dead body. Cotton Mather, himself a physician as well as a minister, used anatomical discourse to make an inventory of the corrupt materiality of the flesh, which becomes especially evident at the moment of death:

. . . it can't be long before the Silver Cord of your spinal marrow will be snap't or before the Golden Bowl of the Membrane that covers your Brain will be broken; . . . before the pitcher of your Arterious Vein be crackt at the right ventricle of your heart, which is the Fountain from whence it fetches your blood into your Lungs; . . . before the Wheel of your great Artery, be split at the left venticle of your Heart, which is the Cistern whereby 'tis carried into and through that noble Bowel; . . . before the circulation of your Blood be fatally and forever stop'd, and that Liquor of Life corrupt in a total stagnation of it.[28]

Flesh here is the inferior mode, subordinate to spirit, which acts something like an chemical preservative. In the absence of spirit, flesh decays, undergoes a proliferating "corruption." But flesh is invested with its own power; bodily desire acts as a contaminant, tempts spirit, pollutes the soul, jeopardizes the possibility of salvation and eternal life. And this antivaluation of the body easily incorporated anatomy—and was itself incorporated into anatomical practice (a matter discussed in the next chapter). Ruth Richardson then is right to focus on animism, but defines it too narrowly and too much in opposition to anatomy and Calvinism: the flesh in seventeenth- and eighteenth-century discourse had a full measure of enchantment. Nehemiah Walter's 1706 sermon to a Boston congregation, "The Body of Death Anatomized," employs an "anatomical" rhetorical procedure (a step-by-step, piece-by-piece, analysis of a subject) to argue that flesh is endowed with a relentless, murderous vitality: "*Original Sin* eats into the *Body*, and diffuses itself through every Member thereof. . . . 'Tis a *Mass* of Corruption, a Collection of Lusts. . . . 'Tis called a *Body of death*, Partly, because it makes Men *dead* unto and in spiritual Duties."[29] In Calvinist theology, Body was the antithesis of value. It had the power to incite; it infested spirit.

Such notions persisted well into the nineteenth century. In her famous 1836 "Appeal to the Christian Women of the South," Angelina Grimké contrasted the transparent disembodied moral ideals of Christian antislavery with the hidden "putrid carcass" of slavery, with its "grave-clothes of heathen ignorance."[30] Grimké was a Quaker who had been raised as a highchurch Episcopalian, but her cultural logic—that flesh is inferior and antithetical to spirit—could easily be mistaken for Calvinism.[31] Only the "life giving command," the Word, can overcome the corruption emanating from "the loathsome body" and bring on a resurrection. The life of the body is an enslavement. Emancipation from the body—accomplished by forcing the public to confront the stench and ugliness of bodily decomposition—is an emancipation from slavery. By equating the "putrid carcass" with Negro slavery, Grimké undermined the proslavery trope that the black man leads a life of the body (not mind or spirit) and therefore deserves enslavement (or that the black body is equivalent to the decomposing body, a thing of all uncleanness). Thus, for both sides of the slavery debate, mind/spirit prevailed over body/matter. And, for both sides, the body was powerful, a prolific generator of corruption.

THE WORLDLY BODY

Methodists and Quakers disparaged the body as the vehicle of original sin, albeit with differences of degree, tone, and practical application. Their essential agreement with Calvinism developed out of a common opposition to Catholicism. Protestants accused Catholics of tolerating, even encouraging, carnality, in the quasi-sexual devotion to images and relics of Jesus, Mary, and the saints, in the Lenten cycle of festival and denial, in the confessional cycle of sinful action and remorseful penitence, and, theologically, in the absolute separation of spirit and flesh. In contrast, Protestants of all varieties promoted the idea that embodied life was inherently suffused with or organized by spirit (again with varying emphasis according to sect and rank): God operated through the material events of history and the regular procedures of natural law (unlike the miracles that interrupted and transcended nature and history in Catholic doctrine).

But differences among Protestant sects and factions, especially the perennial tension between official Protestant practice and "enthusiasm," were also articulated in the idiom of mind/body duality, with a corollary coding that roughly equated those terms with class or rank. Enthusiasts accused religious establishments of being worldly, corrupt (i.e., of the body), or (conversely) too ethereal in their worship style, too disconnected from an embodied divinity—and by extension too eager to serve the interests and salve the guilty consciences of powerful elites. For enthusiasts, redemption could occur only through direct, unmediated contact with God (the entity that fused spirit and matter). An 1840 Mormon hymn privileged body over mind; the Mormon God was embodied, material, palpable, an active agent, unlike the God of religious rivals: "The God that others worship is not the God for me / He has no parts nor body, and can not hear nor see." Protestant religious establishments responded in turn by accusing enthusiasts of taking pleasure in impulsive bodily sensation (shaking, dancing, singing, crying), of violating church discipline that regulated bodily conduct, of being deceived by the Devil (the personification of carnality), of valuing the Body over Scripture. The two positions can be fairly described as key terms in the deep grammar of Protestantism: the same logic that set Quakers in opposition to Congregationalists and the Church of England in the seventeenth century set New

Lights against Old Lights in the eighteenth century, and Disciples of Christ against New Lights in the nineteenth.[32]

But not everyone was a devout Christian, and Christian theology and practice stood in a complex and murky relation to embodied life.[33] In the aftermath of the English Civil War, anti-Puritans revalued flesh as a separate domain which must be given its due; Restoration comedy was worldly, a celebration of the convoluted paths by which desire is consummated or frustrated. Andrew Marvell, a Puritan who made an easy accommodation to the Restoration, depicted the relation between mind and body relation as an ambivalent dialogue. The "soul," Marvell wrote, is "hung up . . . in chains / Of nerves, and arteries, and veins," imprisoned in an anatomical dungeon, "with bolts of bones." But the physical body is just as oppressed: it is "possessed" by an "ill spirit" that needlessly "warms and moves it," cramps it with hope, palsies it with fear, heats it with "the pestilence of love," ulcerates it with hate, and perplexes it with "Joy's cheerful madness." The flesh then justly cries for redemption "From bonds of this tyrannic soul? / Which, stretched upright, impales me so." The phallic soul penetrates the body, takes it over, places uncomfortable strictures on it, makes unreasonable demands.[34]

Body and soul in Marvell's poem are irreconcilable, but in the seventeenth-, eighteenth-, and nineteenth-century Anglo-American world there was a mediating set of gestures, poses, and rituals: manners. Among the aristocracy, gentry, and middle-class risers, manners served as claims on a place in the social and moral hierarchy, a performance that marked one's level of "rarefication" or "refinement." Manners first took shape in the courts and salons of the emergent nation-states of early modern Europe and then diffused widely in some form (or counterform) through much of society, a historical process that took several centuries.[35] Between the two poles of Mind and Body, manners occupied an expansive middle ground, articulating spirit in a set of embodied gestures and practices that grew into an all-encompassing system of social performance. Gentility refused or mediated bodily impulse: public burping, farting, defecation, eating with hands, impulsive movement, unmodulated speech, ecstatic dance, gave way to the concealment of bodily functions, careful poses and postures, choreographed gestures, etc. Elaborate protocols of behavior in every aspect of life demonstrated the work of abstracted spirit on the body. Those without manners—peasants, manual laborers, savages, children—received representation (and to some extent performed themselves) by reference to unmediated flesh. The metaphorology of gentility identified the lower classes with the "body," "meat," "animal," "coarseness," ugliness, stench, impulsive desire, lack of manners, "crudity" of speech and gesture, illiteracy, ignorance, irreligion, etc. The upper crust, conversely, were identified with "mind," "spirit," "delicacy," "subtlety," "humanity," "civilization," "artifice," sweet smell or odorlessness, beauty, grace, discipline, etc.

The precise performances that were linked to these attributes varied from place to place, moment to moment, cohort to cohort, and contradicted or harmonized with each other, depending on the vagaries of fashion, material interest, politics, social position, and religion. Puritanism and the religious "awakenings" of eighteenth- and nineteenth-century America were energized by a critique of gentility as "worldly" and embodied, in opposition to spirit—but also by a critique of genteel artifice as disembodying and false, compared to the unadorned bodily truth imposed, or revealed, by Christian obligation and Christian consciousness. Gentility was a self-making program that put its performers at a distance from bodily impulse, not through denial but through material, embodied practices that produced a heightening of bodily sensation and cultures of connoisseurship. In nineteenth-century America, the vocabulary of gentility was appropriated, with some modification, by a much larger and diverse group of people. The acquisition of gentility was a key procedure in a new social formation and a new class system, a move that precipitated an individual out of the plebeian "million" or "masses" and asserted his or her standing in the hierarchy of "respectable" persons. "Cultivated" manners, home decoration, home architecture, garden landscaping, literary erudition, and dress asserted a claim on a particular version of bourgeois social identity—a claim that was scrutinized and judged by peers and the larger community.[36]

Within the cultural logic of gentility, then, there resided a permanent tension between an ethos and aesthetics of embodiment and disembodiment, a tension that intensified in the middle decades of the nineteenth century. Edgar Allan Poe satirized the contradiction in this speech by the foolish "Miss Clairvoir" in *The Magnetizer* (1845):

> Man, no longer a creature of the elements, no more a slave to the narrow powers excited by mere blood, and bones, and muscles.—man the spirit, not the carcase. . . . It is the victory of science; the triumph of immortal mind over corrupt matter; the exaltation of spirituality over corporality![37]

It was not a coincidence that Poe put such words into the mouth of a female character: the feminine (or effeminate) denial of human embodiedness was an easy mark. Gentility was crucially intertwined with notions of gender. Ancient conceptions of sexual difference that equated the feminine with body and the masculine with spirit continued to circulate, but female refinement could also be signified through a rejection of embodied life. Elizabeth Blackwell, who in 1847 became the first woman to receive the degree of doctor of medicine, remembered how as a schoolgirl she "hated everything connected with the body," and tried to "subdue" her "physical nature" by fasting and sleeping on the floor rather than a bed:

> I had been horrified . . . during my schooldays by seeing a bullock's eye resting on its cushion of rather bloody fat, by means of which one of the professors wished to interest his class in the wonderful structure of the eye. Physiology, thus taught, became extremely distasteful to me. My favorite subjects were history and metaphysics, and the very thought of dwelling on the physical structure of the body and its various ailments filled me with disgust.[38]

Blackwell's sensitivity to anything that referenced the body was part of a complex performance that signified the femininity of a particular social position. From the mid-eighteenth century on, "sensibility" became one of the principal attributes of gentility. Sensibility was defined as a heightened experience of sensation that was the very opposite of the numbed insensitivity (it was thought) of lower animals and uncultivated lower-class "brutes," or, for that matter, the dead body. Such a stance could devalue the cadaver, particularly the lower-class cadaver.[39] But in some hands sensibility might be signified via expressions of empathy for lower (coded as embodied) beings: domestic animals, children, the worthy poor, slaves, and, interestingly enough for our purposes, the dead. To have a cultivated sensibility meant that one had so great a surplus of "feeling" (corresponding roughly to the possession of surplus value) that it could be expended quite extravagantly on one's self (inordinate self-preoccupation) or, benevolently, on inferior beings.[40] For Adam Smith, the harmonious operation of society depended precisely on the operation of an empathic "moral sentiment." Applied to the dead, literary historian Esther Schor notes, such feelings functioned as a "gold standard for the circulation of sympathies within society," convertible into every other kind of moral currency.[41] In his 1759 *Theory of Moral Sentiment*, Adam Smith argues that sensible beings are compelled to identify with the dead:

> It is miserable, we think, to be deprived of the light of the sun; to be shut out from life and conversation; to be laid in the cold grave, a prey to corruption and the reptiles of the earth; . . . to be obliterated . . . from the affections, and almost from the memory, of their dearest friends and relations. Surely, we imagine, we can never feel too much for those who have suffered so dreadful a calamity.

We know that the dead lack the ability to feel, that nothing "can ever disturb the profound security of their repose." But our highly developed empathy overwhelms our reason, and this imaginative identification has far-reaching moral consequences:

> It is from this very illusion . . . that the foresight of our own dissolution is so terrible to us. . . . And from thence arises one of the most important princi-

ples in human nature, the dread of death, the great poison to the happiness, but the great restraint upon the injustice of mankind, which while it afflicts and mortifies the individual, guards and protects the society.[42]

As in Smith's more famous work on political economy, his discussion of empathic fellowship with the dead was empirical, prescriptive, and visionary. In the nineteenth century, identification with the dying and the dead became an insistently recurrent motif in political and religious rhetoric, poetry, and fiction. At its most extreme, this manifested itself as a cultural obsession with premature burial, as in the 1827 first-person tale, "The Buried Alive":

> I heard the sound of weeping at my pillow—and the voice of the nurse say, "He is dead."—I cannot describe what I felt at these words. I exerted my utmost power of volition to stir myself, but I could not move an eyelid. After a short pause my friend drew near; and sobbing and convulsed with grief, drew his hand over my face, and closed my eyes. The world was then darkened, but still I could hear, and feel, and suffer.
>
> . . . I soon after found the undertakers were preparing to habit me in the garments of the grave. Their thoughtlessness was more awful than the grief of my friends. They laughed . . . and treated what they believed a corpse with the most appalling ribaldry.

Premature burial narratives often emphasized the callous indifference of the living and the helplessness of the undefended cadaver.

> When they laid me out, these wretches retired, and the degrading formality of affected mourning commenced. For three days a number of friends called to see me. I heard them, in low accents, speak of what I was. . . . On the third day, some of them talked of the smell of corruption in the room.
>
> The coffin was procured—I was lifted and laid in. My friend placed my head on what was deemed its last pillow, and I felt his tear drop on my face.

The narrator goes on to describe the bolting of the coffin shut, the procession via hearse to the graveyard, the lowering of the coffin into the ground, the long wait alone under ground, and the prospect of a "fall into corruption." But, after a long lapse of time, the natural succession is disrupted: grave robbers who "sing snatches and scraps of obscene songs" exhume the body and convey it to a medical school. The students, after appraising the cadaver as a "good subject," run an electric current through the body, a fairly common experiment in the 1820s. This causes some minor muscular contractions, but only dissection is powerful enough to break the death spell:

> When they had satisfied themselves with the galvanic phenomena, the [anatomical] demonstrator took the knife, and pierced me on the bosom with the

point. I felt a dreadful crackling . . . throughout my whole frame—a convulsive shuddering instantly followed, and a shriek of horror rose from all present. The ice of death was broken up—my trance ended.[43]

KEEPING UP WITH THE FUNERARY JONESES: THE EXPANDING ECONOMY OF DEATH

The late eighteenth- and nineteenth-century preoccupation with death was fed by an emergent and expansionary culture of consumption. Codes of fashionable manners and dress signaled distance from the coarseness of the material world and untutored desire, but also a worldly ambition to outperform, or at least keep up with, neighbors and peers. As social hierarchies grew in size and complexity, and as English-speaking North America became more settled and prosperous, and had more disposable resources, gentility was articulated in ever wider cultural domains: the dinner table, the toilette, the garden, theater, and especially, death. In Tudor England, only the landed gentry had the resources to be buried in their own wooden boxes, the bare minimum for an individualized funeral; the bodies of the lower ranks were buried in a communal "parish" coffin that was shared and continually reused.[44] But over the next hundred years, in the upper reaches of society, funerals became more elaborate. Even the New England ministerial elite, while issuing periodic jeremiads against worldliness, could not abstain from lavish displays: the provision of finely made funeral gloves, scarves, and rings for the mourners; elaborate coffins with beautiful lacquered finishes, ornamental handles, linings, and nameplates; artfully designed and executed headstones; beautiful and expensive mourning clothes; and abundant provisions of delicacies and drink for the mourners.[45] And the passage of (unenforceable) sumptuary laws forbidding funerary extravagance, in mid-seventeenth-century New England, indicates that middling types were also aping their social betters.

Over the course of the eighteenth century, the trend intensified. Funerals became increasingly opulent, a phenomenon only partly checked by the mid-century religious revival. By the late eighteenth century, a new funerary economy had emerged, based on the manufacture and exchange of a new set of death goods and a new aesthetics of death: "beautiful" death. Death's heads gave way to weeping angels and funerary urns; common burial grounds or disorganized, dispersed burial sites gave way to aesthetically regulated cemeteries with precisely apportioned plots and boundaries. Writing in the late 1830s, Harriet Martineau remarked that death constitutes "a large element in [Americans'] estimate of collective human experience, a more conspicuous object . . . than it is to, perhaps, any other people. . . . [A]ll arrangements connected with death occupy much of their attention, and engage a large share of popular sentiment."[46] Lucy Bird, another British tourist, wrote in 1856 that "the citizens of New York carry their magnificence as far as possible to the grave with them, and pile their wealth above their heads in superb mausoleums or costly statues."[47] In Greenwood Cemetery in Brooklyn, a fine burial lot might cost as much as $500, to which might be added the cost of the funeral service, mourning clothes, coffin, food and souvenirs for mourners.[48] Alongside this funerary splendor, a full-blown cult of morbid romanticism flourished in fine art, poetry, and fiction. To outside observers, Americans' social, cultural, and material investment in death goods was extraordinary.

DEATH AND THE STORY OF LIFE

> [W]hen, at last, man is about to take his plunge into the
> abyss of eternity, he strips off all disguise and stands re-
> vealed in his primitive nakedness and helplessness.[49]
>
> ALEXANDER STEPHENS, M.D. (1849)

For present-day middle-class Americans, death mainly occurs in hospitals, nursing homes, funeral homes, and cemeteries, and on television. Commonly shared death rituals are attenuated or have lapsed entirely. Visible and prolonged mourning is regarded as a pathological condition, suitable for medical or psychological intervention, treated by counseling and/or mood-altering drugs. The dying are often treated with drugs that relieve pain, but also quell their consciousness of death.[50] Modern death practice consists of a set of extraordinary measures intended to screen the living from the dead and dying, to help the living and the dying deny the fact of mortality. Death is, for the most part, kept separate from the unfolding meaning of the life narrative.[51]

One or two centuries ago, things were far different. The dead body was then much more material. Dying occurred more frequently—often in the home. Death vigils, usually mounted and managed by the women of the house, were a standard practice. The fact of death provided the occasion for the staging of all sorts of moral sentiments, social meanings. Death provided the space in which people could act out their social identities and invest them with ontological *gravitas*. Death was a performance and even a spectacle: People turned out by the thousands to attend festive hangings of notorious criminals. At the same time, many people had daily experience with slaughtering, butchering, and knackering (disposal of dead horses). Yet this too had a social coding: "refined" or "cultivated" men and women delegated these tasks, to servants or vendors; the ability to do so was a mark of social status. The occupations of butchery and knackery, like that of the hangman, carried a stigma; the dead (uncooked animal or unburied human) body was seen as a contaminant, a threat to moral, aesthetic, physical, and social well-being, not fit to be seen. A newspaper correspondent of 1850 argued that slaughterhouses and butcher shops "ought to be prohibited" from locations within the city, for moral reasons, "because of the brutalizing scenes thus daily placed before the eyes of children," whose delicate and impressionable sensibilities would be imperilled by exposure to "blood bespattered killers, knocking the brains out of" cattle and sheep.[52]

A postmodern truism is that human beings "can only find an identity in self-narration." In the late eighteenth and nineteenth centuries, the philosopher Charles W. Taylor tells us, "canonical models and archetypes" (fables and allegories) were increasingly supplanted by stories "drawn from the particular events and circumstances of this life": "[A]s a chain of happenings in world time, the life at any moment is the causal consequence of what has transpired earlier. But . . . since the life to be lived has also to be *told*, its meaning is seen as something that unfolds through events."[53]

Death, perhaps even more than birth and marriage, had from antiquity a privileged standing within the hierarchy of events. "In order . . . to know the true state of the human heart, we must wait till the closing hour of life; for then only . . . sincerity takes possession: then indeed whatever shows we may have made, if they were false, the prospect of approaching death will soon discover the deceit," explains the narrator of a 1790 allegory.[54] A postbellum Methodist tract makes much the same point: "'A deathbed's a detector of the heart.' We are traveling to the grave; and . . . we shall be honest before God and our own souls when we come to lie upon our dying pillow."[55] Death was regarded as the epitome of life. How one died, and how one's body was treated after death, fixed for eternity one's moral, aesthetic and social status.

This view was fostered by—and provided the impetus for—a proliferation of novels, memoirs, and poems. In sentimental discourse, death provided the occasion for the articulation of a life's definitive moral significance. Samuel Hayes Elliot's 1858 novel, *New England's Chattels: or, Life in the Northern Poor-house*, for example, was a succession of mortuary set pieces: old Joe Harnden (cruelly worked to death); Allanson Boyce (a poet whose excited hypersensibility leads to derangement, debility, the poorhouse, and then death); Boyce's wife (who dies a beautiful death from grief "and she too slept beside him; their graves marked by the purest marble, for their lives had been innocent and good"); aunt Dorothy (a kindly old poorhouse inmate who dies without a proper burial, a death that is a reproach to the community); Polly Tucker (who burns to death, the ugly death of an unrepentant sinner); Mrs. Dodge (missing but not missed, found frozen in the snow).[56]

Such death narratives were not confined to fiction. If social experience provided the material out of which fiction was written, readers (with varying degrees of success) imitated that fiction in enactments and retellings of their own death narratives. The annual reports of the New York Colored Orphan Asylum in the 1830s and 1840s narrated the deaths of the young orphans in consolatory poetry and prose modeled on the death of Little Nell.[57] This was more than just literary styling. The desire to narrate a meaningful death organized the very procedures of death, the performances of the dying, deathbed attendants, mourners, physicians, and ministers.

Consider Harriot K. Hunt's memoir of the death of her father, who passed away during a masonic lodge meeting in 1827:[58]

> [Joab Hunt] observed, "I shall not be here many times more: the way seems longer every time." Having said this, he dropped his head on Major Purkitt's shoulder, who . . . exclaimed, "Brother Joab!" One gasp—it was all over! Not a groan—a struggle—a distortion. It was truly the *sleep* of death! . . .
>
> . . . Every effort was made—warm water was at hand—venesection was resorted to—every thing that brotherly love, combined with medical skill, could suggest. . . . But the soul had gone; the spiritual world had its tenant! . . .
>
> Our family physician, Dr. Dixwell . . . bore the mournful intelligence to us. . . . Many members of the lodge quietly accompanied the bier of our father, and laid it in his own room. We could not believe him dead! He seemed as though in a sweet slumber—a trance. Was it indeed death? It could not be! Life *could*, and *must* be brought back! Thoughts of galvanic remedies rushed to my mind—we would have our father again—but no! Those who have known by experience, the shock caused by a sudden death in a family, will be touched by our condition. They will know it is not to be talked of, but felt. . . .
>
> The deepest darkness of our grief . . . passed away, and now mellow rays of religious faith lightened the heavy gloom. We loved to linger over the body. The countenance gave no sign of its great change. It was natural and pleasant as in its earthly life. It seemed less a death than a translation. He had desired to be removed suddenly—his prayer had been answered. . . . He dreaded leavetakings—he was spared that sorrow. But above all to us, was the consolation of that abiding confidence in divine love which had permeated his whole life, and which had always made his face radiant when he spoke of his Heavenly Father.

As in most sentimental narratives, reconciliation with death and with God was a privileged theme, repetitively signified in the metaphor of death as sleep. That the circumstances of Joab Hunt's passing were outside his control only further affirmed the moral significance of his life, as though God was complicit in the authoring of the final chapter.

But Hunt did not trust his final arrangements to God:

[T]he body having shown the fearful mystery of change which follows its divorce from the spirit, was committed to that tomb on Copp's Hill, which he had carefully built in 1811, and to which he had often taken his children that they might habituate themselves to the spot. . . . My father disliked afternoon burials; he wished the laying of the body in the tomb to be hallowed by connection with a new day and a new morn. On the third day after his death, at early morn, we laid him in the tomb. . . . [I]n the unutterable aspect of desolation . . . my mother asked me to read the fifteenth chapter of Corinthians . . . : "There is a natural body and there is a spiritual body. As we have borne the image of the earthly, so shall we also bear the image of the heavenly." These truths deepened in significance in that sacred moment: a light shone from them and irradiated the tomb; . . . from that moment, our father was ever present to us.

At great expense and effort, he painstaking planned the smallest details of his burial, even the wood for his coffin:

My father's state of mind regarding death, caused him to lay aside Brazilian mahogany for his coffin, which was found just where he said. From the remnant I have a footstool, on which is inscribed, "Durability." My father never knew the fear of dying, or of leaving his loved ones; but amidst his brethren who had known him for years, he passed away. . . . Fifty-eight years of age seems hardly old; but the fulness of years—the completeness of life—has not to do with calendar periods, but with the accomplishment of a *purpose*.

But there could be contention over what moral purpose should be assigned to the dead person's life. In many nineteenth-century death narratives, malign beings (anatomists, bodysnatchers, murderers, traitors, or seducers) seek to impose their own meaning on the death of an innocent. Harriot Hunt remembered how, "during the great anti-masonic excitement, . . . anti-masons called upon us," seeking evidence in support of "wicked and slanderous accusations" that her father's demise was due to a masonic conspiracy. The family rebuked them and her father's lodge brothers swore public depositions as to the true circumstances of his death.

This narrating of death, full of biographical, medical, and moral detail, was a procedure that asserted the bourgeois Christian personhood of both the deceased and the narrator. Such narratives contrasted markedly with the ancient death allegories that were still current among the rural yeomanry and the urban poor. In his memoir of his youth in an early-nineteenth-century Connecticut village, William Alcott mused over the old school primer, with its "alphabet of couplets, with [wood]cuts prefixed," one of which read "Youth forward slips, / Death soonest nips", illustrated by "a representation of a skeleton, armed with a dagger, and pursuing a youth . . . with the apparent intention of striking him through." Alcott remarks that his own "early notions about being struck with death, had . . . a connection with this picture." For young Alcott and his fellow villagers, the difference between life and death was absolute, outside time. Death narrative took the form of a universal allegory; the historical (individual) situation of the person selected was immaterial. Medical intervention was powerless to save persons whom Death had selected: "Death, the personification of Satan or some other demon, has laid hold of the sick or distressed, and . . . it would be . . . useless, not to say sacrilegious, . . . to oppose . . . the grim messenger."[59] Against this superstitious fatalism, Alcott offered a preventative system of medical improvement based on a knowledge of anatomy and physiology (the scientific laws of health), and a knowledge of the particulars of the patient's disease and life history. Alcott's rejection of timeless allegory served to assert a cultural difference between his adult identity as a bourgeois professional and the primitive village life that he left behind.

Working Man's Dead

[The paupers] could not avoid thinking it was a
handsome thing to be decently buried. . . .

Rev. Samuel Hayes Elliot (1858)[60]

If death had to be narrated in its particulars, based on a true accounting of events, then it required a great deal of arranging. Even for middle- and upper-class Americans, an honorable death was no sure thing. Given the boom-and-bust economy of nineteenth-century capitalism, unbuffered by government protections, financial security was hard to come by, even for the relatively affluent. Joab Hunt, pedigreed and prosperous, died with enough resources to ensure a more than decent burial, but upon his death his estate was found to be encumbered, and his daughters were forced to work as school-teachers: a circumstance that probably made his daughter Harriot all the more anxious to narrate his death. If the moral purpose of a life was signified in the manner of death and its attendant funeral ceremonies, then such ceremonies assumed a vast importance.

Over the course of the eighteenth and nineteenth centuries, this cultural logic resulted in the increasingly elaborate moral and material economy of death: the use of the living for the dead (the funerary economy that Benthamite utilitarianism worked to invert; see chapter 4). This in itself was nothing new. In many times and places, death has been the focus of cultural and economic activities: funerary economies are as old as the pyramids. The nineteenth-century Egyptian revival in mortuary architecture—the widely imitated gates and obelisks of Mount Auburn, the nation's first "garden cemetery" (1831)—was a witty allusion in stone to death's growing importance in American cultural life. Death had become the occasion for a (relatively and absolutely) massive expenditure of cultural capital and cold cash (considered on an individual and collective scale), a growing segment of the emerging culture of consumption. As Mrs. Martineau remarked, the burial place was "one of the first directions in which the Americans have indulged their taste, and indicated their refinement."[61] For the American bourgeoisie, the rural cemetery movement that emerged in the 1830s, with its elaborately planned mausoleums, monuments, and pastoral death parks, was a means of marking off the social, aesthetic, and hygienic distance between themselves and the lower classes, a hedge around their bodies that conserved their sensibility in death against the invasion of the body snatchers, and in visible contrast to those who were deemed to have little or no sensibility to begin with, the laboring poor.

The poor, in turn, reacted ambivalently. To the extent that their resources permitted, they attempted to close the social chasm by adopting the conventions of middle-class death discourse and iconography. Nineteenth-century working-class newspapers were full of consolatory poetry and formulaic obituaries, indistinguishable from those of middle-class papers.[62] Most importantly, the working poor tried to assure themselves a place in funerary society by securing burials in cemeteries or churchyards that were equivalent to those of the bourgeoisie, or within bourgeois cemeteries in inferior graves and spaces. The alternatives—to be sold and/or stolen, dissected, and/or displayed in a museum, or to be dumped anonymously in a mass grave in a potter's field—represented social annihilation. The dissected body was nothing but a collection of body parts and waste, a thing; potter's field was a dumping ground, a place of exclusion. Burial there was a risk for a large portion of the population: a sampling of selected years in antebellum New York City shows that potter's field accounted for between 14% and 24% of all burials.[63] For working men and women, burial in the cemetery or churchyard symbolized inclusion in the social order. It also at least potentially signified a leveling of the social order: in death everyone was equal, an ancient trope, but one continually reworked.

This, however, must be set against a process in which the funerary economy of death worked to mark social distinction in fine and invidious detail, even in potter's field. An archaeological excavation of the Uxbridge [Massachusetts] Almshouse Burial Ground, a place where the bodies of "the unworthy" poor were interred in the antebellum period, reveals that many of the coffins had affixed to them small, cheap mass-produced ornamental hinges, plaques, lid fasteners, etc., a trivial investment which served as some recognition of the life lived even if the survivors could not bear the major expense of a proper "decent" burial.[64] In the late 1840s, Nicholas, an employee in the dead house at Bellevue (the New York City almshouse) was "known . . . to stain coffins and receive a perquisite for such from the friends of . . . deceased" paupers who were to be buried at Potter's Field.[65] In his famous 1843 study of the British working class, Edwin Chadwick observed that "[n]othing can exceed their desire for an imposing funeral . . . They would starve to pay the undertaker."[66] The same was true in America: If you accumulated no other capital in your life, your one bit of savings might go to pay for your burial and the burials of your loved ones or, lacking that, perhaps a shroud or a bit of stain for the plain pine box provided by the city. Such small gestures of respect worked to distinguish the very poor from the absolutely indigent and friendless—and, often enough, poor whites from poorer blacks—and thereby attenuated the stigma of an impoverished death.[67] Poor blacks, like poor whites, made every effort to avoid a pauper's death, pooling resources where possible. And the worst fate that might await an unprotected body was anatomical dissection at a medical college.

The gulf between the unmarked graves, and dissected bodies, of the poor and those of respectable persons thus loomed as a vast divide. The middle- and lower-class obsession with burial plots as existential security corresponded to the nineteenth-century obsession with landownership as social security. The emphasis on aestheticized funerary performance and presentation, the costumary of both mourners and the cadaver, the funerary habitat of both coffin and burial plot or tomb, corresponded to the contemporary bourgeois obsession with the aestheticized presentation of self and home. As the absolute quantity of social wealth increased, the middle classes adopted and adapted the funerary practices of the elite. Death became a medium through which class identity (or a critique of class identity) was asserted.

By the late-nineteenth and early-twentieth centuries, working-class men and women were devoting a significant proportion of their resources to death. Commercial insurance companies vied to sell low-cost death insurance to the masses. The proportion of working-class men and women who received a pauper's burial markedly declined (in New York City, from over 360 per 100,000 population in 1867 to 81 per 100,000 in 1915).[68] More prosperous people of working- and lower-middle-class provenance began using funerals as an occasion for the assertion of individual self: an 1890s issue of the *New York World* reported on some "very queer tombstones," a funerary "craze for novelty": a soda pop manufacturer who had a "soda-water tombstone," a butcher who "desired that his tombstone be carved with links of fat sausages," and a baker who wanted a tombstone "in the form of an iced cake."[69] As early as the 1840s, a reform-minded segment of the bourgeoisie began criticizing the working class not for their improvident indifference to death, but rather for their improvident devotion of scarce resources to funerals they could ill afford.[70] Middle-class men and women began agitating for reform of burial practices—cremation, limitation of funeral expenses—which once again set them in opposition to the funerary ethos of the poor. An 1878 editorial in *Harper's Monthly* complained that "the burying of the dead . . . imposes enormous expenses upon those who can not afford them. The savings of a year are often squandered in the idle ostentation of a funeral. . . . [A] living family is often straitened that a dead member of it may lie in a mahogany coffin and be followed by a long train of carriages to his grave."[71] Again, there was a compelling signifying aesthetic: class matters.

S. J. Kleinberg, in a study of working-class death in postbellum Pittsburgh, shows that a barebones funeral with a tombstone, food and drink for the mourners, and a carriage for the widow, might easily amount to $75 or $100, compared to middle-class funeral expenses of $500. Such costs taxed working-class purses. The upper echelons of the working class joined ethnic, fraternal, or veterans' benevolent societies partly or mainly devoted to burial benefits, or trade unions, which also generally offered death benefits. But few workers belonged to unions, which were not generally open to unskilled workers, and even skilled workers had difficulty paying dues during the recurrent and long economic depressions of the late nineteenth century. Many funerals were paid for by passing the hat.[72]

There was still another plebeian option: complete disregard of bourgeois funerary norms. An 1884 New York newspaper reported on an Irish wake where "some rough neighbors . . . emptied the barrels, kegs, and demijohns of alcoholic spirits until the revelry became excessive." During the "ghastly orgie . . . the coffin was thrown from the table and the body rolled out upon the floor, where it remained until some neighbors dispersed the company and restored order." A few years earlier, in the same neighborhood, another wake became so riotous that revelers extracted a corpse from its coffin, "propped it against the wall, and stuck a pipe in the dead man's mouth."[73] In Ireland the wake had long served the impoverished, subjugated Irish as a counterperformance against the English Protestant regime. In nineteenth-century America it served as a counterperformance against bourgeois American culture (and received the censure of the Massachusetts Sanitary Commission). The Roman Catholic hierarchy, seeking a measure of acceptance from the Protestant elite, and trying to impose discipline on its unruly flock, tried to suppress or domesticate the wake. More typically, the working-class Irish adapted the wake

to the dominant funerary forms, turning it into a death ritual that signified ethnic difference, but also inclusion in the larger social order: a "decent burial."

DEATH, THE MARKET, AND THE VOCABULARY OF SELF

Underlying the imperative to secure a decent burial was the assumption
that the dead body was identical with self, and that death should be a
terminus, the telos for the circulation of moral and material goods (a
coffin, stone marker, a bounded plot or tomb), the endpoint of the transmission of wealth and Christian virtue. That is, the honor of the body in
death is what familial wealth is accumulated for. Conversely, the body
should *not* itself be a circulating good—such activities, by definition, dis-
honor the body. The dead body should not be bought and sold, should
not be subordinated to human use. The body should not be the object of
spectatorship, eaten as food, dissected, used for fertilizer. The dead self
should "rest in peace," outside the exchange of goods. If anything, it
should be the *beneficiary* of the system of exchanges. Such a position supplied the definition of mortuary honor and defined a crucial aspect of
the selfhood of the mid-nineteenth-century "individual." Reverend Robert Crowell ended his eulogy with the hope that the memorial marker
over the empty coffins would "bid the hand of avarice [to] beware of
making merchandize of the dead."[74]

This death logic fits nicely within the ideological matrix that came to
dominate nineteenth-century American society, the concept of possessive
individualism, in which the individual has inalienable property in one's
self; the self is excluded from market transactions precisely because in the
grammar of exchange it is assigned the position of *subject*.[75] The bounded
self is the exchanger, not the exchanged (although the sheer weight of
self-making discourse and accessories testifies to the fact that the self
is both producer and produced). In the moral economy of nineteenth-
century capitalism, exactly who was eligible to be a bounded self, or to
come under the protection of that self, was a hotly contested issue. Reform-minded antebellum ministers like Samuel Hayes Elliot deplored the
existence of "a private enterprise in human stocks" and the "traffic in
flesh"—slavery, prostitution, body snatching, indentured labor.[76] The dead
body in its grave was to be sequestered from the market and, like the
home in which the self resided, made into a sacralized object. In Reverend A. B. Winfield's 1846 sermon memorializing the members of the Van
Nest family who had been hacked to death by a casual laborer the coffin
was "a narrow home" where the deceased could regain bodily unity, find
"sepulchral repose." Death was a haven, a place where the travails of production and exchange ceased and harmony reigned.[77] The ending of life

was an emancipation. "We who are crushed to earth with heavy chains, . . . groping through midnight darkness on earth, earn our right to enjoy the sunshine in the great hereafter," wrote Elizabeth Keckley, the former slave who became Mary Todd Lincoln's seamstress and confidant. "At the grave, at least, we should be permitted to lay our burdens down, that a new world, a world of brightness, may open to us. The light that is denied us here should grow into a flood of effulgence beyond the dark, mysterious shadows of death."[78]

"The Arbiter of Life or Death": Funerary Authority and the Production of Death Performances

> The physician must recollect, that he is often the arbiter of life or death.
>
> Robley Dunglison (1837)[79]

If death was a haven in a heartless world, then here the anatomist and the grave robber willfully transgressed. Against the invasion of the body snatchers, the living struggled mightily to protect the honor of their dead, to safeguard the material integrity of their helpless dead selves, to narrate their lives and therefore their deaths. For them selfhood did not terminate with death; rather, death stripped away the duplicitous masks and inessentials of being, leaving an existentially pure residue. Post-mortem photoportraiture, which from the earliest days of photography emerged as one of the most popular genres of the new medium, was intended not so much for spectatorship, but to freeze the self into an iconic last frame—many of the pictures were tucked away as keepsakes, never meant to be displayed, viewed only infrequently or not at all.[80] Nineteenth-century Americans of all classes took this very seriously: how one died fixed symbolically how one lived. For Christians, a deathbed reconciliation with the redeemer—or, even better, a death scenario that featured an imitation of Christ (with the dying person forgiving those who had wronged them, thereby inducing onlookers to repent and accept Christ)—was a matter of urgency, an opportunity to affirm that the end of the life narrative was an eternity in heaven rather than in hell.

But at the same time, while many people continued to hold a belief in a literal hell, death increasingly became a matter of aesthetics and style that thematically articulated the "inner" meaning of the life that had just unfolded on earth. A satisfactory death was a beautiful death, in its plot, performers, staging, setting, accessories, and accoutrements. The unrepentant sinner, the villain—the morally depraved, the hypocrite—could/should expect an ugly, and revelatory, death. A huge number of literary

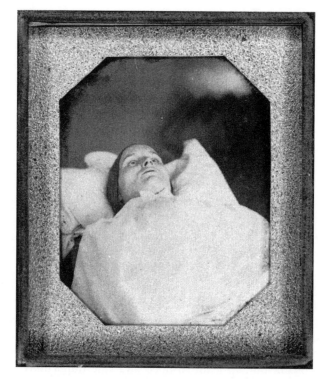

Figure 1.2. Post-mortem portrait. Daguerrotype, ca. 1840–
60. The deceased is posed with open eyes, not in a figure
of repose. The photograph registers the bare fact of a life
ended, without any reference to sentimental narrative.
Courtesy of Steve and Mary DeGenaro.

exercises, celebrated and obscure, worked to elaborate this theme. Take,
for example, "Human Petrefaction," an anonymous 1854 anecdote about
the death of "Deacon Blank":

> The poor of his parish never felt any genial warmth on his approach. . . .
> [I]n our neighborhood his most common and familiar appellation was "Old
> Flint," and well he deserved it, for no species of mineral could be less suscep-
> tible than his heart. Heart—did we say? He had none; and so his doctor . . .
> told him whilst he was in his last agonies. He was dictating his will to his
> lawyer and instructed him to insert a clause providing for the petrification of
> his body, after his decease, according to the newly discovered process. . . .
>
> "No necessity for that[,] deacon!" said the doctor, as he coolly and pur-
> posely mixed the most unpalatable potion in the whole pharmacopeia—"bet-
> ter save your money—you were *petrified long ago heart and all!*"

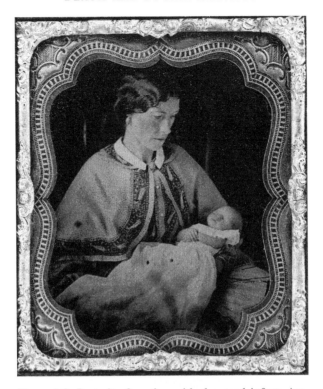

Figure 1.3. Portrait of mother with deceased infant. Ambrotype, ca. 1850–80. This post-mortem photograph implicitly sets the deceased infant in a sentimental narrative of maternal love and infantile innocence. Courtesy of Steve and Mary DeGenaro.

The deathbed is the occasion for the revelatory moment that sums up the life of the dying deacon. With clinical distance and candor, the physician uses his patient's own last request to render judgment on the dying man's life. The story, contrasting the moral hypocrisy of the hardened Calvinist deacon and the moral honesty of the scientific, humanitarian doctor, captures a sociological moment, the passage of funerary authority from one profession (and discourse) to another, but also captures the narrativization of death.[81] Against all efforts to rescript one's life narrative (the deacon's delusionary effort to deny the corruption of the body in death mirrors his denial of the corruption of his soul in life), death would tell the true story, reveal the inner man.

The doctor, then, assumed a key role in the death narrative: he pinned a moral conclusion to the life story of the deceased, and rendered judgment. But he was not the only would-be funerary authority. At the deathbed or the funeral, the minister also asserted moral conclusions about the life lived, and relations between the two authorities were tricky. As autopsyist or as presiding deathbed authority, the physician might complement the minister, find within the deceased's body evidence that corroborated the clergyman's theological assessment. But he also might undermine the minister or render him superfluous; the two professions were potential competitors. Milton Braman, a Congregationalist minister, in an 1830 letter to John Collins Warren, Harvard's eminent professor of anatomy, complained that the physicians in his area were "unitarians" or freethinkers who, "under plausible pretences," prevent their dying "patients being conversed with in respect to the state of their souls" for the sake of "their own eternal good."[82]

Characterizations of physicians as irreligious were common in the middle decades of the nineteenth century. The village atheist, if there was one, was often depicted as "a scoffing and unprincipled physician"; and anatomical medicine was thought to be especially tainted by the materialist heresy of the French revolution.[83] Still, Braman deferred to the local physicians, and for a remedy sought the advice of the highest medical rather than religious authority (albeit one known to be a devout trinitarian). Even at the highwater mark of nineteenth-century evangelicalism, medical authority was gaining.[84]

Conclusion:
"It Makes a Difference How We die"

So it makes a difference how we die! Men should not
allow themselves to say or even think it [does] not.

Rev. Samuel Hayes Elliot (1858)[86]

This chapter has rummaged through a jumble of ancient and contemporary discourses and practices of embodied personhood, of the living and dead body, to see what domains anatomy arose out of, defined itself in opposition to, competed with, assimilated. My aim has been to situate anatomy, death, and the medical profession within a larger sociocultural history. I have argued that a variety of forms, positions, and practices were linked to the development of social identities and the emergent culture of consumption, all of them organized around death: the transition from communal burial grounds (and isolated rural family burial places) to the bounded bourgeois cemetery with enclosed individual plots; the emergence of segmented markets for death products, the mass retailing and commercialization of funerary goods and services, and the intensification of the material and discursive investment in funerary performance and goods; the changing performance of death, from scripted, generic allegory to individualized narrative; and the growing legal and cultural authority of the physician at the deathbed and over the dead body.

In the early modern English-speaking world, death was discursively identified with the body, and bodily desires and functions. The body (living or dead) had an ambivalent relation to the concept and practice of selfhood. But from the late eighteenth century on the body came to be regarded as identical to the self. The language of embodiment, conjoined to the phenomenology of embodied life, provided a stock of images, a repertoire of "metaphors we live by"—and metaphors we die by.[87] Anatomy enriched, disrupted, and drew power from this changing cultural matrix. In the chapters that follow, we will attend to the significance of the anatomical encounter with the dead body. As we shall see, in both discourse and practice, anatomical dissection came to stand for a foundational epistemological principle that authorized professional medicine, but acquired a proliferating array of meanings and countermeanings, with repercussions in disparate cultural domains, including the bourgeois self.

2

"A Genuine Zeal"

THE ANATOMICAL ERA IN
AMERICAN MEDICINE

IN THE LATE 1780s Philadelphia's rival faculties of medicine (the College of Philadelphia and University of Pennsylvania) engaged in a series of fractious disputes. The details of those prolonged controversies are obscure, and for our purposes immaterial: what interests us here is *An Oration Which Might Have Been Delivered to the Students in Anatomy on the Late Rupture Between the Two Schools in This City*, an idiosyncratic nineteen-page satirical poem that urged the reconciliation of the factions, while having some fun at the profession's expense.[1] Its author, Francis Hopkinson (1737–1791), was an eminent figure, a signer of the Declaration of Independence, friend and correspondent of Benjamin Franklin and Thomas Jefferson, designer of the American flag, inventor, judge, composer, poet, and wit. Published in February 1789 and only anthologized once in 1793, *An Oration* plays theme and variations on the ideology, iconology, and social meaning of medical professionalism in late-eighteenth-century America.

The poem takes the form of a plea for unity. The medical "fraternity," the orator warns, is besieged by "num'rous foes." It can't afford internal dissension and bickering; rather, it must close ranks around its "ruling passion": an all-encompassing love of anatomical dissection. The enemies of medicine are rising up against the "brethren of the knife":

> Methinks I hear them cry, in varied tones,
> "Give us our father's—brother's—sister's bones."
> Methinks I see a mob of sailors rise—
> Revenge!—revenge! they cry—and damn their eyes—
> Revenge for comrade Jack, whose flesh, they say,
> You minc'd to morsels and then threw away.
> Methinks I see a black infernal train—,
> The genuine offspring of accused *Cain*—
> Fiercely on you their angry looks are bent,
> They grin and gibber dangerous discontent
> And seem to say—"Is there not meat enough:
> Ah! massa cannibal, why eat poor CUFF?"

The passage makes reference to several incidents: the 1765 Philadelphia "Sailors' Mob" that disrupted Dr. William Shippen, Jr.'s anatomy class and attacked his carriage and house, the April 1788 "Doctors' mob" riot against anatomy students and professors in New York City, and perhaps the June 1788 Baltimore mob that invaded Dr. Charles F. Wiesenthal's anatomy school to reclaim the body of an executed murderer.[2] "[M]assa cannibal, why eat poor CUFF?"—the white man eating the black, an inversion of the usual racist trope—almost certainly refers to the February 1788 public petition of African-American citizens, which called on New York City's Common Council to act against the medical plundering of bodies at the Negro Burying Ground. 1788 was a busy year for anatomists.

In the face of these difficulties, the poet calls out to the quarrelsome factions of the profession and urges them "to engage your high wrought souls . . . / Combine your strength these monsters to subdue / No friends of science and sworn foes to you." The hue and cry disrupts the secret rituals of the medical cult:

> AH! think how, late, our mutilated rites
> And midnight orgies, were by sudden frights
> And loud alarms profan'd—the sacrifice
> Stretch'd on a board before our eager eyes,
> All naked lay—ev'n when our chieftain stood
> Like a high priest, prepar'd for shedding blood;
> Prepar'd with wondrous skill, to cut or slash
> The gentle sliver or the deep drawn gash;
> Prepar'd to plunge ev'n elbow deep in gore
> Nature and nature's secrets to explore. . . .

But dissection is not the only transgressive ritual that binds the profession together. Medical identity is also forged in covert and risky unearthings of the dead, and in the battle to take possession of bodies:

> [W]e have shar'd the toil
> When in Potter's Field . . . we fought for spoil,
> Did midnight ghosts and death and horror brave
> To delve for science in the dreary grave—
> Shall I remind you of that awful night
> When our compacted band maintain'd the fight
> Against an armed host?—fierce was the fray
> And yet we bore our sheeted prize away.

Such secret anatomical activities set the profession apart from the people, but this was not just a matter of social marking. Anatomy had cognitive and behavioral effects: "To me things are not as to vulgar eyes, / I would all nature's works anatomize." The anatomical act is a Faustian procedure that transforms the initiate's relation to the physical world. Via gaze and scalpel, the anatomist comes to dominate the material universe, in toto. In an extended metaphor, the poet converts the geographical world into an anatomical landscape: "I see vast ocean, like a heart in play, / Pant *systole* and *diastole* ev'ry day / And by unnumber'd *venous* streams supply'd / Up her broad rivers force th' *arterial* tide."

But *An Oration* doesn't stop there. Next it becomes a love poem to the poet's "own amour," a "mistress in high taste," named "Brown Cadavera."[3] This obsessive love is figured as an ironic reversal: the dissector is himself dissected, by "Cupid's subtle dart" which "thro' my *pericardium* pierc'd my heart / Brown CADAVERA did my soul ensnare, / Was all my thought by night and daily care— / I long'd to clasp in her transcendent charms, / A living skeleton within my arms." The rest of the poem sings praises of Cadavera's anatomical features, a travesty of the Petrarchan inventory of the beloved's attributes, her "*Os frontis* prominent and bold," her "*alveoli* fix'd secure, / articulated by *gomphosis* sure," "her *carpus, cubitus* and *radius* too," and so on.

Brown Cadavera dies and is buried. The anatomist then "Resolv[es] her precious corse from worms to save": "With active haste remov[es] the incumbent clay, / Seiz[es] the rich prize and [bears] my love away." This elopement leads to erotic arousal, and a desire to penetrate, possess, and annihilate the beloved, anatomically:

> Her naked charms now lay before my sight,
> I gaz'd with rapture and supreme delight,
> Nor could forbear, in extasy, to cry—
> Beneath that shrivell'd skin what treasures lie!
> Then feasted to the full my amorous soul,
> And skinn'd and cut and slash'd without controul.
>   'TWAS then I saw, what long I'd wish'd to see,
> That heart which panted oft for love and me—
> In detail view'd the form I once ador'd,
> And nature's hidden mysteries explor'd.

In an anatomical rapture he boils the bones and wires them together to hang as a skeleton in his cabinet, until "quite inflam'd with passion for the dead / I take her beauteous skeleton to bed— / There stretch'd at length, close to my side / She lies all night a lovely grinning bride." Such is the "extent a genuine zeal will go," the orator comments, to "ev'ry hostile sentiment subdue / and keep the ruling passion [anatomy] still in view."

If this seems ghoulish, the poet insists it isn't, and inveighs against "FALSE delicacy—prejudices strong, / Which . . . Against our noble Science spend their rage." If "the *living* churlishly refuse / To give their dead relations to our use," then surgeons will have no way to rehearse their trade, and will have to make unpracticed, unskilled, movements of the scalpel on the living. What is more, those who accuse the profession of indecency are hypocrites who

> [w]ill pick, and gut and cook a chicken's corse,
> Dissect and eat it up without remorse; . . .
> No where's the difference?—to th' impartial eye
> A leg of mutton and a human thigh
> Are just the same—for surely all must own
> Flesh is but flesh, and bone is only bone.

But, the poet predicts, this squeamishness—manifest in the form of laws against grave robbery—will give way to a rosy, millennial future. "[L]ife and health" will "submit" to the physician's control, and "*death* around him roll." The skulls and bones of the profession's enemies will be collected and publicly displayed "in scientific rows." The "brethren of the knife" will stop squabbling; public objections to anatomy will forever cease; "graves shall freely render up their dead"; "our schools shall wealth in currents flow"; and "physicians . . . shall reign the real sov'reigns of mankind."

In Hopkinson's poem then, the dissection of bodies is medicine's defining practice, the symbol of its commitment to science, its power to transform and control nature—to such an extent as to invite ridicule. An unlimited supply of cadavers ensures a college's success, and is crucial to the progress of medicine. Only anatomy can bind together a profession riven by controversy. Anatomy invites opposition from the superstitious and ignorant populace, an opposition that forges the fraternal bond among doctors. The esoteric, privileged knowledge derived from the transgressive act of dissection elevates the physician above other healers—and the medical profession above other professions.

ANATOMY'S *LONGUE DURÉE*

> [W]ere I to place a man of proper talents, in the most direct road for becoming truely *great* in his profession, I would chuse a good practical Anatomist and put him into a large hospital to attend the *sick* and dissect the dead.
>
> WILLIAM HUNTER, 1784[4]

An Oration documents a particular moment in the history of American medicine. Between 1760 and 1890, diplomaed physicians displaced or subordinated midwives and folkhealers, and—in competition and collaboration with political, economic, and intellectual elites and the clergy—

developed a wide-ranging cultural authority. From a small group, catering to the thin upper crust, the number of practitioners and sites of activity (colleges, hospitals, medical societies, publications) expanded exponentially: physicians became the primary healthcare providers in their communities and American medicine was transformed into a distinctively bourgeois "profession."

The emergence of professional medicine in America is now a familiar story to historians.[5] The canonical account describes the antebellum profession as suffering from a lack of public acceptance, low social status, and an inability to regulate the medical marketplace or enforce standards. The rise of the profession occurs in the 1870s and 1880s, with the triumph of microbiology and laboratory medicine, usually characterized as the onset of American medicine's "scientific era." Anatomical dissection contributes little to the making of medical authority, or is a barrier, given the opposition to the medical appropriation of bodies. In this chapter, I will argue that the cultural authority of antebellum medicine, while never without external opposition and internal contradiction, was considerable—and that anatomy played a crucial role in its formation. Here, much condensed and shorn of some familiar details (the politics of medical licensure, professional organization, educational reform, and competing therapeutic sects and theories), the history of American medicine will be recast as an anatomical narrative.

The period from 1760 to 1860 saw the creation and rapid expansion of the medical profession in America: a proliferation of schools, organizations, sects, practitioners, and publications. In 1810 there were only five medical schools in the United States; by 1860, there were 65, a thirteen-fold increase in a period during which the total population of the country little more than quadrupled.[6] Charles Caldwell, writing in 1834, complained that the profession was afflicted by "the impolicy of multiplying schools": "Within the last fifteen or twenty years, there has broken out, in the United States, a perfect medical-school mania," a mass retailing of medical careers, at the level of both instructor and practitioner.[7] U.S. census figures for 1850 show that there were 176 physicians for every 100,000 persons, a historical high that far exceeded contemporary ratios in Britain and France.[8]

Anatomical dissection played a large part in this mania, and was itself the subject of a mania. As a young medical student in London in 1800, John Collins Warren lauded John and William Hunter, the preeminent anatomists of late-eighteenth-century Britain, for having pioneered "a new era" in surgery, not so much because of "the great discoveries they made" at the dissecting table, "their accurate observations of nature in her healthy & morbid actions, . . . but because they introduced a taste for anatomy—I may almost say a rage for it."[9] Upon his return to the United

States, Warren worked long and hard to propagate that "taste," first as an adjunct professor at Harvard, where his father was Professor of Anatomy and Surgery, then as his father's successor, a position he held for over three decades. A cadre of anatomy professors performed similar services in Philadelphia, New York, Baltimore and elsewhere.

The early-nineteenth-century vogue for anatomy was, of course, part of a *longue durée*, the anatomization of medicine and surgery that flowed from Vesalius's pathbreaking study of the human cadaver, the 1543 *De humani corporis fabrica*, and the subsequent work of Eustachius, William Harvey, Thomas Willis, and others. In the early modern era, anatomical dissection was a domain of special interest to scientific gentlemen who cultivated and collected rare experiences and sensations, and regarded anatomy as both exotic and modern. Fashionable men and women made appearances at anatomical theaters where they could observe (and could be seen observing) dissections. Wealthy patrons bore the costs of printing expensive anatomical folios, via subscription or in toto, and rewarded the most talented anatomists with sinecures and/or the favor of retaining them for medical advice and care. Patronage of anatomy, as of other sciences, redounded to the credit of the sponsor, part of the shared interest in natural philosophy that distinguished certain circles within the gentry and aristocracy.

The social prominence of anatomy was matched by its discursive prominence. According to historian Emily Jane Cohen, "Anatomizing, involving at once an unearthing of hidden mysteries or origins and a dividing into parts so as to reassemble a coherent whole, was *the* paradigm of all philosophical enterprises and was duly reflected in all branches of knowledge and artistic activity."[10] Anatomy was an exemplary science, featured in the court philosophy of middling and high aristocratic circles. In early modern philosophy and literature, references to the intellectual and physical mastery of nature and the body frequently took the form of metaphorical dissections and anatomies.

By the eighteenth century, anatomical studies were being conducted in every intellectual center—Bologna, Leyden, Vienna, even, at a less developed level, in Britain's North American colonies—all part of an international collective project. Edinburgh and London became especially prestigious and productive centers of anatomical training and research. Students from all over the English-speaking world came to study in Edinburgh, where Alexander Monro and his son were renowned anatomists, and in London, where the brothers John and William Hunter carried anatomy to new professional, aesthetic, scientific, technological, and social heights and places—an ascension ratified by William Hunter's appointment as physician extraordinary to Queen Charlotte in 1764 and John Hunter's appointment as surgeon extraordinary to King George III in 1776.

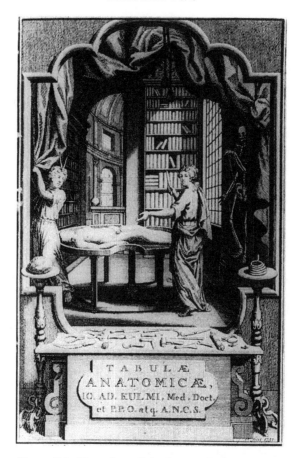

Figure 2.1. Dissection of the human body as an exemplary epistemology that produces textual knowledge. Engraving in Johann Adam Kulmus, *Tabulae An-
atomicae* (Amsterdam, 1732), frontispiece. A body
rests on a dissecting table in the center of a library;
a skeleton stands in an alcove to the right; surgical
instruments are arranged on a pedestal in the fore-
ground. Courtesy of the National Library of Medicine.

The most ambitious, gifted, and well-heeled students made pilgrimages
to both places (and perhaps to Paris and other centers), but the Hunters'
anatomy schools in London were regarded as the most advanced. The
Hunters were celebrated for their skillful dissections, meticulous and
beautiful publications, innovative surgical and obstetrical techniques,
and path-breaking contributions to comparative anatomy and pathology

(and for John Hunter's anatomical collection, which consisted of more than 13,000 specimens). Their obstetrical innovations, in particular, contributed to the entry of male physicians and surgeons into the burgeoning field of "man-midwifery": over the course of the eighteenth century, physicians increasingly attended to the pregnancies of the aristocracy, gentry, mercantile elite, and the upper reaches of the "middling classes" (while learning and developing their techniques on charity cases).[11] Directly and indirectly, the achievements of the Hunters, together with the Monro dynasty in Edinburgh, fostered the proliferation of proprietarial and chartered medical schools (often called "anatomy schools") in Great Britain and the United States. Their students established and operated many of them. Both John Morgan and William Shippen, Jr., founders of the first medical college in America, studied with the Hunters and also in Edinburgh.[12]

Hunterian anatomy characteristically featured highly detailed investigations of gross anatomy, comparative anatomy, and a preoccupation with "morbid anatomy," postmortem dissections that sought to locate specific "seats" of disease in the body, and to construct a narrative of the progress of the disease and cause of death. No longer was it sufficient for medical students merely to attend lectures and witness a dissection performed in the anatomical theater by a professor or demonstrator. The novice had to gain personal, empirical dissecting experience—and this performance was connected discursively and socially to a scientific enterprise that went beyond incremental improvements in surgical technique. "Practical anatomy," as dissection was termed, increasingly came to serve as the prerequisite for a distinguished medical career. A modicum of anatomical erudition, gained from hands-on dissection, became helpful, even imperative, for any young medical man who aspired to establish himself or rise in local, national and international medical networks.

Over the course of the eighteenth century, anatomy transformed physic and surgery. The ambitious physician could not confine himself to the study of texts and materia medica; he also had to dissect the body. The ambitious surgeon could not confine himself to on-the-job training in setting bones, bleeding patients, and amputating limbs; he had to master post-Vesalian texts and techniques. As a particularly messy form of manual labor, surgery originally carried a social taint in the upper reaches of English-speaking society, but advanced anatomical training made surgery respectable: a surgical colleague said of John Hunter that "He alone made us gentlemen."[13] By the 1760s, anatomy had begun to occupy a privileged position in the credentializing process. Anatomy became the essential core of the medical curriculum. Upon his return to Philadelphia in 1765 (after studying with the Hunters in London and Alexander Monro II in Edinburgh), John Morgan worried that some students "seem to imagine if they hear lectures upon Anatomy only, . . . they can easily make themselves masters of all the other branches of medicine by reading."[14] And almost thirty years after that, Francis Hopkinson, as we have seen, made an easy identification of medical study with anatomical study. The "true son of Esculapius" had a "ruling passion": to "plunge ev'n elbow deep in gore / Nature and nature's secrets to explore."[15]

In the early nineteenth century, Hunterian anatomy was eclipsed by the Parisian school, which was even more heavily invested in anatomical study. Those who could afford the expense flocked to Paris, where teachers and students had access to a prodigious number of patients at huge state-run charity hospitals and, at virtually no cost, a large number of cadavers.[16] The highest medical authorities of the age were the great Parisian anatomists—Xavier Bichat, R. T. H. Laënnec, François Magendie, François Broussais, Gabriel Andral, and their students—and they dissected thousands of corpses. The availability of bodies was a point of French national pride, and attracted international attention. By the mid-nineteenth century, the laying out of cadavers at the Parisian morgue was a regular stop on the itineraries of American and British tourists.

Bichat went beyond Hunterian theory to identify and describe the various types of "tissues" in the body. Similar tissues existed in different regions, a fact revealed by pathological conditions that developed only in those tissues, and which therefore were found distributed in various organs, not a single "seat." Bichat's pathological anatomy did not merely establish specific differences between the diseased and healthy body, but became a method for systematically delineating the "general anatomy" of the human body. This emphasis on pathology was further developed by Laënnec, who developed the technique of "percussion" (sounds produced by rapping on the body) and invented the stethoscope ("auscultation"), in order to hear and analyze heartbeat and breathing. Laënnec began to methodically correlate the sounds of percussion and auscultation, and other signs and symptoms, with postmortem findings, a research strategy that bore fruit in advances in physiological theory, diagnosis, and etiology. Some twentieth-century historians have linked the Parisian school to a transformation of the doctor-patient relationship, which became dominated by the physician, rather than being a dialogue between patient and physician. Anatomical medicine was predicated on the metaphorical "death" of the patient, who became an inert object of study rather than an epistemological partner. In the words of a disciple of Laënnec: "We anatomize . . . while the patient is yet alive."[17]

In America, the succession from Hunterian to Parisian anatomy was uneven. J. C. Warren, who was one of the first Americans to study the new anatomy in Paris, attracted many students and physicians to his private "Anatomical Course" given in "rooms over White's Apothecary Shop" in

Boston, which commenced in the fall of 1805, and later to his classes at Harvard.[18] However, in the first decade of the nineteenth century, most of his colleagues were unfamiliar or unimpressed with Parisian developments. Nathan Smith, professor of anatomy at Dartmouth, praised David Ramsay, the eccentric Scottish emigré, as the "greatest anatomist in the world," not Bichat or his disciples.[19] But by the 1820s a small and soon-to-be influential cadre of Americans, many of them sons of prominent physicians, began traveling overseas to study with the Parisian masters, as their predecessors had done in Edinburgh and London, but in ever greater numbers.[20] Anatomy, like all things Parisian, became fashionable. And in Philadelphia, New York, Boston, and Baltimore—even the rural South—a craze for anatomy flourished among medical students. While a passion for anatomy had long flourished within medical circles, medicine now entered a new age of anatomical enthusiasm. The American profession coalesced around a consensus that favored the Parisian research program, notwithstanding the considerable difficulties they experienced in attempting to implement it. Pathological anatomy, many observers agreed, was the exemplary methodology of medical science.

"THE MOST SCIENTIFIC OF ALL SCIENTIFIC SUBJECTS"

> The practice of medicine of the ancients was an art, and not a science, and this dignity it did not acquire until it was based on an acquaintance with anatomy and physiology.
>
> JOSEPH LEIDY, 1858[21]

The rise of anatomy was connected to a transformation of medical identity: a move away from an identification with "trade" and "craft," and toward "profession" and "science"; and an effort to distinguish "art" from "science," and to identify the profession as reliably "scientific." This transformation was linked to the fusion of surgery and physic under the rubric of "medicine." In this merger, first proposed in the 1600s and gradually consummated in the Hunterian and Parisian eras, the old social identities of surgery and physic were recast. *Surgery* was traditionally associated with handwork, the body, and brutality, but also practical effectiveness; *physic* was traditionally associated with spirit and the written word, but also a speculative divorcement from the rigors of hands-on healing. Each had something to give the other, but first the belief in physic's moral and social ascendancy over surgery—and the belief in the moral and social superiority of textual study over practical training had to be jettisoned. Not everyone approved: in an 1823 diatribe, Henry William Ducachet, a conservative New York City physician (and Episcopal minister), complained bitterly of the abandonment of the old moral and social distinctions, and linked that abandonment to the enthusiasm for anatomy:

> expertness in the use of the knife may, by mere dint of practice, be acquired by any one not unconquerably stupid; . . . my remarks . . . apply to those . . . who . . . practise [surgery], not as a liberal profession, but as a *mechanical trade.* . . . [S]urgeons . . . undervalue study [of texts], and . . . attach an unmerited importance to incessant and minute dissection as the only means of acquiring manual dexterity in operating. . . . [A] student of medicine can be much more profitably employed than in the charnel-house; . . . [T]o perform the *highest* operation of surgery, does not require one half the intellectual effort that is necessary for the judicious, speedy, and successful treatment of a fever.[22]

Ducachet was a holdout, a Tory who could not easily abide the national republican ideology. But, in an era when contending schools of therapeutic thought vied for approval within the profession and critics found fault with medical orthodoxy for its dogmatic application of unreliable remedies, physicians and the public increasingly turned to anatomy as a legitimating discourse and a productive practice. Thomas Jefferson, a good barometer of opinion among the scientific gentry (and the leading ideologue of American republicanism), assessed the situation in an 1812 letter to Dr. John Crawford: "While surgery," the domain of medicine most closely associated with anatomy, "is seated in the temple of the exact sciences, medicine [i.e., physic] has scarcely entered its threshold. Here theories have passed in such rapid succession as to prove the insufficiency of all, and their fatal errors are recorded in the necrology of man."[23] Anatomy promised to serve as the vehicle whereby medicine, reconstituted as the fusion of surgery and physic, could remake itself into a reliable science, via a commitment to empirical investigation. Anatomy was a privileged mediator between mind and body, a middle way.[24] To know anatomy one had to read learned texts *and* get one's hands bloody.

The identification of medicine with anatomical science was largely asserted in medical discourse and formal instruction; the proliferation of medical colleges was spurred by the demand for anatomical credentials. The earliest eighteenth- and nineteenth-century medical professorships in America were chairs of anatomy. The first full-time academic position in a basic medical science was the chair of anatomy at the University of Pennsylvania.[25] No matter that most physicians' day-to-day practice consisted of delivering babies, pill pushing, bleeding, plastering, and puking. No medical school was credible unless it offered anatomical dissection, despite all the difficulties schools had in obtaining bodies: students considered anatomical studies to be central to their medical education. Even apprentice-trained physicians (who also styled themselves as "doctor") endeavored to include dissection in their studies and claimed a totemic filiation with Galen, Vesalius, Harvey, and the Hunters. Anatomy conferred epistemological credibility. Insofar as the medical profession could identify with anatomy, it assured its legitimacy. By the 1840s, anatomical medicine's superiority had become axiomatic: James M'Clintock, a medical professor in Philadelphia and Vermont, was stating the obvious when in 1841 he lauded anatomy as the medical discipline that was the "most legitimately deserving the name of a science."[26] Outside the profession, the same sentiment prevailed: an 1850 Boston paper praised anatomy as "one of the most scientific of all scientific subjects."[27]

Thus something referred to as *science*, in the Baconian sense, was present at the birth and infancy of professional medicine in America: the scientific era in American medicine began much earlier than the bacteriological revolution and educational reforms of the 1870s and 1880s. This science was *not* laboratory science, was often passé or provincial, and was always contested at both ends. Critics argued variously that medicine was too scientific or insufficiently scientific. There was always some discontent with the "ideals of science," as too impersonal and dehumanizing, too foreign—or with the profession's failure to meet them.[28] Identification with science was always differential and relational. A poorly educated practitioner might bolster his standing against midwives or botanical healers by claiming possession of the authority of science, but feel insecure when set beside a learned doctor or the latest continental productions of medical knowledge. Based on his greater knowledge of local conditions and the local population, the uneducated doctor might claim that his detailed understanding of his patients' environment and experience in treating their diseases beat out book learning and anatomical studies, but midwives and folkhealers could argue the same. And in the contest between professional and nonprofessional healer, the scientific nature of medicine was the physician's trump card.

The question then is not whether by our standards late-eighteenth- and early-nineteenth-century medicine was "scientific," but rather how did those who claimed the title of "doctor" distinguish their cult from other healing sects, traditions, and practices. And the answer is that they publicly and privately claimed to be practitioners of a "science"—and worked to make good that claim in a variety of venues. They formed distinctive knowledge communities and networks, consisting of colleges, journals, societies, and informal circles. They set aside special spaces where bodies, living and dead, human and animal, could be observed and experimented upon: colleges and hospitals, anatomy rooms, clinics, anatomical theaters. They programmatically encouraged efforts to expand the agency of the medical scientist and practitioner, and these produced tangible results: new techniques, instruments, and diagnoses. They developed agreed-upon procedures for investigation (dissection, observation, experimentation, representation), and for the writing, publication, and demonstration of results. In professional writings and meetings, they encouraged doctrinaire skepticism toward local and received knowledge and practice (although haphazardly applied), matched by an interest in appropriating local or lost knowledge and practice. And they deployed an unstable mixture of rationalist and empiricist rhetoric, including a genealogy of scientific progress that linked medicine to anatomy (and chemistry and mechanics) and to the science of Bacon, Vesalius, Harvey, Boyle, Newton, and Franklin (the most frequently invoked icons). Through all of these activities and claims, the loosely linked corporate body denominated "medicine" derived a common professional identity. From the mid-eighteenth century on, to be a physician or surgeon was to claim membership in an international healing cult whose character was scientific and anatomical.[29]

If the adoption of scientific practices and a scientific identity helped the profession against its outside competitors, it was also useful *within the profession*, particularly for those professionals interested in raising new establishments and razing old ones. This made for characteristic disagreements among schools, factions, authorities, and generations, but also helped settle them. Which is not to say that scientific medicine was received with universal acclaim; far from it. Contemporaries struggled over critical questions: What are the proper procedures, ideology, and institutions of science? Who should practice scientific medicine? What are the limits of scientific medicine? What are its entitlements? Throughout this period, and well into the twentieth century, disputes over the place of science in medicine were common. Often this took the form of a "nature versus art" debate, in which natural healing was counterposed to medical intervention; often it took the form of an "art versus science" debate, in which intuitive, empathic, and experiential healing ability was opposed to techniques derived from book learning and scientific training.[30] And often it took the form of a fierce debate over the social implications of a medicine based on science: was scientific medicine democratic or did it serve to reinstate European social hierarchies?

Clearly, at ground level, a passion for scientific medicine had some disadvantages. The conventional wisdom of the 1840s and 1850s was that too much scientific interest might distract a young doctor from his responsibilities to his patients or create a social and intellectual disparity between him and his patients or colleagues. It was safer to lag behind, to abstain from the latest scientific enthusiasms and attend to the business at hand.[31] But practitioners without formal medical training, without familiarity with the precepts, practices, and rhetoric of scientific medicine, suffered from a far greater handicap. Critics often characterized rural physicians as bumpkins who lacked anatomical expertise. Country doctors defended themselves by claiming expert knowledge of local conditions and individuals, but ambitious risers made sure to be well versed in their anatomy.

"The Health and Happiness of the Human Race": The Power of Anatomical Medicine

> The community at large are fond of the exhibition of activity by the physician or surgeon. . . . Surgery is always a more popular branch with the student—and indeed with the *laity*—than medicine. Treating . . . the *morbi externi* or external diseases, it addresses itself more to the eye; its results are commonly palpable to the meanest capacity, and its agency is *heroic*, and commonly successful, if not in *curing*, at least in *removing* the mischief.
>
> ROBLEY DUNGLISON, 1837[32]

Anatomy's attraction was more than just social or ideological. Anatomy enabled doctors to perform, or take credit by association with, complicated amputations and excisions, spectacular operations on the body's interior (lithotomies, caesarians), resuscitations, galvanic experiments, postmortem dissections, the use of novel medical instruments—a variety of astonishing public feats involving the dead and living body. Most of these were first performed in isolated instances by highly educated medical men. But in time lesser practitioners came to adopt the new techniques, instruments, and ideas. This is not to say that these were necessarily used "correctly." In many cases the new medical science and technology functioned as a legitimating device and a placebo (as it still does), one that served to assure the patient that the physician had realistic knowledge of the body and was effective. The dissecting scalpel, microscope, stethoscope, and hypodermic syringe were icons that referred back to a narrative of scientific progress that was already familiar to patients. Accounts of new medical techniques and discoveries, and instructive essays on anatomy and physiology (sometimes accompanied by a brief history of medical progress), circulated in both widely read and obscure newspapers, journals, and books. Thus, it was widely believed, among doctors and the laity, that anatomical medicine had exerted a "beneficial influence upon the health and happiness of the human race," long before the bacteriological revolution that replaced it as the paradigmatic instance of medical progress.[33] "[I]t is well known," historian George Bancroft noted in an 1831 issue of the *North American Review*, "that more and greater improvements have been made in surgery in the last half century, than in any two centuries that preceded, and . . . these may all be traced to the minute and thorough acquaintance with anatomy possessed by those that made them."[34]

Medical students demanded training in anatomical science; patients demanded anatomically trained healers. Such healers could offer an authoritative narrative of bodily sickness and disease, and could point to a long-lived and ongoing series of improvements in technique and knowledge. Although the eighteenth and early-nineteenth centuries also saw advances in chemistry and botany, medical progress before the bacteriological revolution was typically linked to anatomy and surgery. Between 1750 and 1845, surgeons revived plastic surgery, began to tie the great and deep arteries for aneurysms, learned to resect the lower jaw, repaired large hernias, and became comfortable with performing difficult amputations at the ankle, shoulder, or hip. And Americans contributed to the advancement: Ephraim McDowell, a Kentuckian, developed the technique of surgically removing ovaries; Frank H. Hamilton pioneered the use of skin grafts and medical statistics; Valentine Mott, the New York surgeon, was renowned for performing the difficult feats of successfully tying the common iliac artery at its origin and both carotids simultaneously (but with fatal result).[35] The introduction of anesthesia in 1846, which was celebrated as the greatest and most distinctively American surgical innovation, vindicated public belief in medical progress and in anatomy; anesthesia facilitated the application of surgical techniques developed in dissection of cadavers to living bodies.[36] But even before ether, nitrous oxide, and chloroform came into common use, the programmatic expansion of medical knowledge and technique was a well-known centuries-old work in progress.

As the Mott example cited above indicates, the advance of surgical, pathological, and physiological anatomy did not necessarily benefit patients. "[T]he public," Robley Dunglison complained in 1837, were "imperfect judges of professional merit," and "infinitely more impressed with the success of an operation—which, perhaps, ought never to have been undertaken—than by the skilful and humane exertions of the surgeon to render such operation unnecessary."[37] Dunglison worried that surgeons were performing flashy but unnecessary procedures, but enthusiastically endorsed the larger project of anatomico-physiological medicine. More critical contemporaries charged that anatomical doctors were indifferent to their patients, inappropriately eager for deaths to occur so as to have the opportunity to perform the autopsies that would produce some insight into the causes and nature of the disease, and perhaps an interesting anatomical specimen for display and study.[38]

Anatomy's appeal therefore came from the ways in which it conspicuously expanded what doctors could do and say, and the areas and behaviors of the body susceptible to medical intervention. Anatomical medicine encouraged belief in the unique powers of the physician and surgeon.

Otherwise patients and students would not have sought out healers who deployed anatomical rhetoric and techniques (and healers would not have increasingly sought anatomical training and credentials). This is not to scant the ambivalence that patients felt in seeking help, or their frustration with the limited number of conditions that medicine could reliably cure. Patients rightfully feared the pain and damage the doctor could inflict: before anesthesia, physicians bled, blistered, and puked; surgeons performed their operations on screaming struggling patients. The necessity of causing pain, and the ability to heal through procedures that caused pain, were part of the vocabulary of curative authority. Visible and painful effects were identified with the performance of healing.[39] Anthropologists tell us that shamans' healing powers are derived from an initiatory journey in which the shaman consorts with the dead and is ritually "killed," an ordeal that is sometimes connected to a demonstration of the shaman's power to withstand painful tortures. In some cases, shamans are respected as much for their power to kill as to heal, and the two powers are believed to be closely related.[40] By a similar logic, the commonly told jokes that historians have cited as evidence of the low esteem in which the nineteenth-century profession was held—that the doctor could as likely kill you as cure you—may, on the contrary, be taken as evidence of the power that the profession was thought to possess.

"THE POPULARITY OF DISSECTIONS": STUDENT DEMAND FOR ANATOMICAL TRAINING

By the 1820s a mania for anatomy was in full swing in Paris, London, and Edinburgh—centers of medical education which attracted students from all over the Western world—but also in Boston, Philadelphia, New York, and obscure towns like Lexington, Kentucky and Fairfield, New York, any place where medical colleges or preceptors trained ambitious students. The faculty of the University of Pennsylvania, then the most prestigious medical school in the United States, reported in 1824 that private "dissecting rooms have multiplied to an injudicious extent"; the next year, in recognition of the increasing "popularity of dissections," they made plans to expand their own anatomical facilities.[41] In the largest American cities, the demand for instruction in anatomical dissection along Parisian lines greatly exceeded the ability or willingness of existing schools to provide it; many new diploma-granting and non-diploma-granting schools arose to fill the void. In the years 1820–1822, more than 40% of University of Pennsylvania graduates—the most ambitious students—attended extracurricular dissecting courses, had private instruction, or voluntarily took the mandatory course of instruction a second time.[42] By the early 1840s, in addition to the three main medical colleges and private preceptors, Philadelphia boasted three unchartered schools that offered anatomical dissection, one of which, the Philadelphia School of Anatomy, had classes of about 100 pupils (more than most chartered schools). Students could also attend the practical anatomy rooms of the University of Pennsylvania and Jefferson Medical College, without having to enroll as matriculants.[43]

The enthusiasm for dissection was not limited to medical colleges: anatomical training was often undertaken prior to formal courses, in a variety of locations. After fighting on the losing side in the Canadian Rebellion of 1837, Dr. John Rolph fled Toronto and settled in Rochester, New York. Two of his apprentices, H. H. Wright and James H. Richardson, followed him there to continue their anatomical studies, taking up residence in the attic of his home. (The cadavers were shipped across Lake Ontario in whiskey barrels: an early instance of international trade in bodies.) On his return to Toronto, Richardson carried out further anatomical dissections with other students in a room that adjoined a stable. Later, he went on to a course of formal study at King's College in Toronto and then Guy's Hospital in London.[44] This pattern of nonsystematic medical education, varying combinations of private and scholastic instruction, was common to both Canada and the United States.

To attract students, established medical institutions and newer schools alike were forced to intensify their commitment to anatomy. Those that did not, or could not, risked extinction. Medical schools proliferated and what they were selling—what students demanded—was training that featured anatomical dissection as its centerpiece. Thus in 1810 Harvard Medical School was forced to relocate to Boston, because cadavers were "utterly unattainable at Cambridge." In his petition to the president and fellows of the university, John Warren argued that "one of the great objects" that attracted students to the school was the chance to dissect cadavers. Without cadavers (which Warren planned to obtain from the nearby Boston Almshouse), Harvard would never succeed in its goal of becoming an eminent medical institution, and would be overshadowed by "other establishments, even in the remote parts of the Country."[45] In the antebellum period, schools competed for students and invariably promised them an abundance of anatomical material.[46] Rival faculties publicly clashed over the veracity of such claims—even though such controversies called attention to the illicit means through which schools obtained their cadavers (see chapter 4 below).

MAN-MIDWIFERY AND THE EMERGENCE OF THE ANATOMICAL PHYSICIAN

I was Calld . . . to see the Desection of the Son of Esquire Davis which was performd very Closly. The left lobe of the lights were found to be much inflamed, the

intestines allso in which were 4 intersections, an inflammation of the kidneys and Blather. There were not a single worm Contained in the boddy but a small quantity of
what the operators supposed to be the bed in which they
resided. The gaull blather was larg and very full. The
opperation was performd by Doctors Colman and Page.
Judg North, Son Jonathan & myself were attendants.

DIARY OF MARTHA BALLARD, FEBRUARY, 1801[47]

Professional medicine's intensified commitment to anatomy, and anatomical training, was fueled by changing patient demands and expectations.
These changed demands in turn fueled a change in the composition and
identity of medical practitioners, from midwife to physician. A suggestive
account of this transition appears in Laurel Thatcher Ulrich's *A Midwife's
Tale*, a microhistorical study based on the late-eighteenth- and early-nineteenth-century diaries of Martha Ballard.[48] Mrs. Ballard, a farm wife and
midwife, served as the principal healer for her remote Maine locality, but
was outranked by physicians who attended the elite families in the area,
and who were consulted in difficult cases by the rest of the community.
Ulrich shows that the two types of practitioner worked cooperatively and
hierarchically (although with some tension), the midwife deferring socially and occupationally to the physician—a gentleman whose income
derived mainly from landholdings and mercantile activity, not medicine.
Between the book-learned, anatomically trained male physician and the
orally and experientially trained midwife, there was a settled division of
labor based on gender and social class, a relationship ceremonially enacted in the ritual of autopsy. Where the cause of death was not self-
evident or "natural," the leading medical authority, the gentleman-
physician, was called on to perform a postmortem dissection—a formal
opening of the body in which the examiner searched for signs that only
he could read, in order to render a definitive explanatory narrative of the
death, a ceremony solemnly witnessed by midwives.

    In the eighteenth and early nineteenth centuries, however, a new kind
of physician emerged, one who competed with and eventually supplanted
the midwife.[49] This physician sought to become the principal healer for
the entire community, and derived the better part of his income from his
practice (though still usually not all of it). "Man-midwifery" (a term supplanted by "obstetrics" in the 1810s and 1820s), while exhausting and
generally poorly paid, was essential to the building of a successful medical
practice—the act of delivering a baby established a decisive, durable
bond between physician and patient (both mother and child). The doctor's claims to medical competence and cultural authority in delivering
babies rested upon his familiarity with authoritative medical texts and,

above all, on unmediated knowledge of the body via dissection. In order to displace midwives, the medical professional argued that he had a superior knowledge of the female body not available to midwives.[50] He had science, not ancient lore and superstition; he was educated and had dissected—a practice that women were forbidden to undertake until a few gained admittance to a handful of medical colleges in the late 1840s.

Women had long been barred from dissecting, but in the early decades of the nineteenth century physicians also stopped using midwives to witness autopsies, and began to actively set out the logic behind the ban on women's admittance to medical school and dissecting room.[51] Dissection of the body, male physicians emphasized again and again, was injurious to the fragile sensibilities and frail health that were defining characteristics of feminine "refinement."[52] An anonymous 1820 pamphlet commented that women could not be instructed "in the science of medicine":

> we cannot carry them into the dissecting room and the hospital; many of our
> more delicate feelings, much of our refined sensibility must be subdued, be-
> fore we can submit to the sort of discipline required in the study of medicine;
> in females they must be destroyed; . . . a female could scarcely pass through
> the course of education requisite to prepare her . . . for the practice of mid-
> wifery, without destroying those moral qualities of character, which are essen-
> tial to the office.[53]

The transition from female midwife to male physician is thus linked to the emergence of a new definition of womanhood in the nineteenth century, the familiar angel of the house, whose delicate moral character and health would be jeopardized or insulted if she were exposed to the naked body. The cadaver, with its stench, gory disorder, and unveiled genitalia, was the antithesis of domesticity's aesthetic and ethos, of femininity itself. Such a conception of womanhood, it should be emphasized, was a defining feature of "refinement," the bourgeois social identity of the early nineteenth century.[54]

Refinement was signified in a variety of ways: by dress, posture, vocabulary, home design and furnishing, and also by mode of healthcare. Attendance in the home by a scientifically trained, diploma-bearing, male medical practitioner was in earlier times a privilege accorded only to the elite. The displacement of midwives (along with other non-Hippocratic healers) was fueled by the demand of patients and their families for a refined social identity—typically the demand of middling, socially ambitious women. Adrian Wilson argues that in eighteenth-century Britain manmidwifery originated among the upper classes, and

> offered a bridge by which those of intermediate or ambiguous status could
> symbolically climb the ranks and "ape the quality." The artisan's wife might

not be able to afford a carriage, but every couple of years . . . could afford a man-midwife. Man-midwifery thus became an area of conspicuous consumption; the new men-midwives cashed in, and the loser was . . . the traditional midwife.[55]

The same logic extended to the broader demand of patients, especially female patients, for scientific medical practitioners and remedies, but more as a matter of social performance than conspicuous consumption. Resort to a nonscientific practitioner—the type of healer that tended to the everyday needs of the common folk—was a hazard to social credibility, an unrefined thing.

In the final instance, the trend toward physicians and away from midwives and folkhealers was a matter of resources. In the eighteenth century, care by a physician was too expensive for all but the prosperous; the primary level of healthcare was some form of "domestic medicine," provided by mothers or experienced women of the neighborhood. In the nineteenth century, as a large group of people with disposable income developed into a middle class, care by a physician became more affordable and desirable. But the performance of healthcare always had a social coding: in novels and plays, the attendance of a physician, for less than grave illness, suggested hypochondria, an affliction of over-refinement, wealth, and effeminacy.

"A LIBERAL PROFESSION": MEDICINE, SOCIAL IDENTITY, AND THE DEMAND FOR BOURGEOIS CAREERS

The female market for scientific practitioners was one that male physicians worked hard to cultivate. The profession, especially the beginning practitioner, was frequently criticized for pandering to women: "Everyone knows that no young physician can succeed without the approbation of the maids and matrons of his particular precinct."[56] The need to secure a practice was paramount in the making of a professional career, and what female middle-class patients wanted was a genteel practitioner. On the other side of the equation, what socially ambitious young men wanted was a "profession," not a "trade": there was a tremendous demand for income-generating occupations that signified one's bourgeois social identity. The occupation had to generate income, but in a way that somehow elevated the earner above the cash nexus, the sordid grubbery of the market economy, and especially above manual labor. As Alexander H. Stephens, president of the New York State Medical Society, proudly proclaimed in an 1849 address: "We claim to constitute . . . a liberal profession; and the very . . . essence of a liberal profession, as distinguished from a trade, is that the acquisition of money is not its primary object."[57]

This was the bon ton that professional medicine promised to supply. Thus, in response to the twin markets for genteel medical practitioners and genteel careers, the learned and disinterested profession of medicine emerged as a sought-after line of work, signifying respectability (or a reaching for respectability) among its practitioners, all the more popular in that it did not necessarily require a particularly large capital or labor investment.

But social standing was relative: a medical career might signify an improvement in gentility only in relation to what went before. For the son of a poor farmer to become a doctor, as William Alcott did in Connecticut in the mid-1820s, was to gain a foothold in the emerging bourgeois order, but Alcott could scarcely claim any high authority within the medical hierarchy. As a practitioner, and later as a medical popularizer and reformer, he drew on the existing stock of medical knowledge, which he added to only marginally and gesturally in the form of an occasional short report to the *Boston Medical and Surgical Journal*—and his contributions were frequently mocked by the editors, who had a higher and more secure standing in the medical and social hierarchy.[58] Alcott's career path was determined by a unique set of particulars: membership in overlapping (medical, kinship, evangelical, and educational) networks; temperament; talent; entrepreneurial ability; and luck. John Godman, a young orphan, served as a printer's apprentice, became a sailor, and then at age 21 a medical apprentice. By virtue of his determination, intellect, talent, scientific publications, and location in Baltimore, Philadelphia, and New York, Godman became one of the most distinguished American anatomists of the 1820s and 1830s, and won acceptance in some high social and intellectual circles. There were many different locations within medical and social networks, many different career trajectories; resources had to be mustered, niches to be found, established, or conquered. Study in Europe with the masters, a course of instruction that included a prodigious amount of dissecting, might cost a few thousand dollars. Study in Philadelphia, Boston, New York, or Baltimore might cost several hundred dollars, with varying opportunities for dissection, again depending on one's pocket, aptitude, location, connections, and resourcefulness. Least expensive of all was study in a rural school or with local physicians (with scholastic medical studies deferred to a later date, or not undertaken at all), with far fewer opportunities for dissection, and a lesser credential at stake. But strata within the medical hierarchy were not rigidly segregated. It was possible to rise: an apprentice might, after a short or long duration of time, go to a medical college; a rural student might make his way to the city for more intensive instruction; a physician might, after a few years of practice, raise the money for European studies.[59]

The fluid sociology of the profession tends to complicate any assess-

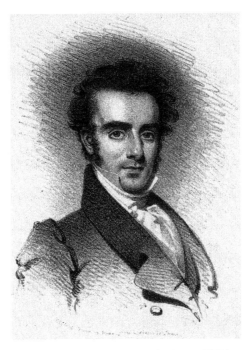

Figure 2.2. John Davidson Godman (1794–
1830). Courtesy of the Library of the College
of Physicians of Philadelphia.

ment of its changing status. Antebellum jeremiads about the low quality
of practitioners, the meager income derived from many medical practices, and the ephemerality of many medical careers have led some scholars to characterize medicine in the 1820s, 1830s and 1840s as a low-status
occupation, practiced by a lackluster, impoverished bunch of rural or plebeian illiterati.[60] But this interpretation conflates the status of the lowest
practitioners within the medical hierarchy with the status of the hierarchy
as a whole. Anatomical science was culturally prestigious and the medical
profession's expansion was based on an identification with anatomical
science. Critics within the profession felt that this expansion was too
rapid and the coinage of medical authority had become debased by the
easy entry of new men. But these new men sought out the profession
precisely because the role of "doctor" represented not just a job, but affiliation with the world of science, learning, and gentility. The social meaning and success of medicine's claims to cultural authority can perhaps
best be gauged by its enemies. Samuel Thomson denounced the regulars
for their aristocratic pretensions and latinate textual tradition, not for

their illiteracy and shabbiness. Class *ressentiment* played a key role in the rise of the Thomsonian movement; and the movement ultimately fractured when some Thomsonians tried to ape the regular profession by establishing formal schools that granted medical degrees and provided training in anatomical dissection (see chapter 5 below).

The medical brahminate (many of them sons of doctors) attained high places within the professional hierarchy by a combination of connections, expensive training, social ability, medical competence (however that was defined), and commitment to anatomical medicine. Pedigreed and wealthy, they were the profession's standard-bearers. At the same time, many rural physicians—the bulk of the profession—generated only a bare competence from some combination of doctoring and farming or trading, and perhaps not even that. But they too were served, in their competition with midwives, folkhealers, herbalists, and other irregulars, by asserting their connection to elite medical science, the anatomical Great Tradition. It might be only some modest gesture or display, a few anatomy books on the shelf, a skeleton in an open closet, or an anatomical preparation in a glass jar on his desk, but the humblest country doctor claimed descent from the line that stretched from Hippocrates through Galen, Harvey, and Hunter, right down to the great medical professors of the day.

Antebellum observers frequently remarked on the social transformation of medicine. According to Dr. Edward H. Dixon, editor of *The Scalpel*, a popular medical journal of the 1850s and 1860s, in the late eighteenth century,

> a doctor of medicine was as rare as an orange tree in a hot-house. He wore a three-cornered hat, a powdered head or wig, with a pig-tail, a court-cut vest, a white neck-cloth, a frilled front to his shirt, black small clothes, with silver or gold buckles at the knees, black silk stockings, and shoes with large silver buckles, a pair of venerable gloves on his hands, and a gold-headed cane in one of them. His fee was a guinea, and invariably paid on receiving his advice.

Such a refined healer had a select clientele, although he might bestow some patronage upon the poor. He "was not to be had by every body, nor for every thing":

> He prescribed in real medical Latin, and could read some Greek. He counted the pulse by a gold repeater, looked at the tongue through gold spectacles, and asked the usual questions about other matters with unusual gravity. Every word was medical, every look was learned.
>
> The wealthy, of course, always employed him, for they had the guineas to pay, and their health was of consequence enough to spend guineas upon it. The middle class, and the poor, could not afford guineas, for their health.

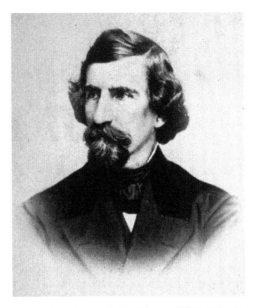

Figure 2.3. Edward H. Dixon (1808–80), in
E. H. Dixon, *Back-bone; Photographed from "The
Scalpel"* (New York, 1866), frontispiece. Courtesy
of the National Library of Medicine.

Back then the common people consulted folkhealers, midwives, or no
one at all. But now the old aristocratic "class of doctors is dead"; the
demand for refined occupations and refined healers has led to the mass
marketing of medical careers. These "modern M.D.s" lack refinement, are
"as common as blackberries":

> A young man, having worked on a farm, or loafed in the city, or having been
> a carpenter, or a clerk in a grocery store, or a letter-carrier, or a clerk in the
> Post-Office or Custom-House, or a bar-tender, or a member of Assembly—all
> at once conceives the thought of being an M.D.[61]

Dixon cast a jaundiced eye on the aspirations and abilities of these plebeian risers, but also mocked the gentleman doctor of the past, whose authority (and clientele) comes from his dress, elite birth, and showy performance of erudition rather than an anatomical understanding of the body.

In a memoir of his student days in New York City in the early 1830s,
Dixon emphasized that he and other middling students took anatomical
studies more seriously than the sons of the gentry:

> [The] . . . deprivation of college [dissecting] privileges was not very distress-
> ing to most of the students, who were travelling the scientific highway in silk

stockings, and felt the intimate relation between a rich father's pocket and their sheep skins proper and prospective; but there were a few of us who looked to our profession only for advancement.[62]

Students like Dixon had to make their way on the basis of medical expertise and skills, rather than inherited social standing. Their professional and social success grew out of a command of, and publicly avowed allegiance to, the latest trends in anatomical medicine.

The career of Nathan S. Davis (1817–1904) provides an example of how anatomy might figure in the rise of a medical man. An autobiographical letter tells us that Davis was born in 1817 in sparsely populated Chenango County in upstate New York, "in a rough log-house." As a boy, he received primary schooling at a district school and only six months of secondary education at a seminary in a neighboring county. At seventeen, he began a medical apprenticeship with a local physician. At eighteen, he attended the College of Physicians and Surgeons of the Western District of New York in rural Fairfield, a respectable but not stellar school. After graduation at 20, he got married and set up practice in Binghamton, New York. Davis describes his activities as an ambitious, newly diplomaed, young doctor:

> [I] gradually acquired a good practice in all the departments of Medicine, Surgery and Midwifery. I occupied every leisure moment in study, making myself familiar with the Medical Botany of all that region—working in practical chemistry . . .—every winter refreshing my anatomical knowledge by dis-

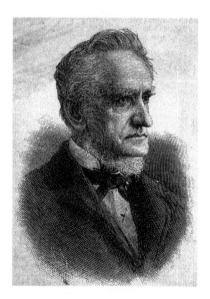

Figure 2.4. Nathan S. Davis (1817–1904). Portrait, 1887. Courtesy of the Library of the College of Physicians of Philadelphia.

secting one or more subjects in the work-room over my office and instructing students (generally had to get the subjects with my own hands).

Expertise in scientific medicine attracted patients and medical pupils. It also helped to underwrite a broader professional authority: Davis gave lectures on "physiology or some department of Natural Science" in local elementary and secondary schools. The vogue for anatomy extended even to remote western New York: Davis made sure to keep up his dissections and to instruct local medical pupils. The requisitioning of bodies was illegal and risky (Davis doesn't divulge details), but scientific and professional advancement required anatomical acumen. In the 1840s, Davis presented papers and wrote articles for professional journals, some of them commentaries on recent developments in British anatomy and physiology. He also began actively participating in the Broome County Medical Society and New York State Medical Society, making a name for himself as an advocate of greater rigor in medical education, especially a greater emphasis on practical and pathological anatomy. Eventually his labors bore fruit: In 1847 he moved to New York City to assume the position of demonstrator of anatomy and lecturer on forensic medicine at the city's College of Physicians and Surgeons and became a key figure in the founding of the American Medical Association (a forum for those who advocated the reform of medical education and the raising of professional standards). Two years later he moved to Chicago, where he became a professor at newly formed Rush Medical College and a pillar of the city's social and medical establishment.[63]

Davis's success, it may be argued, was exceptional, but the recipe for self-improvement in medical knowledge and advancement within the medical hierarchy was no secret. All over the nation, ambitious young physicians and their pupils were similarly seized by anatomical enthusiasm. Ashbel Smith, a well-born North Carolina physician, reported to a colleague in 1834 that "I am collecting medical observations . . . for *my own* improvement. Last winter I dissected with great care 7 bodies. I neglected my patients and they grumbled; this winter my scalpel has not tasted dead flesh."[64] Smith had studied in Paris a few years earlier, but many aspiring doctors lacked the resources for study, even in an American medical school. In isolated Jefferson County, in western Pennsylvania in the 1850s, J. C. Simons, a young doctor who was "ambitious to become a surgeon" and "believ[ing], like all intelligent doctors . . . , that a knowledge of anatomy was the foundation of the healing art," set up his own informal course of anatomical instruction. Simons and his pupils stole their own cadavers, at some risk to themselves: after they were discovered, they narrowly escaped tarring and feathering by a mob.[65]

By the standards of contemporary New York and Philadelphia, the western Pennsylvanians were not very polished, but within their own communities they might become leaders. One of Simons's students, W. J. McKnight, went on to build a successful rural medical practice and served many years in the Pennsylvania state legislature. Physician-legislators, while always outnumbered by lawyers, could be found in every state.[66] The successful physician was well placed to become a politician; he played a key role in communities and connected together diverse persons and geographical locations. If medical practices did not always produce great profit, physicians derived income from farming, real estate, manufacture, and other activities that might be helped along by the contacts maintained through a medical practice.

Conclusion: "The Importance of a Knowledge of Anatomy in a Medical Education"

We hardly need to dilate upon the importance of a knowledge of Anatomy in a medical education:—it is the ground-work, the very alphabet of that education.

Massachusetts Medical Society pamphlet, 1829[67]

In mid-eighteenth-century America, the possession of a diploma was a title: bearers claimed the rank of gentleman, attended to the elite, and almost automatically claimed the respect of medical colleagues. With the proliferation of medical practitioners, by the middle decades of the nineteenth century, a diploma no longer sufficed. Physicians gained the respect of colleagues and patients through the quality and quantity of their training and researches in anatomy, physiology, and other subjects, and through a rhetorical commitment to scientific medicine.

There was an internal dynamic that furthered the anatomization of professional medicine. Training with the eminent Parisian anatomists and physiologists, a demonstrated knowledge of the latest theories, techniques, and methods, assured respect within the American medical hierarchy, and a place within the medical professoriate. To take the most prominent example, the 1836 cohort of Americans who clustered around the great anatomist Velpeau at La Charité hospital in Paris—Henry I. Bowditch, Oliver Wendell Holmes, Sr., George C. Shattuck, William Wood Gerhard, Alfred Stillé—all became medical professors in Boston and Philadelphia, the leaders of the profession. Their students in turn spread far and wide, and generated their own students. If some elders still warned that an identification with anatomy was injurious to the maintenance of a practice—the linkage between therapeutic skepticism and anatomical empiricism seemed especially dangerous for practitioners—this should not obscure the larger anatomical gestalt that dominated and defined early- and mid-nineteenth-century American medicine.

The picture I have drawn, then, is of successive and intensifying waves of anatomization as anatomical practitioners displaced, or succeeded, less anatomical and nonanatomical practitioners. These waves, beginning in the mid-1700s, diffused widely and unevenly from Britain and France to various cities and regions of North America (with Germany and Austria displacing France for medical eminence in the 1860s). Over time, medical training increasingly emphasized anatomical dissection, physiological experimentation, and postmortem examination, even if (in American conditions) such training was difficult to stage, requiring hospitals, clinics, access to large numbers of cadavers, and eventually endowments to fund research.

This trend was not merely a "top-down" effect: a few elite institutions in the 1840s and 1850s did try (unsuccessfully) to mandate more rigorous standards, which included requirement of more practical, pathological, and "microscopic" anatomy, but in the 1820s, 1830s, and 1840s, it was students who demanded advanced instruction (even as they resisted mandatory requirements) from a balky establishment. The demand of patients must also be kept in view here, but, while patients sought out scientific healers, the standards for what made a healer scientific, and what qualified a healer for a diploma, teaching position, or office in the county medical society, were negotiated largely within the institutional structures of medicine. Tellingly, the 1830s is also the decade when physicians began to vigorously promote the idea that patients and the public needed to be educated in anatomy and physiology, arguing that such knowledge would help them discern the difference between scientific healers and quacks (see chapters 5 and 6 below).

It should be emphasized that the cultural and material benefits derived from the position of "professor" of anatomy (or any medical subdiscipline) were not negligible. A commitment to anatomical medicine was typically connected to the rising trajectory of a young medical man, not only a large and lucrative practice but also relocation to the metropolis— think of James Marion Sims, the surgeon whose gynecological experiments on slaves served to elevate him from an obscure practice in rural Alabama to social eminence, and his own hospital, in New York City (where he continued to perform gynecological experiments on Irish immigrants). If in some cases and at some times (particularly early in the century) professors subsidized their schools or scientific work, such work, in the long term, served to elevate one's social, cultural, economic, and professional status, with the highest cultural goal perhaps being "immortalization" in the pantheon of medical giants via the naming of body parts, syndromes, operations, buildings, chairs, rooms, museums, etc.

Finally, the authority that accrued to practitioners of anatomical medicine was not confined to medicine. Physicians attained prominent posi-

tions in church organizations, government, private associations, philan-
thropies, and reform movements. John Collins Warren, for example,
helped found the Massachusetts General Hospital, the McLean Asylum
for the Insane, and the American Association for the Advancement of
Science, actively participated in the Massachusetts Agricultural Society,
Bunker Hill Monument Building Committee, and Boston Atheneum, and
was at various moments a Justice of the Peace, President of the Massachusetts Medical Society, Boston Society of Natural History, and Massachusetts Temperance Society. He addressed the state legislature on several occasions and frequently corresponded and dined with members of
the political and social elite. He also vigorously promoted measures to
improve public health, such as the relocation of burials outside the city
limits, and to incorporate "physical education" (instruction in anatomy,
physiology, and hygiene, as well as exercise) into the public school curriculum.[68]

Warren occupied the highest tier of American medical and social eminence, but such wide-ranging activities were not unusual among physicians. Even at lower levels, doctors gained in status by adverting to their
membership in the larger medical hierarchy and, by the very nature of

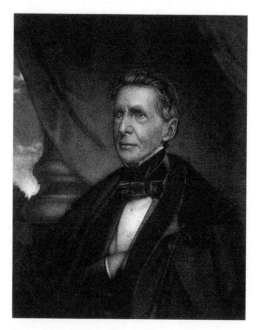

Figure 2.5. John Collins Warren (1778–1856).
Courtesy of the Library of the College of
Physicians of Philadelphia.

their work among a dispersed clientele, formed a social nexus that facilitated participation in public affairs. "In your native states," J. W. Draper told the University of New York Medical Department class of 1842, "you stand in the position of men, who can advise for the body politic as well as the body corporeal; and in a hundred cases can advise with enlightenment those whose means of observation have been less extended than yours."[69] Thus, while antebellum medical writers typically complained that an influx of unqualified and unrefined practitioners was degrading the profession, Daniel Drake could still plausibly assert that "medical men exert more influence on the manners of society, than any other class, except the rich."[70]

3

"Anatomy Is the Charm"

DISSECTION AND MEDICAL IDENTITY
IN NINETEENTH-CENTURY AMERICA

> The day when the medical student enters the dissecting
> room is the time of dedication to his profession; for then
> he puts his hand to a task that other men dread, and
> joins the company of those who have laid aside the deep-
> est fears and prejudices of mankind. . . . [T]he student
> of anatomy . . . is one of that profession whose history is
> an endless record of hard-won progress from darkness
> toward the light.
>
> G. W. CORNER, 1930[1]

ON 16 MAY 1825, Jerome Van Crowninshield Smith, professor of anatomy
at the Berkshire Medical Institution in Pittsfield, Massachusetts, composed a letter to John Collins Warren, professor of anatomy at Harvard.
Faced with perennial difficulties in obtaining cadavers, Smith proposed
that they petition the Massachusetts legislature for a bill that would permit the medical colleges to take the bodies of prison and almshouse inmates. The problem, Smith reckoned, was getting the profession to unite
behind the petition: some doctors would support the measure only if it
entitled "any regular surgeon, in town or country," to obtain "a convict's
body." But this, in Smith's view, would defeat the purpose of the bill:
cadavers must be reserved solely for the use "of our medical Colleges, or
the number of students will certainly diminish. Anatomy is the charm,
and if physicians can accommodate their pupils at home, it will be a finishing blow to the anatomical theatres."[2]

Thirty-five years later, in an address to incoming students at the Medical College of the University of Pennsylvania, D. H. Agnew, the eminent
surgeon and anatomist, explained the appeal of dissection, again using
the word "charm," but as a kind of meditative internal housekeeping, a
celebratory inventorying of the body:

> What a charming task, to sit quietly down in the apartment and take apart
> this master-piece of workmanship; to call each piece by its proper name;
> know its proper place and work; to wonder over the multitude of organs so

compactly pressed together, so diverse in operations, yet each executing its appointed task in the grand confederation.[3]

"Anatomy is the charm," "what a charming task": the phrases are striking. We customarily regard the dissection of dead bodies as necessary but repellent, astonishing but grotesque. In contrast, eighteenth- and nineteenth-century medical students and physicians were drawn to anatomy, charmed by it. "To the young student, the department of *Anatomy* is decidedly the most attractive," Robley Dunglison reported in an 1837 manual for new medical students.[4] Anatomy provided the physician with real advantages in his competition with midwives, folkhealers, clergymen, and other physicians, helped him to filiate his occupation with learned texts and productive science. But the above passages hint at something more. What was anatomy's charm? How did it confer epistemological, healing, and cultural authority? How did it comport with, and even come to define, the professional and personal identity that students, teachers, and physicians worked so hard to shape and perform, and that patients demanded? What were the social conditions for anatomy's success?

In chapter 2, I argued that the period from 1760 to 1880 was the anatomical era in American medicine (actually several successive anatomical

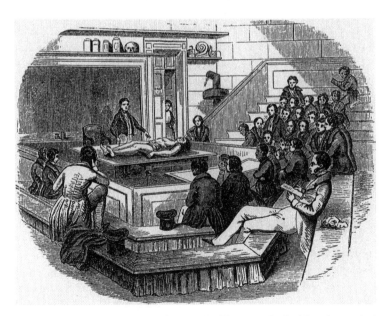

Figure 3.1. Anatomy class. Henry Hollingsworth Smith, *Anatomical Atlas, Illustrative of the Structure of the Human Body, under the supervision of William E. Horner* (Philadelphia, 1849). Courtesy of the National Library of Medicine.

eras). Here I will try to decode the metaphor-laden cultural poetics of anatomy.[5] I will show that, in the late-eighteenth and nineteenth centuries, membership in an authoritative cult of medical knowledge was established and asserted via anatomical ritual and performance; and that the emergent profession, patients, and lay public were impressed, fascinated, and even obsessed by anatomy. In the anatomical theater and the dissecting room, in lectures and textbooks, at the deathbed and the graveyard and in the doctor's office, physicians defined themselves and their reliable knowledge of the body in opposition to magic, charms, and powers (some of them originating from the dead body)—and against the force the dead body itself exerted on the professionally immunized medical initiate. Given this opposition, the profession claimed anatomy as a kind of magical antimagic. In cutting open, displaying, and experimenting on the dead human body, the anatomist legitimated himself and his profession, trumped competing healing and funerary practices. Dissection, body snatching, anatomical iconography, and the history of anatomy were venues in which physicians staged rituals and exhibitions and told stories that constituted the profession as an authoritative cult, a male fraternity of dissectors. Within sequestered professional spaces in medical colleges, and, extramurally, before ticket-buying audiences and coroner's juries, anatomy generated emblems and performances that asserted the cultural power of orthodox medicine as a profession, and the physician's standing within the cult of medical knowledge. Such was the message implicitly staged in the mid-nineteenth-century physician's office, which was likely to have one or more prominently displayed anatomical charts, office skeletons, anatomical preparations, anatomy books, diplomas, and memento mori.

ANATOMIST VERSUS CADAVER

In his 1765 address to the first graduating class of the College of Philadelphia, Dr. John Morgan (recently returned from anatomical study in Europe) made sure to mark anatomy's priority in the medical curriculum. "In studying the art of healing we commonly begin with Anatomy, and very justly. . . . It is Anatomy that guides the doubtful step of the young votary of medicine through an obscure labyrinth, where a variety of minute objects . . . perplex his imagination." The young physician was a "votary" of a healing cult that had anatomy as its chief mystery, its foundation.[6]

In the century that followed, such sentiments became a staple of American medical oratory. Anatomical dissection was depicted as an authoritative epistemological procedure, a spiritual rite that transcended the mundane world of embodied labor and exchange, an operation that elicited from the dead body a revelation, a "natural theology." According to John F. Sanford, a mid-nineteenth-century professor of anatomy: "the Scalpel . . . can reveal the most beautiful and profound structures" of the body, "its intricate and noble fabric."[7] To the untrained eye and hand, a dead body might be a meaty, decomposing, even dangerous, mess; to the anatomist it was "the wonderful machinery of man," "the tenderest tissue," and so on. This transvaluation of the dead body required that the dissector have heroic (and implicitly masculine) personal qualities, "a steady hand," "acute vision," a "strength that subdues a world to his will."[8]

The encounter between anatomist and cadaver was linked to a larger narrative. In lectures and textbooks, the history of anatomy was a tale of medical origins. This was an epic, centuries-long battle between reason and superstition, of "light" versus "darkness," in which "the natural horror which attends meddling with human dead bodies" was gradually overcome through the heroic efforts of a line of anatomists stretching from the ancient Greeks to Vesalius to the moderns. This could be narrated as a triumphalist tale of medical progress, but also as a recurrent and neverending struggle between empirically-based reason and delusionary, irrational folk beliefs. The battle still raged. Frank Hamilton, an upstate New York anatomy professor, warned the incoming class of 1837 that

> a large proportion of our fellow-citizens consider the human dissector . . . an enemy to his species, a rude and unnatural wretch, who can only find amusement in violating the sanctity of the grave, and disturbing by wanton slaughter the repose of the dead. That in the early ages, when the dead were embalmed, preserved, and even deified; held as the sacred abode of departed spirits; anatomy should have been neglected and despised, viewed as a kind of hell-born necromancy, we cannot wonder; but our wonder is, that in these later days, when the light of reason and revelation unite to teach the lifeless corse to be nothing more than the clay tenement of a departed spirit, the same bitterness of feeling against dissections in a great measure exists.[9]

Lecturers often connected the contest between anatomical medicine and an ignorant public to the millennial progress of Christianity against pagan superstition. Reason's most profound victory came through the illumination of the interior of the dead body. Xavier Bichat, the most influential anatomist of the dawning nineteenth century, urged his students to "Open up a few corpses: you will dissipate at once the darkness."[10]

To the image of the interior of the human body lit up was joined a striking auditory image. "The triumph of modern medicine begins," announced John Godman, the eminent American anatomist of the 1820s, "the voiceless dead are interrogated."[11] W. W. Keen, in an 1870 introductory lecture to his anatomy class, paid homage to a historical, and entirely male, succession of "bold innovators who first forced the dead human body to disclose its secrets for the benefit of the living."[12] The knowledge of the mysteries of the recalcitrant human body had to be extorted by force majeure.

This seizure could only be accomplished by a technician of the sublime: in the nineteenth century, the anatomical narrative was linked to the romantic cult of genius. In the dissecting room, the student was asked to retrace the explorations of the anatomical greats, and in doing so invested himself with their greatness.[13] Vesalius was compared to Columbus, as a discoverer, geographer, and conqueror of a New World, a masculine force of will. By extension, so were all dissectors.[14] "[T]he anatomist," a well-known antebellum physiology professor happily reflected, "now travels unhesitatingly into regions, half a century ago unknown to the scientific world."[15] Such rhetoric evoked the intellectual, professional, and social opportunities opened up by anatomy, especially pathological anatomy. George Eliot noted that "About 1829, the dark territories of Pathology were a fine America for the spirited young adventurer."[16]

Obviously, the primary function of training in anatomical dissection was to give medical students a knowledge of the internal structure and topography of the body, a methodology for investigating that structure, and practice in surgical technique. But socially and professionally it was also designed to transform the student, to inure him to the body and to death. This was a difficult procedure, emotionally and cognitively.[17] "A human corpse," William James wrote in his 1890 *Principles of Psychology*, "seems normally to produce an instinctive dread."[18] In the presence of death, the living are typically moved to tears, trembling, weakness in the limbs, goose bumps, loose bowels, even vomiting and fainting. The dead body acts on the body of the anatomical initiate, tests his poise and courage.

Reminiscences of eminent nineteenth-century physicians often touched on this theme. The autobiography of James Marion Sims, the celebrated gynecological surgeon, contained two anecdotes of dissection room experiences during his student days in South Carolina in the 1830s. Significantly, both occur after dark. The first was his own encounter with a cadaver, the second that of his friend, William Sims Reynolds, who "alone at ten o'clock at night," dissected some "parts concerned in an inguinal hernia":

> Reynolds's only candle was . . . resting on the epigastric region of the subject. . . . He started to pass round the lower end of the table for some purpose, when he . . . jostled the body so as to knock loose the chain at the upper end of the table. . . . [T]he body . . . was, by the weight of the lower limbs, suddenly jerked to the floor in the upright posture, and its arms were forcibly thrown over Reynolds's shoulder. The light was of course put out. I

think I should have left that body to the force of gravity. But Reynolds took it under the arms and replaced it on the table.[19]

In the absence of illumination (a reworking of the "Enlightenment" trope of light versus dark), the dead body becomes "uncanny," threatens to overwhelm the reasoning self.

Nineteenth-century observers often remarked on the power of the cadaver. The cadaver's invasive smells and fluids offended the principles of refined aesthetics and taste, but, more perilously, "deadly effluvia" and "putrid emanations" could poison anatomy students and the surrounding community.[21] More dangerous still was the prospect of direct bodily contact with "the terrible poison of the putrefying human body": before the advent of antisepsis, anatomists often contracted fevers and infections, sometimes fatal.[22] Jacob Bigelow warned that "what is most formidable in dissecting, is the poisonous effects of a slight wound, or crack in the skin, which is made by the dissecting knife, or otherwise, so as to apply the putrid solid or fluid material to the wound . . . I knew a young student, who cut his finger in dissecting a subject that had been too long kept, who died in three days after, in a distressed and feeble state . . . attended with a mortification of the whole arm."[23] Those who died in this way were often eulogized as martyrs to the cause of medical progress. Edward H. Dixon, a usually hardboiled literary stylist, offered this tribute to his classmate, Abel J. Storr, who "died . . . from phthisis, developed by a wound received in dissecting":

> That noble heart, that clear intellect, intent on ambition's most holy return— the knowledge of curing disease—has ceased to beat. . . . I recall with a tear and a sigh that one so true should have been cut down on the threshold of the temple, whose corner stone had laid so securely on the foundation of anatomy.[24]

At the same time, the critics of nineteenth-century anatomy—and anatomists themselves—cautioned that familiarity with the cadaver could have deleterious moral effects.[25] The dead body could incite desire (necrophilia), inspire contempt for humanity, or lead students to reject Christianity entirely in favor of "materialism" (atheism), and so jeopardize their immortal souls. In an 1854 polemic, theologian Tayler Lewis warned that "the air of the dissecting room is unfavorable to a belief in the doctrine of the resurrection."[26] The dead body was corrupting: in political and theological rhetoric, the term "corruption" identified immoral behavior with the repulsive image and smell of decomposing flesh.

Such were the assumptions underlying the anatomical rite of passage. The cadaver was powerful. The beginning medical student was initiated into a cult of dissectors who appropriated, cut into, worked on, and produced knowledge from, the interior of that body. In undertaking this hazardous and intellectually demanding initiation, the medical novice was trained to see the body in a new way, was transformed himself into an instrument, a *scope:* "To me things are not as to vulgar eyes, / I would all nature's work anatomize."[27] The medical gaze, acquired through the act of dissecting the dead, was the scalpel's cognitive equivalent. The gaze had a certain killing quality. The body, so full of force, must be divided, colonized, and drained of agency, made over into a "subject" or "matériel."

The struggle between anatomist and cadaver, therefore, was first of all an act of self-affirmation, a test of courage and power. If the training progressed to a higher level, the body became a canvas; the dissection became a work of art, the student an artist. As a beginning medical student in Philadelphia in the late 1810s, Solomon Mordecai initially dreaded the dissecting room, but after some weeks of practice he reported that he began to avidly "devote days to it instead of hours." Two months later, he sent his sister Ellen a letter boasting of the "apparent nonchalance" with which he "appl[ied] the dissecting knife": "[Y]ou can form no idea of the beauty of a masterly dissection."[28] The best students, ambitious young men, often made a specialty of dissection, acting as "prosector" or "demonstrator" for the professor of anatomy and surgery; their quick, perfect cuts expertly opened up the body for exhibition, with the parts finely delineated. Like fresco, such artistry was regarded as a particularly masculine accomplishment.[29]

The Homosocial Meaning
of Anatomical Mayhem

In the anatomical encounter, then, the medical student acquired and demonstrated a powerful mastery of both the subject and himself. An 1830s journalist celebrated the new generation of young medical men as "death-daring aspirants" who

> wallow in the filth of the dissecting room, with a cheerful and animated countenance, and sustain the most offensive effluvia without a qualm, for the sake of unravelling the morbid condition of some rotten viscus. They will hazard their own lives to detect the cause of death in others. Nor can infection nor contagion deter them from living examination, or *post mortem* investigation. The risk of *exhumation* [body snatching] is to them trifling, when compared to the advantages of a laboured investigation of the human frame by the dissecting knife. Their thirst for the acquisition of knowledge is as ardent and craving as the appetite of a drunkard. It is to such *spirits* as these that our profession owes its elevated rank.[30]

The passage speaks in the idiom of mind/body duality: the "death-daring" anatomical students are disembodied "spirits" whose fearless operations on the decomposing corpse "elevate" the profession and themselves, that is, raise it above the level of the purely material. At the same time the writer conjures up a kind of anatomical intoxication, the "appetite of a drunkard," and a moral impunity to dirt, disease, and corruption, a license not accorded to members of the public (and certainly not women), a promethean giddiness.[31]

The passage also alludes to the high-spirited camaraderie of medical students, who often enough performed rituals of professional and scholastic solidarity via copious consumption of alcoholic beverages and tobacco, in addition to their dissections. According to Arthur Hertzler's memoir of student life in the 1880s, smoking was part of the dissecting experience: "Many a properly raised young man blew his first tobacco smoke across the dissecting tables. Tradition had established that it was impossible to endure the odors of the dissecting room unless one smoked."[32] This too served to exclude women; cigar smoking, public consumption of spirits, uproarious pranks, were all emblems of manliness.

In the eighteenth and nineteenth centuries, alcoholic jollity, morbid humor, dissecting-room antics, and body snatching were very much part of a fraternalist medical school culture. At Harvard in the 1770s, William Eustis wrote John Warren a letter (in conspiratorial schoolboy Latin) alluding to their participation in a body-snatching "Spunker's Club" (also known as the "Anatomical Society").[33] In such conspiratorial clubs and less formal associations, one can see a homosocial logic at work.[34] Dissection and grave robbery were rituals, mysteries, that served to bond a group of young men together in opposition to those outside, rituals that marked a passage from protected youth to masculine adulthood. As such, they bore a familial resemblance to the sometimes bloody, and often transgressive, "hazings" prevalent in nonmedical fraternities and secret societies.

Homosocial groups of men are often held together by a shared (real or imaginary) traffic in women. Medical students substituted or added to this a traffic of dead bodies. Samuel Craddock, Jr., in an 1847 letter to his sister, described student behavior at a medical school in upstate New York:

> If a student does not carry himself just so, he is hissed and cheered (by stomping) in a manner that is not at all pleasant. . . . Last week . . . a drunken Irishman . . . struck his head on the pavement and killed himself, and the night after he was buried, some of the students . . . went to the grave yard to dig up his body for a subject to dissect; but . . . they were shot at by some one who was there to watch the grave—they have tried every night

since but have not been successful, for the grave has been watched by other Irishmen—last night just before I went to bed I heard a number of guns fired off in the direction of [the] grave yard, but I have not heard the result.[35]

To falter in the dissecting room or fail to "carry himself just so" was dangerous; to excel in dissecting and body-snatching activities helped to cement one's status within the band of student dissectors.[36] Craddock, in confiding to his sister about such matters and in abstaining from the quest for the Irishman's body, signals an anxious ambivalence about his place in the homosocial order of the student class.

Students needed bodies to dissect, but the persistence with which Craddock's fellows sought their prey testifies to a transgressive group ethic that goes beyond bare necessity. In both the dissecting room and the graveyard, jokes and sport with corpses were devices that allowed students (many of whom were in their late teens and twenties) to playfully test their newly acquired inurement to the power of the dead body—and to

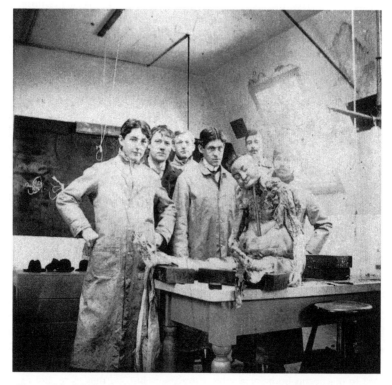

Figure 3.2. Medical students with a propped up, partly dissected cadaver. Mounted photo, ca. 1890. Courtesy of the Dittrick Medical Center.

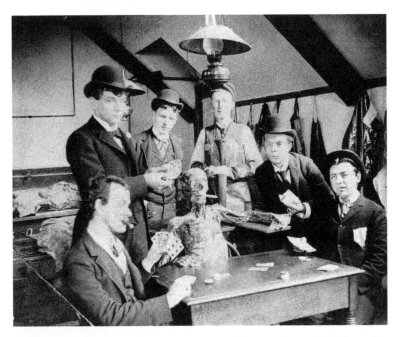

Figure 3.3. Medical students playing cards with a cadaver, which has a lit cigarette in its mouth. Mounted photo, ca. 1890. Courtesy of Steve and Mary DeGenaro.

playfully assert their newly acquired right of eminent domain over the dead, and especially the working-class (or Irish or black) dead. An 1854 editorial in *Harper's Monthly* condemned the "spirit that pervaded the dissecting-room," where a "trifling levity" was combined with "indifference" to the respect due the recently deceased.[37] Medical students, a postbellum journalist observed, were "apt to be lawless, exuberant, and addicted to nocturnal disorders."[38] Late-nineteenth- and early-twentieth-century souvenir photos and medical-school yearbooks conserved and perpetuated this anatomical fellowship. Students stare into the camera around the dissecting table; their cadavers and skeletons are propped up in casual poses, with caps rakishly askew or cigars in their mouths.[39] Hertzler fondly remembered the climate of tomfoolery that prevailed in his 1880s anatomy class:

Curiosity brought many visitors to the dissecting room. The policeman on our beat was greeted by a shower of whatever happened to be at hand on the occasion of his visit. He had been called several times to quell class riots. . . . One evening a number of students from the theological school paid us a visit. To them, medical students were a terrible bunch of rowdies. They all wore

Prince Albert coats and many of them received in their tail pockets, free donations of the various available appendages.[40]

The anatomical mayhem defined a homosocial band—the medical students asserted their masculine power and group solidarity by putting the effeminate theological students in their place. And the publication of the story in a doctor's memoir of the 1930s—well into the era when bacteriology had overthrown anatomy as medicine's most prestigious epistemological model—suggests the continuing importance of anatomy as a narrative the profession lived by.

In the eighteenth and nineteenth centuries, pranks involving body parts were common. Students courted disaster by throwing pieces of their dissections at visitors, displaying severed limbs in windows, or taking bodies and body parts home. Class mates dared each other to snatch bodies from graveyards or even from death vigils. In a published memoir, Valentine Mott, the eminent antebellum surgeon, recounted his student "resurrection adventures" and the "trophies" (bodies) he collected.[41] The danger was that such antics might provoke the local populace, which always suspected medical schools of appropriating and mocking their dead, into rioting against the school (the 1788 "Doctors Riot" in New York City is said to have been precipitated in this fashion). School administrators, with varying degrees of success, attempted to police student behavior. In 1822, the faculty of Transylvania University Medical Department in Lexington, Kentucky issued a rule that prohibited anatomy students from "raising subjects for the purposes of dissection" and required them to pay an extra fee of $5, to fund the activities of more discreet professional body snatchers.[42] Over time, the increasing use of agents, the passage of laws that allowed medical schools to requisition the bodies of the indigent poor, and a tightening of discipline by scholastic authorities put an end to student body snatching, but this trend occurred unevenly, varying widely by state and region. Student pranks attracted the notice of newspapers into the 1880s.

But, far from being an embarrassment, such escapades became part of the lore of the profession, featured in the published reminiscences of elite physicians and lesser lights. Samuel Wakefield Francis triumphantly recalled how James Anderson, John Godman's anatomical demonstrator and later president of the New York Academy of Medicine,

> went forth in the manner of "Cruncher" [the body snatcher in *A Tale of Two Cities*] . . . with some six medical students, to procure a body for the use of Professor Godman. . . . Not a few have praised his daring in endeavoring to dig up a body in Potter's Field, while others of his party called on the keeper and endeavored to arrest his attention while they continued their labors. Memory also laughs over the roused suspicion of the keeper and his son; the

sudden accelerated ejection of the two callers at midnight; their chase by
bull-dogs, and sudden secretion in the company of five hundred hogs; as
though, like evil spirits, they had been cast into the swine; and the return of
the disappointed party![43]

Out of such dangerous escapades emerged what might be termed a professional esprit de corps(e); body snatching became as much a medical
rite of passage as dissection itself. And, in the memoir and after-dinner
anecdote, served to renew and celebrate identity and solidarity.

In its most extreme form, the anatomical narrative could verge on
transgression in the telling itself. In an unattributed humorous anecdote,
purporting to be a true reminiscence of student life, published in several
1835 papers, three young medical students are roommates in a boarding
house; two of them are in the habit of playing tricks on the narrator,
often stealing his food. One night, when the narrator has gone out drinking, they plant a female cadaver in his bed: "having no light to guide me
to my bed, I groped my way as well as I could in the dark. I threw off my
duds, and was about turning down the bed-clothes, when my hand came
in contact with something cold and clammy . . . it was a corpse!" In such
narratives, the extinction of light typically poses a threat to anatomical
reason. But after the student quickly lights a candle, he experiences a
second shock: the woman is black. Death and negritude here are paired
equivalents, equally polluting. "Not exactly admiring either the color or
the temperature of my bed-fellow," the narrator regains his composure,
places the cadaver under his bed, and goes to sleep, "not even dreaming
of ghost, corpse, or any thing else relating to raw heads or bloody bones."
The next day, the roommates "get the laugh upon" the narrator, "for
having had a black corpse for [his] bed-fellow." But an answering prank is
not long in coming: the narrator cuts "some fine large steaks from the
buttocks of black Sue," has his landlady cook them, and then leaves the
premises so his friends will have the opportunity to steal his "breakfast
steak." When they heartily consume the meat, the narrator returns to
inform them that they have eaten human flesh and has the last laugh as
they rush to take medication to help them puke out their breakfast.[44]

The story is almost certainly fiction, a fiction that played on the fact
that medical student life was marked by bantering, stag humor, and practical jokery—and often enough a flirtation with cannibalism and necrophilia. But it suggests that the anatomical body had an erotic valence,
whether positive or negative, and usually gendered female, which even
the highest medical authorities might make reference to. Oliver Wendell
Holmes, Sr., in one of his medical essays, imagines a scene in which Giles
Firman (who is said to have performed the first dissection in Puritan New
England) takes up a "giant folio . . . in which lovely ladies" display their

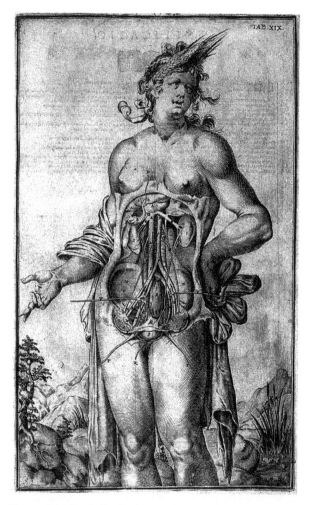

Figure 3.4. Genitalia feminarum, Adriaan Van de Spiegel
(Spigelius), *De Humani Corporis Fabrica Libri Deem* (Amsterdam, 1627), pl. 19.8. Courtesy of the Library of the College
of Physicians of Philadelphia.

viscera with a coquettish grace implying that it is rather a pleasure . . . to
show the lace-like omentum and hold up their appendices epiploicae as if
they were saying, 'these are our jewels'."[45] Adding to the erotic *frisson* is
the presumption that the "lovely ladies" were likely to have been deceased
prostitutes. In the nineteenth century, the anatomy room could serve as
the setting for art that verged on pornography: "The Post-Mortem," a
lithographic plate, appears in a late-nineteenth-century volume of poetry

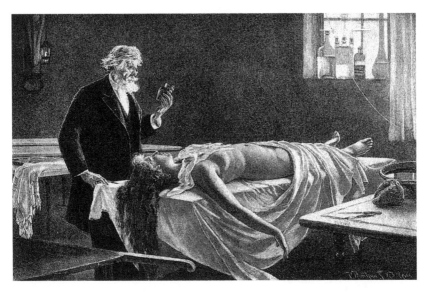

Figure 3.5. "The Post-Mortem," in Ina Russelle Warren, ed., *The Doctor's Window* (Buffalo, 1898). Courtesy of the Library of the College of Physicians of Philadelphia.

on medical topics, intended for a medical readership. The dissection of beautiful young women constituted a small erotic subgenre of medical illustration.[46]

Body snatching and dissecting-room jokes and narratives often had a sexual, class, ethnic, and/or racial coding, as in W. J. McKnight's memoir of body snatching as a medical apprentice in the 1850s in western Pennsylvania, entitled *How I Skinned the Nigger*.[47] The performance of dissections and grave robberies asserted and reinforced professional identity and solidarity, but also privileged other social identities, in this case whiteness. In robbing graves and dissecting their subjects, medical students asserted a ghastly seigneurial privilege: they freely transgressed the funerary customs and honor of working men and women, blacks, Indians, convicted criminals, and immigrants. Complicating this was the erotic potential of the cadaver, which was identified, via anatomical discourse and illustration, with the "animal economy," the site from which desire emerged, and also as the object of desire. For both dissector and dissected, body snatching figured as a rape of the grave, while dissection was a public undressing, a rape of the dead body. Cadavers, like women, were regarded as vulnerable, in need of male protection. Critics of medicine often denounced the desecration of bodies on the dissecting table and in the graveyard as an "unnatural act," equivalent to sodomy. The affront to sexual/funerary honor was even more forcefully suggested when the body in question was that of a woman. "Who," the narrator of an 1880 poem asked, "would want the mortal remains of / Wife, mother, daughter, sister, / Upon the block, with veins, arteries, / Nerves, muscles, exposed to view?"[48]

"[S]HE ENTERS THE FOETID LABORATORY": HOMOSOCIALITY AND THE PROBLEM OF THE FEMALE DISSECTOR

Nor would any man want "wife, mother, daughter, sister" to view the dissected body, or to herself dissect. Dissection of the body, male physicians emphasized again and again, endangered the "delicate" sensibilities and health that were the defining characteristic of refined womanhood.[49] Femininity at mid-century was discursively unstable: it could be figured as a morally redemptive ethereal spirit, or as a morally endangered object of erotic desire, or as an active and morally endangering erotic subject. When middle-class women began actively seeking admission to medical schools and the dissecting room, in the 1840s and 1850s, critics warned that anatomy was corrupting. Intimacy with the innards of the body taints the female dissector, destroys her sexual honor:

> The female arm was never intended to wield the sledge or swing the scythe, nor her hand to grasp the dissecting knife. . . . In her own sacred home, amid her domestic duties, or in her parlor surrounded by . . . friends, . . . she shines the ornament and glory of the race. But when she enters the fœtid laboratory of the anatomist, and plunges her hands into the gore of dead men, she loses all her feminine loveliness, and appears like a fallen angel, an object of universal horror and disgust.[50]

The opening of the profession to women therefore posed a challenge to the masculinist coding of anatomical dissection—and medicine in general—and met with fierce resistance in orthodox medical circles.[51] Women who sought medical careers were pilloried in the popular and medical press, and in popular fiction. In Mark Twain and Charles Dudley Warner's comic novel *The Gilded Age* features as one of its main characters, Ruth Bolton, a medical student who devotes herself to dissection. Bolton tests herself against the cadaver's power, risking mental and physical collapse (to which women were assumed to be especially susceptible). If Bolton survives this test, it will transform her into something more than a woman. Anatomical training forecloses the normative progression from young woman to young wife, makes marriage impossible. (In part, this is what draws Bolton to a medical career; she is ambivalent about the prospect of marriage to her fiancé.) Working late at night in the dissecting room (the liminal time when anatomical illuminism is vulnerable to a return of the repressed), Bolton is shocked when presented with a black cadaver that wears a "repulsive . . . scowl," "an ugly life-likeness that was frightful" and "that seemed to say, 'Haven't you yet done with the outcast persecuted black man, but you must now haul him from his grave, and send even your women to dismember his body?'" Dissection is quintessentially phallic. A woman who undertakes it jeopardizes the very basis of feminine identity: she is "desexed."[52] The postbellum racial narrative is premised on the notion that the black male body is a contaminant that threatens the sexual purity of white women; white men are therefore honor-bound to castrate or destroy black men who transgress. By assuming the role of dissector, Ruth Bolton loses her need, and waives her right, to protection against the phallic/contaminating black male body. She becomes a surrogate castrator.

The "desexing" effects of dissection could also carry a positive valence. For women, anatomical studies offered the possibility of escape from relentless gender codings and obligations. The female dissector is exempt from marriage, becomes a kind of taboo object to men. In her autobiography, Elizabeth Blackwell places her desire for a medical career precisely in this context. Averse to "a life association" that required intimate contact with the male body, and uncomfortable with her own erotic feelings, Blackwell writes that she sought to "place a strong barrier" between herself "and all ordinary marriage." Her decision to assume an occupational role that heretofore had been reserved for men helped to erect such a barrier. Yet her career decision paradoxically required that she conquer her "disgust" for "the physical structure of the body and its various ailments." A decisive episode enabled her to overcome her feelings. While teaching school, a colleague offered her a dead insect, a "cockchafer," as "a first subject for dissection":

> I . . . placed the insect in a shell, held it with a hair-pin, and then tried with my mother-of-pearl-handled penknife to cut it open. But the effort to do this was so repugnant that it was some time before I could compel myself to make the necessary incision, which revealed only a little yellowish dust inside.

From that moment on, her fear of the body dissipated: afterward, she records that she "never had so serious a repugnance to" undertaking dissections on humans.[53]

Given this complicated ambivalence, catalogues of nineteenth-century female medical colleges toed a very careful line on anatomy. Anatomy occupied a central role in the curriculum—they had to offer it (otherwise they would not be credible as medical schools), but they did so discreetly, allusively.[54] Harriet Belcher, an anatomy student in the class of 1875 at Woman's Medical College of Pennsylvania, noted that "dissection as managed by women is a very different matter from one taken under the charge of male attendants. Every precaution is taken to spare the senses."[55] Female colleges may have downplayed anatomy, but women medical students performed their own version of dissection antics. With a bit more circumspection, they also posed for anatomy photos, sometimes in comic poses with dressed-up skeletons—and tried to constitute themselves as a sorority of dissectors. In coeducational settings, female dissecting-room behavior was governed by a parallel homosocial order whose power was challenged only with the rise of feminism in the 1970s.

Pauline Stitt, who attended the coeducational University of Michigan Medical School in 1929, describes how things worked:

> I guess I might have been the only girl . . . that landed with the men at the dissection table. . . . The other girls were practically all in a medical sorority. I wasn't asked to be in it. . . . They thought me insufficiently dedicated to medicine . . . because they knew I really enjoyed the boys and other interests they regarded as trivial. . . . "We are not trivial people. We are forthright, up-and-coming women working for our careers. We do not associate with the flibbertigibbet over there who puts ruffles on her blouses and laughs." The men were the in-group, and those women were outside, so they were cutting their hair more like the men and doing all kinds of things to join [emulate] the "in-group." The classic cliché about women doctors in those days was that they were very masculine. . . .[56]

The "in-group" men were imitated by a female "out-group" who wore their hair short like men, were "serious" (eschewed female frivolity and feminine dress), who abandoned the normative female role. The male homosocial order excluded women. The female (quasi-masculine) homosocial order excluded Stitt precisely because she refused to forgo the markers of femininity: long hair, frilly dresses, makeup, a "sweet" voice, flirting with men.

Anatomical Performances

With the exception of Stitt's reminiscence (an early-twentieth-century oral history), the body-snatching and dissection memoirs discussed so far date from around the mid-nineteenth century and were written primarily for physicians, but also haphazardly circulated among the general population. But from at least the mid-eighteenth century medical practitioners also aimed anatomical writings, advertisements, performances, and displays at patients and the public. If physicians dissected in order to improve their surgical and diagnostic skills, to enter, establish, and/or elevate themselves within professional networks and hierarchies, and to contribute to the progress of medical science and technique, they also sought to publicly broadcast (and were glad to have others broadcast) their anatomical commitments and expertise.

This was demonstrated in a variety of public performances. These might be something as simple as the "anatomic figure commonly seen in the shops of apothecaries," which Horace Walpole mentions in a 1762 book on painting (in England, apothecaries combined the roles of pharmacist, general practitioner, and surgeon).[57] Or they might be more spectacular productions. In the eighteenth century, anatomists occasionally put on anatomical shows for the education and entertainment of the public. In the 1760s William Shippen, Jr. caused the first North American anatomical theater to be constructed in Philadelphia, for the instruction of his medical students, but his theater was also used to stage a dissection of Siamese twins for a public, ticket-buying audience.[58] A very different sort of performance was the dissection of suicides or criminals hanged for capital crimes. In such cases the anatomist was a highly visible associate of the hangman: the requisition and dissection of criminal or pariah bodies was a form of "overkill," an added punishment dispensed to particularly heinous criminals, blacks, Indians, prostitutes, and friendless beggars. A 1734 Boston paper reported that "Several Surgeons of the town are now curiously dissecting" the body of a black man who had been executed for rape.[59] In the eighteenth century, when full anatomical dissections were relatively infrequent and popular interest ran high, newspapers and broadsheets often reported on the dissections of offender.

The practice of dissecting certain criminals convicted of capital crimes continued well into the nineteenth century. John Johnson, an Irishman and the father of five children, was convicted in 1823 of having "barbarously murdered" a man in the course of a robbery in New York City. His sentence was death by hanging, to be followed by delivery to the surgeons for dissection. The *New York Gazette* estimated that between 50,000 to 70,000 people witnessed the execution.[60] The handing over of bodies for dissection and subsequent printed reports of the autopsies were part of a public spectacle which accrued to the cultural gravitas of the dissector.

If notorious enough, an executed person's body might be mined for anatomical "curiosities," or serve as a template from which to manufacture copies; the anatomist then assumed the role of collector and exhibitor—a stance that combined proprietary ownership and cultural authority. A criminal reliquary was a regular feature of anatomical museums, both those attached to medical colleges and freestanding popular museums. The body of Charles Gibbs, a pirate who was hanged in New York City in 1830, was turned over to David L. Rogers, professor of surgery at the New York College of Physicians and Surgeons.[61] Some twenty-odd years later, a "Fac simile [*sic*] of the Penis of the celebrated Gibbs the Pirate, in perfect health" [!] turned up in the Grand Anatomical Museum

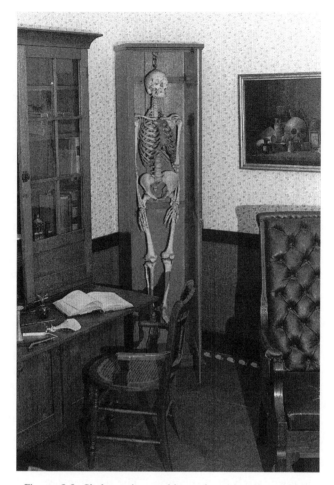

Figure 3.6. Skeleton in a cabinet, doctor's office, 1880s.
The skeleton and cabinet are genuine, but the room is a
composite "period room," put together by a mid-twentieth-
century curator; some details are inaccurate. Courtesy of
the Dittrick Medical History Center, Case Western Reserve
University.

at 300 Broadway, New York City, while in the mid-1870s a cast of his skull
(with a phrenological analysis appended) appeared in Dr. Baskette's Gallery of Anatomy in Chicago.[62] Anatomists similarly collected unusual
pathological cases, to present in whole or in part in private and public
anatomical "cabinets" and museums. And there were, on a few occasions,
public dissecting spectacles. In 1836, P. T. Barnum arranged for David

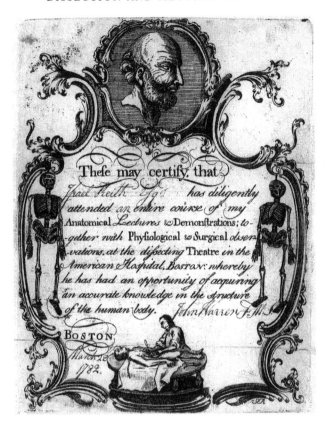

Figure 3.7. Certificate of attendance of anatomical lectures and demonstrations, awarded to Israel Keith by John Warren, Boston, 1782; engraved by Paul Revere. Courtesy of the Francis Countway Library, Harvard University.

L. Rogers to dissect the body of Joice Heth, the aged black woman who Barnum exhibited as the 161-year-old former nurse of George Washington. A crowd of 1,500 at the City Saloon attended; Barnum collected 50¢ a head. (Rogers found that the body could not be more than 70 years old and pronounced the whole thing a hoax.)[63]

The most common anatomical display was the physician's skeleton. In a 1773 notice in the *Providence Gazette, and Country Journal,* Daniel Hewes advertised his intention to go into medical practice, and invited the public "to see the Frame of Bones," a wired skeleton prepared from the body of an "executed negro."[64] Given the belief that the bones of hanged men and "negroes" had mysterious powers or were innately "curious," the identification of the bones served to attract spectators but also to reassure

viewers that the funerary honor of members of the (white) community
had not been violated.

By the early nineteenth century, the physician's skeleton had achieved
iconic status (and its social origins and provenance were not usually advertised). In his autobiography, William Holcombe fondly recalled his father's office with its

> imposing shelves of portly volumes, . . . big jars of hideous specimens pre-
> served in alcohol, the pervading odors of paregoric and lavender, the bloody-
> looking map of the 'great sympathetic' on the wall, the long white skeleton
> grinning in the closet, and the mysterious box, containing the detached
> bones of a baby's skull. . . .[65]

Toward the end of the nineteenth century, the stethoscope, microscope, and examination table began to supplant the physician's skeleton
as medical icons.[66] But as late as 1882 D. W. Cathell's manual was still
advising physicians that in their offices, they should display (in addition
to books, microscopes, and diplomas) "anatomical plates" and "professional relics and keepsakes whose history is connected with your medical
studies, such as the human skeleton, either entire or in parts, pathological or anatomical specimens, and mementos of your dissections."[67] Many
diplomas also featured anatomical iconography.

If the physician's skeleton, anatomy books, and specimens were the
most familiar anatomical displays, the autopsy was the most familiar dissecting performance, witnessed by members of the community (the coroner's jury), and sometimes the family of the deceased. The most unusual
and dramatic postmortem performance was the galvanic experiment.
Luigi Galvani's eighteenth-century experiments—making the muscles of
dead frogs contract through stimulation by electrical current—had been
widely reported all over the Western world. The phenomenon, also called
"animal electricity," seemed to substantiate and make visible the "vital
spark" or *élan vital* that animated living things. In the early nineteenth
century, Giovanni Aldini, Galvani's nephew, put on shows of medical electricity in a tour of western Europe. In a widely publicized 1803 performance, he amazed an audience of Londoners by running an electrical
current through parts of an executed criminal's body, producing twitches
and spasms in the dead man's face and extremities. This helped to inspire Mary Shelley's *Frankenstein* (1818), the novel that virtually invented
the mad scientist genre (the mad alchemist was an earlier gothic precedent), and the 1818 galvanic experiments on the body of a hanged man
by Dr. Andrew Ure of Scotland.[68]

An account of Ure's experiments, reprinted in an 1820s New York
newspaper, suggests how deeply affecting such demonstrations could be:

In the third experiment, when the supra orbital nerve was touched, the muscles of the face were thrown into frightful action and contortions. The scene was hideous; . . . many spectators left the room; and one gentleman nearly fainted, either from terror, or from the momentary sickness which the scene occasioned. In the fourth experiment, from meeting the electric power from the spinal marrow to the elbow, the fingers were put in motion, and the arm was agitated in such a manner, that it seemed to point to some spectators, who were dreadfully terrified, from an apprehension that the body was actually coming to life. . . . Dr. Ure seemed to be of the opinion, that had not the incisions been made in blood-vessels of the neck, and the spinal marrow been lacerated, the body of the criminal might have been restored to life.[70]

American doctors eagerly took up galvanic experiments on the dead. After the 1835 hanging of pirate Manuel Fernandez, the body was brought to the anatomical theater of the New York College of Physicians and Surgeons where David L. Rogers made a series of incisions, attached "galvanic wires" to various nerves and got the dead man's cheek, lips, and little finger and toe to twitch.[71] Such experiments fostered belief in the prospect of a nearly miraculous expansion of medical agency. Power over the living and power over the dead were paired—the profession, according to an editorial in an 1854 issue of *Harper's Monthly*, would soon "extract the elixir of life and health from mortality."[72]

CONCLUSION: ANATOMY AND CULTURAL AUTHORITY

The impact of anatomy thus becomes evident when the ensemble of anatomical activities is considered in its entirety. Anatomy conferred authority and legitimacy because it *worked*: it expanded the technical repertoire and proficiency of medicine; it provided a detailed and plausible narrative of bodily processes to patients, physicians, surgeons, and the laity. To the public, the anatomist, and by extension all physicians, demonstrated mastery over the welter of emotions, beliefs, and regulations associated with death and the dead, and wielded shocking powers. Only the physician could penetrate, dissect, and stage performances with the dead body; only the physician could read the body and render a definitive assessment of the body's physical/moral condition. In medical discourse, the transaction between physician and cadaver was identified with a metahistorical battle between life and death, health and disease, reason and unreason, light and darkness.

Yet critics also condemned anatomy as a "dark science" and medical students reveled in that identification, using the dissecting room and the graveyard to stage a carnivalesque anatomy.[73] Entrée into the profession entailed a journey into the upside down netherworld of dissection and

body snatching. Once initiated into the fraternity of dissectors, the rules
and loyalties that governed everyday conduct were superseded by those
(mostly unwritten) rules and loyalties that governed professional conduct.
In later life, these bonds persisted: physicians maintained (or even
strengthened) their anatomical identity through the performance of autopsies and dissections, as a means of medical "self-improvement." And,
long removed from medical school, doctors sometimes acted as infor-
mants, covertly providing professors, students, agents, or school employees with intelligence on the death of patients whose fresh bodies
could be harvested.[74] Not surprisingly then, the profession acquired a
quasi-Masonic conspiratorial aura, the nuances of which are usually
missed by historians who have not brought an anatomical perspective to
bear on the heated antebellum debates over medical licensure.

Patients, it should be apparent, were deeply ambivalent about anatomy
and the medical profession. To the degree their resources permitted, they
demanded treatment by anatomically trained medical practitioners, a cult
that could powerfully manipulate and affect the body. But anatomical
"magic," like all magic, held the possibility of catastrophe: variations on
the idea that the cure was worse than the disease, that physicians might
kill you with their treatments, and that the best treatment was often none
at all, peppered the pages of antebellum newspapers and magazines.

Therefore, popular opposition to anatomy, based on the perception of
anatomy as a death cult that derived power, even necrophiliac or canni-
balistic pleasure, from the violation of the dead—anatomy as an amalgam
of unnatural acts and social pretension—was, in a certain way, realistic.
The venues through which students were inducted into the medical profession, the practices that served to define the boundaries of the profession, the rhetoric of anatomical discourse and practice, confirmed the
"prejudices" of the public, and in some sense were even intended to do
so. Anatomical performances signified a bold and contentious appropriation of the body and of death. The establishment of a distinctive medical
identity and authority over the living and the dead depended on the
deployment of a cultural poetics set in the physician's office, medical
school, hospital, deathbed, dissecting room, and graveyard, with a distinctive cast of performers and vocabulary of symbols: the professor, student,
body snatcher, the outraged or morally instructed public (maybe several
different "publics"), the "worthless" or "beautiful" cadaver.

This reading then challenges the progressive narrative of anatomy's triumph over superstition by arguing that (1) popular resistance (if not too
severe) was, at least foundationally, useful to the bourgeois learned profession, as that which it defined itself in opposition to; but also that (2)
anatomy's "charm" lay in the production of a distinctive professional cha-
risma, a command over the body, that deliberately transgressed the

boundaries between life and death, purity and contamination, and (in some readings) the sacred and the profane. Medical distinctiveness and respect for the medical profession were enhanced if the physician did what no lay person dared or was able to do, and so depended on a coding of the dead body as powerful rather than as a disenchanted, inert collection of inoperative mechanisms.

Then too they also depended on a coding, multiple codings, of the body as Other: as black, as female, as worker, as matter. And they materially depended on a complex series of economic and political transactions. A purely discursive claim on the body would never have sufficed. The profession needed to requisition actual bodies, to take them and move them from one place to another, to deploy them and transform them, and to dispose of the remains. In the next chapter, I will consider some of the social and professional consequences of those transactions, the traffic in dead bodies.

4

"A Traffic of Dead Bodies"

THE CONTESTED BIOETHICS OF ANATOMY
IN ANTEBELLUM AMERICA

IN MAY OF 1847, physicians from all over the United States gathered in Philadelphia to form a national medical organization (which would ultimately become the American Medical Association). The association, they hoped, would do a number of things. It would exclude botanical and homeopathic physicians from medical societies. It would regulate competition between physicians, referrals to consulting physicians, and the setting and collecting of fees. And it would require that physicians conduct themselves with diligence, confidentiality, and sexual propriety. The organizers compiled all these measures into a proposed "Code of Ethics" that enumerated the "duties of physicians to their patients," to each other, and to the public. The Code, however, contained no provision that even remotely resembled the standards of "informed consent" and "patients' rights" which form the basis of medical ethics in the last quarter of the twentieth century.[1] It certainly did not regulate anatomical practices. But one paragraph—"Obligations of the Public to Physicians"—did allude to dissection:

> The benefits accruing to the public . . . from the active and unwearied beneficence of the profession, are so numerous and important, that physicians are justly entitled to the utmost consideration and respect. . . . The public ought . . . to make a proper discrimination between true science and the assumptions of ignorance and empiricism—to afford every encouragement and facility for the acquisition of medical education—and no longer to allow the statute books to exhibit the anomaly of exacting knowledge from physicians under liability to heavy penalties [anti-grave-robbery laws], and of making them obnoxious to punishment for resorting to the only means of obtaining it [body snatching and dissection].[2]

The passage obliquely refers to the facilities needed "for the acquisition of medical education"—knowledge of the body's interior is the "qualification" that distinguishes physicians whose practice is based on "true science" from those whose practice is based on "assumptions of ignorance and empiricism"—but refrains from uttering the words "anatomy," "dissection," and "cadaver." However, as we have seen, even if they dared not speak its name *here*, elsewhere physicians used anatomy to legitimate their claims to medical authority and healing effectiveness. At the same time, the provision of cadavers for medical schools was clearly practically troublesome and a morally troubling problem in ethics, as physicians then defined it: the good of the profession.

For one thing, anatomical practices undermined the profession's claim to gentility. In the 1820s, John Gorham Coffin, an eminent Bostonian physician and medical professor, wondered how it was possible "that any medical practitioner should . . . engage in a traffic of dead bodies":

> Will it be credited that numbers of dead bodies should be obtained for no other purpose than to strip off the flesh in order to make the sale of the bones to the highest bidder? . . . Is it credible that men of the profession can have so wholly forgotten what is due to . . . their brother practitioners, among whom they live, and whose safety they are bound to regard, as to engage to supply subjects for dissection, to persons at a distance, whenever they are called for? . . . An odium has thus been brought on the whole profession, and serious consequences have been threatened.[3]

Coffin was perturbed by the vilification, physical attacks, even criminal prosecution, to which the profession was recurrently subject on account of its requisitioning and cutting up of bodies. But the "odium" also had social ramifications: a learned professional should not soil his hands in trade or "traffic," certainly not in anything as distasteful, as corporeal, as dead bodies.

This, to be sure, was not the only ethical issue that anatomy posed to the profession. Despite the delicacy of the Code's language, in an era of fierce competition between medical schools, physicians participated in private and public discussions about discretion, methods of provision, and allotment of bodies. However, the larger ethical issues were raised by the laity, and especially the groups of people whose bodies were likely to be taken for dissection. There were heated debates, and on many occasions physical struggle, between the profession and the public over the anatomical treatment of the dead.

Despite a large literature detailing the particulars of body snatching, riots, and anatomy law, the practice of anatomy in nineteenth-century America is not well known or well understood. Complicating matters is the fact that the form and duration of the conflicts over anatomical dissection varied from state to state and region to region, stretching from the eighteenth century into the twentieth. The discussion that follows will give a brief overview of the legal, legislative, and business history of anatomy in nineteenth-century America, focusing primarily on antebellum New York. As in other states and other times, in antebellum New York, a politics of class was conducted in the idiom of anatomy. And, as in ante-bellum battles over slavery, prostitution, and temperance, the clash over anatomy provided the occasion for a critique of the market.

ANATOMICAL PRIVILEGE AND THE LAW

[T]he bones—of substance firm and hard
Long they remain th'Anatomist's reward.
Wise nature, in her providential care,
Did, kindly, bones from vile corruption spare,
That sons their fathers' skeletons might have
And heav'n born science triumph o'er the grave.

FRANCIS HOPKINSON, *An Oration Which Might
Have Been Delivered to the Students in Anatomy*

In late-eighteenth-century society the anatomically trained physician was regarded as a gentleman. His place of privilege was demonstrated and asserted in the confiscation and dissection of the dead, and in the production and reproduction of anatomical knowledge, a cultural matrix that, in succeeding decades, became the basis for the formation of the bourgeois medical profession. Anatomical dissection and body snatching were rites of professional passage that established medical identity and authority.

This, however, was problematic in a number of ways. For one thing, the scope of the profession's exemption from funerary discipline was asserted more in professional discourse and practice than in law: the legal status of anatomical appropriation and rendering of bodies was ambiguous, a matter of custom and common law as much as statute. The regulation of dissection was introduced into English law by the Act of 32 Hen. 8, c. 42 (1540), which allotted an annual ration of four hanged felons to the Barber-Surgeons of London. Similar statutes were enacted under Elizabeth and Charles II, and in the 1641 Massachusetts "Body of Liberties" which decreed that no man who was put to death shall be unburied for more than 12 hours, except in cases of "anatomy."[4] A 1647 resolution of the Massachusetts General Court further stipulated that medical and surgical students be allowed, once every four years, "to reade anotomy, & to anotomize . . . some malefator, in case there be such as the Courte shall alow of."[5] In the English colonies generally, common law precedent was regarded as sufficient to permit the dissection of the body of an executed criminal. A "request from several young Students in Physick, Surgery, &c." sufficed to obtain "The Body of *Julian* the Indian Man, who was Executed" in Boston in 1733.[6]

In 1752, Parliament passed "An Act for better preventing the horrid crime of Murder" (Act of 22 Geo. 2, c. 37) that *required* the hanging in chains or dissection of the bodies of *all* executed murderers so that "some further Terror and peculiar Mark of Infamy might be added to the Punishment of Death." This remained English law until 1832. But in practice, even before the 1752 act, dissection was meted out as extra punishment for capital offenses, in an age in which the death penalty could be applied to cases of arson, theft, attempted rape, as well as murder, in both Britain and the colonies. Thus a 1734 Boston newspaper reported that "skilful Surgeons in this Town" were dissecting the body of John Stoicks, who had been executed for burglary.[7] In the postrevolutionary period, state legislatures replaced English law with their own statutes explicitly permitting judges to sentence men convicted of capital crimes to be dissected by anatomists. In some states other transgressions were also made punishable by dissection. A 1784 Massachusetts act provided that men killed in duels, as well as men executed for killing someone in a duel, could be given over "to be dissected and anatomized" and deprived of a "Christian burial."[8]

The other relevant body of law concerned the status and disposition of dead bodies, including the prohibition against graverobbery. This was ambiguous insofar as the precedents and governing statutes had been originally designed to apply to nonmedical exhumations. A 1604 English law made it a felony punishable by death to disinter a dead body in order to remove parts for use as charms or sorcery in witchcraft. In the absence of specific laws by colonial legislatures, this statute was applied to cases of medical body snatching in Massachusetts, Pennsylvania, South Carolina, and elsewhere.[9] After the Revolution, British statutory law was no longer in effect, but British court decisions still influenced American courts, especially the case of Rex v. Lynn (1788) which ruled that the theft of a body was not a felony because the body was not property: a principle which also theoretically barred individuals from willing their bodies to medical schools.

In the early decades of the nineteenth century, this legal ambiguity was partly resolved through a series of laws passed in response to the proliferation of medical schools and, consequently, grave robberies. Thus, as soon as Dartmouth College proposed to offer a course of medicine, the New Hampshire General Assembly passed a state law prohibiting the unauthorized disinterment of bodies, punishable by a fine not to exceed $1,000, imprisonment of not more than a year, and a public whipping not to exceed 39 lashes; Vermont passed a similar law in 1804. In 1810, when the Connecticut legislature passed an act chartering the medical school at Yale, it also passed an act prohibiting secret disinterment of bodies for the purpose of dissection, or to knowingly "assist in any surgical or anatomical experiments therewith or dissections thereof." On the question of how Yale should supply its medical school, the law was silent. In 1815 Massachusetts passed a law "to protect the sepulchres of the dead" that made unauthorized *possession* of a dead body a crime punishable by fine of $1,000 and imprisonment for a year, with the same penalty for disinterment—thereby putting anatomists, and not just body snatchers, in legal jeopardy. Connecticut followed suit with a nearly identical law in 1817. By 1818, every state in New England had a similar statute against body snatching.[10] New York followed with an anti-grave-robbery statute in 1819, and Maine in 1820. In 1831, Ohio passed a law making illegal the commission, aiding, and abetting of body snatching, with a fine of up to $1,000 or 30 days in jail with only bread and water; its legislature at the same time failed to act on the petition of a convention of surgeons and physicians to permit dissection of persons convicted of capital offenses or who die in jails or penitentiaries.[11] In 1838, Michigan made grave robbery a crime punishable by a fine and one year in prison; and so on.[12]

For most of the seventeenth and eighteenth centuries, common law precedent served as a hazy license to disinter and dissect, and anatomy law was not a big issue. With dissections fairly infrequent and few statutes to prohibit medical grave robbery, anatomists appropriated and dissected bodies where they could, but typically requisitioned only certain kinds of corpses: Indian prisoners of war, people hanged for capital offenses, prostitutes, suicides, and slaves (paupers seem to have been exempted until the last quarter of the eighteenth century). Judge Samuel Sewall of Massachusetts noted in his 1676 diary that he and some other men "Spent the day . . . dissecting the middlemost of the Indian executed the day before," a prisoner captured in King Phillip's War.[13] We don't know whether Sewall dissected to punish and terrorize his enemies, to improve his knowledge of human anatomy, or merely to satisfy his "medical curiosity," but an ambivalent, ill-defined, and quasi- or extralegal mixture of punitive and medical purposes was characteristic of seventeenth- and eighteenth-century anatomy.

So was the criminal, nonwhite, or non-Anglo-American identity of the dissected. The selection of cadavers was determined in large part by the public's response to the anatomical appropriation of bodies. In 1763 Samuel Clossy, an Irish anatomist of some distinction, emigrated to New York. Unable to secure an appointment as professor of anatomy at King's College—funds were low and his supporters "were partly out of Favour"—he determined to brighten his prospects by doing "something more than common" to attract attention. Clossy commenced a course of anatomical lectures, probably the first such course ever given in the city. His first subject was a 20-year-old white woman (probably stolen from a church burial ground) and then "a female black" who bore a "beautifull carving on the Neck breast and belly. . . . Hieroglyphics possibly of the kingdom of Angola." But for the third part of the lecture series, he was unable to obtain a body: he and his confederates were so well known "that we could not venture to meddle with a white subject, and a black or Mulatto I could not procure." Unable to complete the curriculum, the course ended after 44 evenings.[14] (Clossy ultimately succeeded in obtaining an appointment to lecture at King's College and in 1767 was named its first professor of anatomy.)

It is important here to emphasize that dissection for the purposes of medical instruction or "curiosity" was stigmatizing, but autopsy had an entirely different social meaning. The cutting open of the body in autopsy was limited to the parts believed to be involved in the cause of death; and the autopsy was performed in a private room, often before a coroner's jury, and not by medical students in dissecting rooms or an anatomical theater. Public autopsies were judicially mandated in cases where foul play was suspected. There was no shame attached to the authorized cutting open of a victim's body.[15] At the same time, members of the aristocracy and gentry sought out private autopsy almost as a matter of privilege—their bodies were important enough to warrant some medical explanation of the death. In a few instances respectable people invited autopsy as a philanthropic contribution to medical understanding. A 1736 Boston newspaper recorded that Margaret Fisher, who died of "a Pulmonary Phthisis" at age 26, showed an "exemplary publick Spirit and Benevolence to Mankind": "[w]hen a dying, she earnestly desired, that her Viscera might be Anatomically inspected, for the Benefit of those, who may be afflicted with the like Disorders."[16]

In contrast, full-body dissection had punitive associations. This linkage was made explicit, with increasing frequency in the latter part of the eighteenth century, in sentencing in murder cases. The usual pronouncement took this form, as in the 1792 case of Whiting Sweeting, an Albany man:

> Your sentence is, That you be taken back to the place when you came, and from thence to the place of execution, and there to be hanged by the neck until you are DEAD, and that your body be delivered to the surgeon for dissection:—and the LORD have MERCY on your SOUL.[17]

According to Sweeting's published last testimony, the two parts of his sentence affected him in different ways: "[O]n my receiving the sentence of death I was not terrified, yet to hear of the DISSECTION of my body, seemed disagreeable to nature." His hopes for clemency focused on the dissection rather than the hanging:

> [When m]y wife and children and other friends took their last farewell from me in this world; the tears and heart-breaking sorrows of parting I cannot describe. It having been proposed that my wife and friends should apply to

the doctor to whom my body had been given for dissection, and beg that it might be delivered to them for burial; which they did; and being refused, it so exceedingly affected them that I could not help taking a part in their extreme sorrow on my account; and having been advised to try to make my escape, I attempted and effected it, and with my irons got some distance . . . but was soon taken and brought back.[18]

Sweeting was hanged on 26 August 1792 and his body given over to a surgeon for dissection. Posthumously, his plea for mercy succeeded: "the surgeon . . . had the humanity to deliver [the body] to a brother of the sufferer's, who took it to . . . Stephentown, where it was decently interred."[19]

Judicial dissection, then, was perhaps more feared than capital punishment itself. Medical dismemberment and exhibition of the human body was seen as the inverse of a Christian burial that deposited the body whole into the ground and placed it safely out of view. The dissected human was demoted to the status of slaughtered meat, in the words of one commentary, "a raw head and bloody bones" taken up by a "Tribe of Dissectors."[20] Even worse, the exhumation and dissection of bodies rendered them risible: a New Yorker of the 1790s complained that corpses were "being violently dragged" from the grave "to become a subject of mirth to a licentious set of men and the laughter of fools . . . who cut and mangle the body."[21] And worse still, dissection was seen as having affinities to necrophilia, cannibalism, and satanic ritual.

Given the small number of felons who were sentenced to be hanged and dissected, anatomists were forced to obtain bodies through other means. As the need for cadavers grew, medical students and their agents grew bolder and commandeered the bodies of people who had friends and supporters in the community. This was an altogether riskier proposition. Funerary customs were ultimately enforceable by crowd action; violations could provoke the formation of angry mobs. In 1765, a group of sailors "mobbed" the home of Dr. William Shippen, who had just commenced a series of anatomical lectures; the mob believed that he had "taken up" bodies from a church burial ground. Shippen hastened to assure the populace through the *Pennsylvania Gazette* that the bodies he dissected were "persons who had willfully murdered themselves [suicides], or were publickly executed, except now and then one from Potter's field, whose death was owing to some particular disease," and that he never stole any bodies "from the church or any private Burial Place."[22] But even the appropriation of the bodies of executed criminals could have repercussions. In Worcester, Massachusetts in 1771, a mob formed to demand the return of an executed man's body from Elijah Dix, an apothecary. After receiving it, they displayed the remains as they marched through the street, as though in effigy. Later that evening, the crowd marched to Dix's home and hung a dead dog in his doorway.[23] In this incident, as in some others, the rioters showed little regard for the cadaver. Their intent was to publicly brand the dissector as an offender rather than restore the honor of the dead.

The Doctor's Mob, the 1789 Act, and the John Young Case

The chronology and geography of "great excitements" against anatomists and medical schools reflects the expansion of medical education in North America, the growing importance of anatomy in medical discourse and practice, and the intensity of opposition to grave robbery and dissection. A full examination of anatomy riots, the provision of cadavers, and the legal history of anatomy in North America, would require a book rather than a chapter. The discussion that follows, with a few digressions, focuses on anatomy in New York City. New York had a prestigious medical establishment (second only to that of Philadelphia) and was connected commercially and culturally to other regions. In some accounts, New York is credited as the first state to establish a legal mechanism to supply schools with bodies, in 1789 (most writers credit Massachusetts with priority for its more comprehensive and workable 1831 law), but the passage of the New York "Bone Bill" of 1854 was another significant milestone. That law, and the debate surrounding it, provided an influential model for other states.

Formal anatomical instruction in New York City began in the mid-1760s, when Samuel Clossy began teaching anatomy at King's College. As an institution bearing the charter of the colonial governor and legislature, King's College had the privilege of granting the degrees of bachelor and doctor of medicine. These were marks of gentility that most healers did not have, even if many of them were referred to as "doctor." A formal degree signified that its owner possessed a certain degree of literacy and some capital—not necessarily a huge amount of either, but more than the majority of the population possessed. A diplomaed doctor, in the eighteenth-century Anglo-American world, and especially in the colonies, was in "society."

After the Revolutionary War, King's College revived under the name of Columbia College and its medical department resumed. Demand for anatomical instruction grew: the number of medical students (although still relatively small) increased, and so did the emphasis on anatomy in the medical curriculum and enthusiasm among students for anatomical studies. In October of 1786, Dr. Richard Bayley, a respected surgeon who had studied with John Hunter in London, began teaching an extracur-

TABLE 4.1 CROWD ACTIONS AGAINST AMERICAN MEDICAL COLLEGES:
1765–1884

1765	Philadelphia: Sailors' Mob
1771	Worcester, MA: Crowd protests the dissection of a hanged man by a local apothecary
1788	New York City: Doctors' Mob
	Baltimore: Crowd sacks Dr. Charles Wiesenthal's anatomy school, seeking to retrieve the body of an executed murderer
	Boston: Crowd invades Dr. John Jeffries' anatomy lecture in Boston
1807	Baltimore: Crowd destroys "Anatomy Hall" at the University of Maryland
1811	Zanesville, OH: Riot against medical apprentices
1824	New Haven: Riot against the medical department of Yale
	Hartford: A "group of citizens" reclaim a body from an anatomist
1830	Pittsfield, MA: Riot against the Berkshire Medical Institution
	Woodstock, VT: Riot against the Vermont Medical College
	Castleton, VT: Riot against the Castleton Medical College
1839	Worthington, OH: Riot against the Reformed Medical College
1840	Pittsfield, MA: Second riot at the Berkshire Medical Institution
1844	St. Louis, MO: Riot against McDowell Medical College
1845	Painesville, OH: Mass meeting of citizens to protest body snatchings
1846	Philadelphia: Crowd gathers in front of the Franklin Medical College
1847	Willoughby, OH: Riot against local medical college
1848	Jacksonville, IL: Rioters force a local medical school to close, due to a lack of cadavers
1849	St. Charles, IL: Riot against the Franklin Medical College
1852	Cleveland: Riot against the Homeopathic Medical College
1854	Rome, NY: While putting out a fire at the Eclectic Medical College, volunteer firemen find dissected bodies, riot, throw remains out the windows, and wreck the school
1857	Brookville, PA: Riot against medical apprentices
1882	Philadelphia: Mobilization of the black community (including an "indignation meeting") to protest the plundering of graves at the Lebanon Cemetery
1884	Des Moines, IA: Swedish immigrants invade medical school to reclaim a body

ricular, non-degree-granting course of anatomy and surgery at the New York Hospital, unconnected to the Columbia Medical Department.

New York City in the late eighteenth century had a population of about 25,000.[24] Even with a mortality rate that by our standards was high, only limited numbers of bodies were available for dissection. "There was a hierarchy for the eighteenth-century dead as surely as there was one for the living," historian Steven Wilf has observed, with the ranking ritually delin-eated by the manner of burial.[25] A gravesite's proximity to the church was linked to the social standing of the deceased: the higher the standing, the closer to the church. In colonial New York, as in Europe, members of the elite were traditionally buried under the church floor or on the church grounds. Such bodies constituted a funerary community, symbolically protected by their enclosure and physically protected by wardens and hired watchmen. Those outside the church burial ground, buried in a variety of circumstances, had a lower standing in the community, and lesser or no protection. Eligibility for burial on church grounds de-pended on wealth, occupation, family ties, and social connections.

There was also a racial determinant. Black men and women, even those who were not indigent, were buried in the Negroes Burying Ground, a segregated section of potter's field, which was adjacent to the almshouse. In the late 1780s, roughly 15% of New York City's population was black. Slavery was still legal, but there was a sizeable group of free blacks. Bayley's dissecting tables, as well as those of Columbia College, were sup-plied mainly from the Negroes Burying Ground. On 14 February 1787, a group of free blacks petitioned the common council of the city to ban medical students from "making a merchandize of human bones."[26] The students, they complained, "under cover of night . . . dig up the bodies of the deceased, friends and relatives of the petitioners, carry them away without respect to age or sex, mangle their flesh out of wanton curiosity and then expose it to beasts and birds." To stop these "most wanton sallies of excess," the petitioners proposed that dissection should be limited to people convicted of capital crimes, the traditional source of bodies.[27]

The petition was ignored. The black community could not muster the political and social resources to protect their dead. The plundering of bodies from the Negroes Burying Ground continued. A year later, on 16 February 1788, another letter of protest, to the *New York Daily Advertiser*, complained that "few blacks are buried whose bodies are permitted to remain in the grave. . . . [S]wine have been devouring the entrails and flesh of women, taken out of a grave, which on account of alarm, were left behind: . . . human flesh has been taken up along the docks, sewed up in bags."[28]

The grave robbers, were growing more audacious, and began to range beyond the Negroes Burial Ground. On 21 February 1788, it was reported that the body of a white woman had been stolen from the graveyard of Trinity Church; the rector of Trinity publicly offered a reward of $100 (a hefty sum) for information leading to the arrest of the perpetrators.[29] The city was in an uproar. The *Daily Advertiser* printed a stream of correspond-ence on the subject of grave robbery, including a defiant and inflamma-tory letter by "A Student of Physic." A retort, published under the pen name "Humanio," bluntly warned the body snatchers: "lives may be the forfeit . . . should they dare persist."[30] But the resurrectionists did persist and their activities provoked a fierce response—the Doctors' Mob of 13 April 1788.

The immediate events that triggered the uprising are obscure. Contemporary accounts differ in key details and almost certainly contain embellishments or misinformation on some points. According to newspaper reports, the riot began when a group of boys playing outside the City Hospital tried to peer inside the window of one of the rooms where dissections were taking place. In some tellings, a medical student responded by waving a severed arm at the children to scare them away; in other tellings the children merely saw the arm "impudently hung out of the window to dry."[31] In still other accounts, one of the boys, whose mother had recently died, then ran to his father, a mason, and told him what had happened. The woman's grave was inspected and her body found to be missing.[32] Whether any of these tales is true or not, what is certain is that a group of workmen assembled in front of the hospital, entered forcibly, and found some half-dissected bodies which they removed and publicly displayed. As the crowd grew larger and angrier, the hospital was sacked; some medical students were seized and roughed up. One escaped, but the mob took four men captive until Mayor James Duane, the sheriff, and a group of prominent men succeeded in rescuing them, by the expedient of arresting the students and locking them in jail.

The next day the mob, out in force, searched the city for physicians, medical students, and cadavers. When 300 to 400 men marched down Broadway toward the city jail, intent on rousting the students held there, Governor George Clinton, Mayor Duane, Chancellor Robert R. Livingston, John Jay, Baron von Steuben, and "a number of . . . Citizens"—the political elite of the city—stood up before them and urged them to go home. The crowd refused to disperse and began swelling with more supporters, leading to a standoff that continued throughout the day. The magistrates countered by mustering a detachment of eighteen armed men. When these wilted under the pressure and dispersed, they mustered another more resolute detachment of twelve. Finally, the mob, now numbering perhaps 5,000 and carrying wooden staves, rocks, and clubs, surged toward the jail and its handful of defenders. After a siege of several hours, Governor Clinton ordered out the militia, consisting of 50 to 150 armed men. The crowd responded with a hail of bricks and stones: von Steuben was struck, receiving "a wound first about the corner of his left eye & nose" and Jay "got his scull almost crackd."[33] In danger of being routed, the militiamen opened fire and charged with bayonets. Three rioters were killed and six others wounded; the militia suffered three deaths. The crowd dispersed, but after the killings sympathies for the protesters ran high: the local militia was unable to muster its men. Clinton then called up another militia, composed of men from surrounding counties, who marched through the streets the next day and quelled the disturbance.[34]

In the riot's aftermath, the old status quo was no longer tenable. The Federalist establishment of the city was shaken and, anatomists were forced to become more discreet and to forgo indiscriminate plunder of graves. The next year, the state legislature passed an "Act to Prevent the Odious Practice of Digging up and Removing for the Purpose of Dissection, Dead Bodies Interred in Cemeteries or Burial Places," the first law to sanction dissection in the United States. The 1789 act had two main provisions: First, "in order that Science may not . . . be injured by preventing the Dissection of proper Subjects," judges were empowered to add the sentence of dissection to that of hanging for the crimes of murder, arson, and burglary, as long as a "Surgeon . . . , or some other Person" appointed by him, "shall attend [the execution] to receive and take away the dead body." Second, body snatching was outlawed and made punishable, at the judge's discretion, by a fine of an undetermined amount and/or imprisonment for an undetermined duration of time, or by a sentence of publicly standing in stocks for an unspecified length of time.[35]

The New York act gave statutory legitimacy to the dissection of executed criminals.[36] But if its purpose was to forestall popular uprisings against anatomy by putting an end to objectionable anatomical practices, it quickly proved unsatisfactory. Just a little more than four years after the riot, a newspaper published a letter complaining that "the inhuman practice" of body snatching for the purposes of dissection had resumed, and that another public uprising was brewing.[37]

The inadequacy of the law became especially evident in the events that attended the 1797 execution of John Young.[38] A music publisher and musician who had just been released from debtors' prison, Young had killed a deputy sheriff who was attempting to return him to jail. As a known member of the community (just prior to the incident, he had provided entertainment at the house of Aaron Burr) and as a debtor, Young garnered considerable public sympathy: a large portion of the city's population was in debt and had direct or indirect experience with debtor's prison. This sympathy only grew after Young was sentenced to be hanged and dissected—and in his printed "confession," rather than the usual repentance, directly attacked creditors and the credit system as an assault on the honest working man. As the time of the execution drew near, with the prospect of another riot, Governor John Jay called out the militia and ordered it to march in formation through the streets. Young's fate then became enmeshed in party politics. Jeffersonian Republicans rallied the city's debtors and denounced the sentence and the law. Federalists supported the sentence and the law, and the need to penalize debtors who defaulted on their loans. Republicans identified anatomy with aristocratic privilege and pretension.[39]

After his hanging, Young's body was not given over to the surgeons, as his sentence stipulated, but instead buried in Potter's Field. At a late hour, it was secretly disinterred, delivered to the anatomical theater, and hastily dissected. During sentencing, the judge had ordered that Young's remains be interred at Potter's Field after the dissection, but the workmen, fearing discovery by the aroused public, dumped the dissected body parts into a sack and threw it into the East River. When news got out that the sack had washed up on shore, another riot seemed imminent, but a further display of force from Jay's troops dissuaded the crowd. A poem published after the incident, "The Ghost of John Young," condemned the anatomists, the judiciary, Jay, and by extension all of Young's detractors, for their insensibility. Young committed a crime of passion, "by rage propelled," but "Say *cool deliberate* actors, *what are ye? / . . .* Who can pass sentence with a tearless eye." No moral principle could justify the dismembering and mangling of Young's body "by the *Greedy Knife.*" The sentencing of John Young was a betrayal of republican ideals: "Shame on the Country . . . Where *Power* from *Justice* wrests the trembling scale, / And cooly dips in human gore his hands."[40]

Thus, despite the dissection of Young's body, the 1789 anatomy law failed in its several purposes. It had not detached anatomy from the jockeying of political factions and from the ideological contest over elite rule versus democracy, the shaping of the new political order. It had not deterred the heinous crime of murder; it had not made midnight disinterments unnecessary; and its application caused too much disturbance and risk to make it a useful procedure for supplying bodies to medical schools. But even had Young's dissection gone smoothly, long-term trends would have rendered the act inoperable. First, there were not enough people hanged to supply the dissecting tables, especially after 1796, when the New York State Legislature made arson and burglary noncapital offenses. Second, over the next half century, the number of medical students increased markedly within the region and nationally, as did emphasis on anatomical dissection within medical education, leading to a far greater demand for cadavers. So that, even with New York City's huge population increase, the supply of bodies could not keep pace with regional demand. Third, over the next half century, Americans gave increasing priority to efforts to obtain a "decent burial," consisting of a respectful funeral service, memorialization in the form of a gravemarker, an embellished coffin, and an enclosed plot of land. Exhumation and dissection were the antithesis of a decent burial, and fiercely resisted.

The Underground Economy

In 1792, both Richard Bayley and New York Hospital became associated with the Medical Department of Columbia College, but the college's medical school failed to thrive, in part because of the legacy of the Doctors' Mob and the John Young affair. In 1807, a new and more robust medical school, the College of Physicians and Surgeons (P&S), began operations under a state charter (Columbia's medical department, by then a shell, was dissolved into P&S in 1814). P&S was fairly successful in its first few decades, rapidly attaining a student body of close to 200 students, but labored in the shadow of the University of Pennsylvania, which was universally regarded as the finest American medical college, with an enrollment of more than 400 students per year. This was the post-Napoleonic period in which Parisian anatomy achieved new heights and epitomized a scientific approach to medicine, in part because the French famously had access to an unlimited supply of bodies through the giant charity hospitals of Paris. Medical education and research in America lagged behind, but, as we have seen, the rage for anatomical dissection did cross the Atlantic. Philadelphia, Baltimore, and New York vied for the title of locale most conducive to the pursuit of anatomy: the city most bountifully endowed with bodies.

How did P&S get its cadavers? A few bodies were obtained under the provisions of the 1790 federal law that applied to capital crimes committed in military garrisons and at sea. Other bodies—mainly foreigners or blacks convicted of murder—came to the college under the provisions of the 1789 act, in the absence of supporters who could mobilize to prevent the dissections. But these made up only a small portion of the cadavers dissected at P&S. The rest, according to an 1811 report of the New York State Regents, were "furnished by the state prison, without the violation of law," an assertion reiterated sporadically by P&S, and other New York City medical schools, for the next forty-odd years.

The evidence, however, tells a different story. For one thing, the bodies that P&S obtained from the state prison included those who died of disease or other causes (but who were not sentenced to be executed), in direct violation of the provisions of the 1789 act. Even then, supply could not keep up with demand; not enough people died in prison (and presumably some deceased prisoners had family members or friends who managed to successfully claim their dead). By 1826 a report of the Regents admitted that "the provision made by law, for delivering over for *dissection*, certain convicts, who are executed, or who die in the state prison, furnishes an insufficient number of '*subjects*,' even for the regular course of surgical and anatomical lectures."[41]

But, by then, dissections performed *outside* the "regular course" were proliferating wildly. Enthusiasm for anatomy, the Regents noted, had induced large numbers of medical students, and not just prospective surgeons, "to assemble in the dissecting room, out of lecture hours, to participate in actual [dissecting] practice"; mere observation of a dissection was not enough. "[T]hese volunteer associations," the report made clear, required an additional supply of cadavers. "[A] usage has, therefore, been introduced, that each student . . . shall contribute the sum of *five dollars*, to constitute a common fund, from which to *provide other subjects*, to operate upon," plus an additional two dollars from each student to hire "a *servant*" who "waits upon the students at the *dissecting room* . . . ; provides water, soap, and towels, . . . and attends to the removing the offals and useless parts of the *subject*, and cleaning the room."[42] Although the Regents worried that such practices might lead "to evil consequences," they sanctioned the extracurricular anatomical activities, so long as they were officially regulated by the College. The Regents refrained from considering how the additional bodies, so readily purchased with five-dollar contributions, were obtained, but the unhappy response of the P&S faculty to the Regents' report supplies the answer: "exhumation, at which every feeling of the human heart revolts, which is alike odious to the enlightened and the ignorant . . . , with all the horrors which the imagination associates to its practice"—language that betrays anxiety about the public reaction to promiscuous body snatching, and perhaps a guilty conscience as well.[43] Evidence from other sources confirms that P&S students and faculty had been directly and indirectly engaged in grave robbery from at least the mid-teens and probably from the very inception of the college. The minutes of a January 1814 meeting of the P&A faculty, for example, refer to "rumors of an unpleasant nature . . . that Bodies from the Cemeteries of the City have been brought to [P&S] for dissection."[44]

Even at that early date, P&S was not the only consumer of dead bodies in the region. In 1812, the state legislature had chartered another College of Physicians & Surgeons, at the village of Fairfield "in the Western District of New York" (the lower Finger Lakes region). Alexander Ramsay, a well respected Scottish anatomist and a prodigious dissector, assumed the chair of anatomy, and took on a number of private students. At the same time, private preceptors in all parts of the state were also taking up anatomical activities. By 1819, with body snatching activity rising, the New York state legislature made grave robbing a felony, with a penalty of five years in prison. Shortly thereafter, the legislature granted Fairfield the same right to bodies from the new state prison at Auburn that P&S had at the state prison in New York City.[45] These, however, were not sufficient to answer to the purpose. An 1824 letter from W. E. Horner, professor of anatomy at the University of Pennsylvania, reveals that an emissary from Fairfield was in Philadelphia, seeking to purchase bodies.[46]

Under such circumstances, fear of body snatching diffused widely. In Palmyra in upstate New York in that same year, Joseph Smith (the father of Joseph Smith, Jr., who would go on to become the founding prophet of Mormonism) placed a notice in a local paper stating that he and a few neighbors had dug into the grave of his recently deceased son Alvin and opened the coffin to prove that the body was still there. According to a local rumor, the grave had been robbed and Alvin's body dissected. Smith, who presided over a debt-ridden farm family that was often in danger of losing its land or falling below subsistence, felt compelled to expend scarce capital to advertise to the community that the rumor was false. Alvin's exhumation and dissection would carry a stigma: it would rank the Smiths with indigents, criminals, blacks, and Indians as people who were unable to protect their dead, whose dead deserved no protection.[47]

The rumor, in this case, was unfounded but not farfetched. Resurrectionists were at work in upstate New York, especially in the fall and winter, when the weather retarded the decomposition of bodies and permitted their transport over long distances. As the demand for anatomical instruction increased, professional grave robbers were increasingly called upon to assure that medical colleges were supplied with bodies. The use of such men provided a buffer against critics and the law: with paid agents, anatomists could claim to be unaware of how bodies were obtained. An 1820 letter by N. P. Wiley describes an encounter with a body snatcher at his business:

> I spent a dull day on the road . . . We had but one incident worth mentioning. A scoundrel looking fellow with us had a large box, containing as he said, *venison*. He was very careful to keep it in a cold place whenever we stopp'd and talk'd a great deal about his anticipated steaks—but unfortunately it fell from the driver's hands at Poughkeepsie while taking off the baggage & the lid flew open & discovered—a dead man! [The man] was a resurrectionist and had got [the body] . . . at Utica. He made quite a joke of it, & gave us all the particulars without any compunction. He inquired at all the towns about the sick, wanted to know their size, proportions, &c.—the most hardened villain I ever saw.[48]

The 1819 New York statute increased the penalty for the act of grave robbery, but failed to penalize those who received the stolen bodies and who commissioned the act. It did not, in any case, serve as much of a deterrent. At $5 to $25 per body, grave robbery was too lucrative to resist: a skilled journeyman in the mid-1820s might only earn $20 to $25 for an entire week's work.[49] And when body snatchers were caught, the statutory

penalty was rarely enforced. Solomon Parmelee, convicted in a New York
City court in 1824 for entering Potter's Field to obtain corpses, was sentenced only to six months in the penitentiary, not five years. (The conviction did not hamper him in future dealings; he went on to own a Great
Lakes steamship and an upstate salt works.)[50]

In the 1820s and 1830s, more medical schools were established, and
there was growing competition for students. Many of the new colleges
were rural schools that charged lower fees and offered a lower standard
of instruction—less anatomy and clinical medicine. But some were urban
and sought to attract ambitious students by aligning with the latest currents in European anatomical medicine. Such was the case in New York
City in 1826, when a good portion of the P&S faculty defected and set up
a competing school. Unable to secure a charter from the New York legislature, the seceding medical professors used a dormant New Jersey state
charter, issued years earlier for the never viable Rutgers Medical College,
to set up shop in New York City.

The schism was caused by personal conflicts, but also dissatisfaction
with P&S's laggardness in embracing Parisian anatomy. For its professor
of anatomy, Rutgers imported John Godman of Philadelphia, then perhaps the most sophisticated anatomist in the United States, and an avid
supporter of French pathological anatomy. The sudden and fierce competition between Rutgers and P&S undoubtedly worked to stimulate increased interest in "practical anatomy" among medical students, at both
institutions.

How did P&S and Rutgers get their bodies? The answer, in part, is
contained in the confidential correspondence of John Collins Warren,
professor of anatomy at Harvard. In the 1820s, Harvard had difficulty
getting bodies, and looked to other cities to make up the shortfall. Warren first turned to W. E. Horner, professor of anatomy at the University of
Pennsylvania. But Horner wrote back that, while the Philadelphia police
were "fortunately . . . not disposed to interfere" with body-snatching activity, he was having his own difficulties: student enrollment was up to 475,
of whom almost 200 were taking anatomy, and not enough people were
dying.

> [S]ince the opening of our lectures, the town has been so uncommonly
> healthy, that I have not been able to obtain a fourth part of the subjects
> required for our dissecting rooms. The scarcity is felt with still greater sever-
> ity, in consequence of the influx of students, exceeding that of any former
> year. . . . While this scarcity continues, I am left in an incessant state of anxi-
> ety, by the eagerness of the new students to commence operations, and thus
> disappointment at postponement. Anatomically speaking when the times be-
> come more propitious, I shall then be able to turn my attention to the wants

of friends. I have no expectation of being free on this point, at the time mentioned by you.

To make matters worse, Horner reported, other schools were also trolling for bodies. A professor from the medical college at Fairfield, New York had sent his brother to Philadelphia on a similar mission, but for the same reason, was also sent home empty handed.[51]

Unable to adequately supply his anatomy course, Warren kept casting around for a solution. A few years later, he wrote to an old family friend, Dr. John Revere (the youngest son of Paul Revere), asking for help.[52] Revere arranged a shipment of bodies from New York to Boston, and referred Warren to John Godman. Godman, in turn, referred Warren to James Henderson, a "trusty old friend and servant" who could, for "moderate compensation, . . . at any time, and almost to any number, obtain the articles you desire" from New York burial grounds, and "take upon himself all charge of procuring, packing and forwarding to any designated address."[53]

Godman was not completely accurate here: in the summer, when bodies were apt to quickly decompose, long-distance transport of bodies was impractical. Godman also erred in his estimate of the cost: in December of 1828, with the weather getting cold, Henderson shipped Warren 14 to 16 bodies "well pac[k]ed and in good order" and "the best quality" at $25 per body—a discount, he claimed ("I have been offered 30 Dollars for them but on account of my freind [sic] Dr Godman and as you have depended on mee . . ."). This was a considerable sum for 1828, but not pure profit for Henderson who reported to Warren (how truthfully is uncertain) that he paid "ten Dollars for each subject my self exclusive of the expence of Bringing them in, . . . the packin and Box and other expences."[54]

Looking to mitigate the cost and trouble, Warren then wrote to Godman for advice on setting up a cadaver provision system in Boston. Godman answered forthrightly: In both New York and Philadelphia, anatomists bribed public officials and burial-ground employees to gain unhindered access to the paupers buried in Potter's Field. In New York, the superintending official divided the bodies into two categories. Those "most entitled to respect, or most likely to be called for by friends" were buried in Pit No. 1 and exempted from dissection; the rest were buried in Pit No. 2, which was plundered to supply the medical colleges. In Philadelphia, however, the anatomists were entitled to "all the subjects buried in the two public grounds." If schools or physicians differed over who should get an allotment of bodies, the dispute was to be settled by the mayor—a high-reaching conspiracy that resulted in a harvest of about 450 bodies per school year, enough to supply most of the needs of the

University of Pennsylvania, Jefferson Medical College, and the other schools.[55] In fact, there was a secret treaty among Philadelphia anatomists, signed 22 November 1828, agreeing to a fair division of bodies, "to sustain the medical interests of Philadelphia, and to prevent the public scandal and excitement incident to the cultivation of anatomy."[56]

For obvious reasons, such arrangements were kept under wraps, but a few decades later Edward Dixon published an account of his days as God-man's pupil at Rutgers in the early 1830s. He and his fellow students, Dixon reminisced, made "diligent use of the shovel and the scalpel." On such forays, they always "unearthed common clay" and never "gentle clay," never dug up the graves of middle- or upper-class persons. The students made sure to observe social distinctions between bodies.

Dixon's memoir emphasizes the competition between colleges for ca-davers: a school's reputation rose or fell on whether it could provide stu-dents with "abundant anatomical material." There was also an element of fraternal rivalry in this; students playfully jockeyed for bodies as a kind of secret intercollegiate sport. Thus, according to Dixon, in 1831,

> when the feud between the old Barclay Street College [P&S] and the Rutgers Faculty . . . was at its highest, among the . . . methods they contrived of an-noying each other . . . was that of cutting off the supply of material for the dissecting room. Whoever bid the highest to induce the keeper of Potter's Field to tie up his dogs, get drunk, and go quietly to bed, was allowed to monopolize the pauper bodies.

For ambitious but less well-off students like Dixon, whose "surgical anat-omy" was "imperative in its requisitions," but "who could not forget the charms of whiskey punches and choice Havanas, with an occasional the-atre or opera ticket," the cost of such bribes "drew . . . deeply on the pocket." Dixon and his friends therefore resolved "to turn resurrection-ists" and find other locations where they could rob graves at some risk to themselves, but without the need for payoffs.

A favorite place was a U.S. Navy burial ground. Sailors were eminently eligible for dissection. Many seamen died in port, with few or no local connections or resources, and so no one to discover or oppose the rob-bing of their graves. Even better, "Uncle Sam's men," Dixon reported with characteristic sarcasm, "were in high repute with us as subjects, from their fine development of muscles." They were also not hard to exhume: "when the poor fellows would 'slip their wind,' after returning from a cruise, they were . . . planted in a very convenient place, in rows, on a certain side hill."[57] It is also likely that many of them were nonwhite—as any reader of *Moby Dick* knows, the antebellum sailing ship was a multira-cial workplace—and this perhaps also made them safer targets for body-snatching activities.

"The Use of the Dead to the Living":
Anatomical Bioethics and the State,
1820–1840s

Student exploits were perilous—Dixon's memoir, like many medical reminiscences, featured a comic account of an episode in which he and his friends were nearly apprehended. The carefully constructed schemes of anatomy professors, students, demonstrators, and agents, were easily upset: an attempt by instructors at the University of Pennsylvania to deny bodies to instructors at nonchartered schools led to the public disclosure of the secret treaty in Philadelphia and difficulties for all parties.[58] As the vogue for dissection intensified, anatomists increasingly risked exposure, censure, and mob attack, all of which could lead to disruptions in supply—shortages of bodies and rising prices. And if the body trade was a seller's market, medical education was a buyer's market. Medical faculties perennially worried that students would desert them for better-endowed colleges.

The price of bodies was highly unstable. G. S. Pattison, a Scottish anatomist who taught in the United States in the 1810s and '20s, testified before the 1828 British Parliamentary Select Committee on Anatomy that bodies from Potter's Field went for $2 to $4 in Baltimore and $10 in New York, where they were easily procured, but "not so ample as in Philadelphia and Baltimore." Boston was subject to recurrent difficulties: a report of another Select Committee on Anatomy in the Massachusetts House of Representatives lamented that the price of subjects had risen from $5–$10 in the early 1820s to $15–$20 in 1831. But shortages occurred even in New York and Philadelphia, favored locales for the harvesting of cadavers. It seems clear that bodies represented a considerable expense, and were sometimes unobtainable at any price.[59]

Anatomists and their allies in New York, Massachusetts, and Connecticut (after rioters attacked Yale's medical department in 1824) responded by lobbying for measures that would ensure a steady supply of bodies and set anatomy on a legal basis. In February 1826 the P&S faculty called for an extension of the 1789 statute that would permit them to take the bodies of those who could not pay their burial expenses, plus the bodies of those who died in the city prison. "Then would exhumation . . . cease for ever. . . . The public mind would be tranquilized, the dead would rest undisturbed, and the sepulchre be sacred." It would also seal their advantage over rural schools. The city had unique resources for anatomy, the immigrant poor, if only they could be tapped: "It is only in this part of our state that . . . we find multitudes from all nations unclaimed and unconnected, without relatives or friends to defray the expenses of their interment, . . . who might therefore be used, without offence to the most delicate emotions of our nature, to promote the safety and happiness of the living."[60]

Such proposals echoed those being made in Great Britain, where prices for cadavers were notoriously high and anatomists had even greater difficulties in getting bodies. With the end of the Napoleonic wars, the low cost and easy availability of bodies in Paris lured many British students to cross the channel to study with the French masters, so that British medical schools suffered a loss of prestige and income. Thus, beginning with John Abernethy's Hunterian Oration of 1819, the British profession beat the drum for a law that would allow anatomists to take the bodies of paupers.[61] A succession of body-snatching scandals and riots against medical schools fueled the clamor for legislation—which reached a crescendo after the 1828 Burke and Hare scandal in Edinburgh, in which the murderers suffocated ("burked") their victims and then sold the bodies to medical colleges.

This call for an anatomy bill was linked to a larger social agenda. In the mid-1820s Jeremy Bentham, the utilitarian philosopher, promoted anatomy legislation as a stalking horse for a New Poor Law.[62] In Bentham's welfare reform scheme, the indigent poor would be incarcerated in poorhouses where they would be forced to work for food and shelter, rather than supported at home by payments of money, food, and firewood. The operation of a free market in labor would be linked to a disciplinary regime of reformatory institutions that would teach the moral discipline and "habits of industry" required by the burgeoning capitalist order. The poorhouses would be punitive: inmates would perform long hours of tedious and uncompensated work, be fed meager rations, sleep in overcrowded dormitories, have no privacy and no personal liberty. The poor had to be dissuaded from preferring public assistance to wage labor (even if wages were below subsistence level and the work hazardous to life and limb), and from regarding public assistance as a right.

Anatomy would play a disciplinary role in the new regime. The fear of death in the poorhouse followed by dissection would compel working people to defer to the dictates and exhortations of employers, ministers of the faith, politicians, magistrates, and reformers. Dissection would be a fitting end for those who indulged in the moral vices associated with indigence—promiscuity, impulsiveness, laziness, insubordination, intemperance. In life, a drain on the public purse; in death, they would be made to serve the public good.

But Bentham was interested in an anatomy law for symbolic, ideological reasons that extended beyond its usefulness to the medical profession and the larger capitalist order. He saw the theory of moral sentiment, in which the dead were icons of moral value and attractants of sympathy, as an obstacle to the rationalization of society and culture. If a utilitarian calculus was to govern society—that the good consists of the greatest benefit to the greatest number of people—then it was necessary to dispel funerary sentiment. The dead body would have to be valued solely according to its usefulness to the living. This might perhaps include an ennobling but limited empathy for the dead (if subjected to careful cost-benefit analysis), but also the use of pulverized human bones as fertilizer, and dissection of cadavers for purposes of medical instruction, to cite two favorite examples. To dramatize the point, Bentham made an elaborate testamentary provision for the disposition of his own body. Upon his death in 1832, the aged philosopher was publicly dissected and then transformed into a morally instructive "auto-icon," a wax likeness sculpted on the frame of his own skeleton, dressed in his own clothes, with his actual preserved head sitting on a table beside him (to be displayed, as it still is, at the University College in London)—a famous gesture that Bentham dubbed the "further uses of the dead to the living."[63]

This last was a reference to "The Use of the Dead to the Living," a closely reasoned 1824 polemic from the pen of Dr. Thomas Southwood Smith, a Bentham protegé (and the man entrusted with the task of carrying out Bentham's funerary instructions). "The Use of the Dead" had a long shelf life in America, where it was quoted and paraphrased in debates over anatomy legislation well into the 1890s.[64] It argued that anatomical dissection of the dead was necessary to save the living. Physicians and surgeons who had precise knowledge of the body's interior could assess the condition of patients and perform the actions required to save them. Ignorance of the body gave rise to unsound theories, which medicine, from antiquity to the present, was prone to. But sentimental attachment to the dead body stood in the way of anatomical study.

Tender regard for the deceased, in Smith's view, was laudable but not rational: "Veneration for the dead is connected with the noblest and sweetest sympathies of our nature: but the promotion of the happiness of the living is a duty from which we can never be exonerated" (81). In any case, it was "ignorance," "bigotry," and "superstition," rather than empathy for the dead, that motivated the "multitude" (86) to rise up against body snatchers and the schools that employed them. Such attacks directly reduced the number of bodies available for dissection in Great Britain. As a result, British anatomy schools were declining drastically. Students had to go through the course of anatomy without obtaining enough practical experience or, even worse, were flocking to Paris and other locales where bodies were more easily obtained.

Yet, the hue and cry, Smith contended, was "not against anatomy," but against grave robbery (87). This actually was untrue. Opponents of anatomy typically objected to both body snatching and dissection. But "The Use of the Dead" elided this key point in order to draw a moral and social distinction between the refined, morally sensible anatomist and the vulgar, morally insensible body snatcher—ignoring the fact that anatomists commissioned and sometimes took direct part in grave robberies. The argument pivots on the social logic of the funerary economy (and not classic economic principles, which approve the law that supply arises to meet demand), paradoxically endorsing something very like Adam Smith's theory of moral sentiment: Coarse, brutal, animalistic resurrectionists have no sentimental regard for the dead, and are therefore outside the moral order. Body snatchers act on the principles of the market, principles that trespass on funerary custom and law. Contact with such "odious" persons taints the anatomist and the medical profession. Even worse, in exploiting their leverage in a seller's market, grave robbers invert the social order that places cultivated and respectable gentlemen over the illiterate rabble. They feel free to insult and tyrannize their betters. They even, on occasion, have the audacity to steal the bodies of respectable folk, who have the standing to deserve something better than exhumation.

Smith proposed to solve this distressing situation through "legislative interference." Judges should no longer be allowed to sentence criminals to be dissected; logically, dissection was a positive thing, not a punishment. The robbing of graves should be made a felony. Diplomas should be awarded only to persons who can show that they have dissected at least five bodies (considerably more than required anywhere in Britain). Deceased inmates of "hospitals, infirmaries, workhouses, poor-houses, foundling-houses, houses of correction, and prisons," if "unclaimed by immediate relatives, or whose relatives decline to defray the expenses of interment" (93), should be directly given over to institutions of medical education upon payment of a small handling fee. Then, after 28 days, the remains of the dissected bodies should be "decently buried."

To forestall the objection that the proposal was class-interested legislation which unfairly garnished only the bodies of the poor as "public property," Smith replied that "those who are supported by the public die in its debt": "their remains . . . might, without injustice, be converted to the public use."[65] But, given the overwhelming moral imperative to honor the dead, Smith retreated from asserting this position too rigorously: the measure would not lead to the dissection "of the bodies of all the poor: but only . . . that portion . . . who die unclaimed and without friends" (94); no living person would have cause to feel distress. This, of course, conveniently neglected the fact that would-be claimants, who could not bear the expense of a funeral, would be greatly distressed. And, as poor people suspected, the provisions for notification, mandatory waiting period, and "decent" burial of the remains, were carelessly administered in the actual implementation of the bill.

No matter, Smith concluded. Whether or not the bill passed, given the unequal medical resources commanded by the rich and the poor, class power would ultimately rule:

> if the dead bodies of the poor are not appropriated . . . , their living bodies will . . . be. The rich will always have it in their power to select . . . the surgeon who has . . . signalized himself by success: but that surgeon, if he have not obtained [his] dexterity . . . by dissecting and operating on the dead, must have acquired it by making experiments on the living bodies of the poor [in charity institutions]. (94)

Thus the poor would be no worse off, and the anatomy bill would "tranquillize the public mind," meaning in this instance the middle and upper classes who would be assured that "[t]heir dead would rest undisturbed: the sepulchre would be sacred: and all the horrors which the imagination connects with its violation would cease for ever" (95)—the very words borrowed by the P&S faculty (unattributed) in their petition to the Regents. But a considerable portion of the populace would lack such assurance. Given the wild oscillations of the capitalist economic cycle, the progressive substitution of low-paid factory work for skilled artisanal labor, and the dangers of incapacitating disease or accident or bad weather, the lower middle and laboring classes might find themselves driven into destitution for longer or shorter periods, and then put at risk of dissection.

Anatomy bills on the Benthamite model were highly controversial. They fared badly in parliament and the Massachusetts legislature in the late 1820s, but modified versions passed in Massachusetts in 1831 and Britain in 1832. Victory, in both places, was achieved by emphasizing the goal of the bill as the elimination of body snatching—and by limiting the application of the bill to large cities (in Massachusetts, only to Boston), a tactic that defused the objections of rural legislators. The other provisions closely followed the measures advocated by Southwood Smith. The class of bodies eligible to be dissected was defined not as the indigent but as the "unclaimed" (a category consisting entirely of those who died in the poorhouse and other institutions who had no money to defray the costs of funeral and burial; for practical purposes this would be nearly all the bodies). There was to be a short waiting period in which bodies could be claimed, and an exemption for respectable "strangers" who might die while passing through a locality where they were unknown (and so have no claimants). By defining the bodies as "unclaimed," rather than paupers, the discriminatory intent of the legislation was partly disguised; technically, a wealthy person could also be unclaimed. The successful bills also mandated that the remains, after dissection, be given decent burial, increased the penalties for grave robbery, and outlawed the use of dissection as a punishment in capital cases.

In Britain, the passage of the 1832 anatomy bill pretty much resolved the controversy, but in America the results were much less conclusive. Despite passage of the bill in Massachusetts, opposition in other states ran high. The Connecticut legislature passed an anatomy act in 1833, but repealed it in 1834. The New Hampshire legislature passed an act in 1834, but repealed it in 1842. (In Massachusetts, the legislature strengthened the anatomy act through revisions in 1834 and 1845; an 1846 repeal effort was defeated.)[66] In Maine, Pennsylvania, Ohio, and Vermont, anatomy legislation could not get off the ground. Attempts in the New York legislature in 1831, 1832, 1843, and 1844 failed dismally. In the same period, several states passed laws that increased penalties for body snatching, without making any provision for the legal acquisition of cadavers.

"Considerable Trouble":
The Body Trade in the 1830s and 1840s

> The means of high medical education are accessible in
> many country institutions. Every intelligent man . . .
> knows that the *materiel* of Anatomy is abundant and can
> be transported any where . . . that Railroads, and Steam-
> boats, and Transportation Lines, and Expresses . . .
> make the movement of the *materiel* . . . a matter of the
> least difficulty.
>
> Chester Dewey, M.D., 1847[67]

In the 1830s and 1840s, American medical colleges continued to multiply—there were 38 chartered schools in operation in 1849—and, despite the rash of statutes increasing penalties for grave robbery, so did body snatching. Allegations of malfeasance beset every school and colleges were at risk of being set upon by angry crowds: rioters shut several schools down. In New York, Rutgers Medical College (1826–1831) lost its war against P&S, and the College of Physicians and Surgeons in the Western District also lapsed out of existence, but new medical schools sprang up in Geneva, Albany, Buffalo, Brooklyn, and briefly in Auburn (located conveniently next to the state prison). In New York City, the Medical Department of the University of the City of New York (UNY), the ancestor of New York University Medical College, was the most prominent and successful newcomer (staffed in part by survivors of the Rutgers debacle). There were also a number of small, nonchartered anatomy schools that prepped students or augmented the training given by the city's chartered institutions.

Although collegial courtesy sometimes obtained between schools, competition for students was intense. Urban schools invariably boasted of

TABLE 4.2. SELECTED AMERICAN ANATOMY LEGISLATION, 1789–1944

Laws giving bodies of the indigent poor to medical schools for dissection, unless otherwise noted.

1789   New York: "An Act to prevent the odious Practice of Digging up and Removing Bodies . . . for the purpose of dissection" provides bodies of executed prisoners, at discretion of the judge

1790   Congress gives federal judges the right to add dissection to the death penalty in murder cases (only federal law on anatomy in the nineteenth century); similar New Jersey law

1810   Connecticut: legislature establishes Medical Department of Yale, prohibits secret disinterment of a body (or aiding and abetting of) for purpose of dissection, or to knowingly "assist in any surgical or anatomical experiments therewith or dissections thereof"

1815   Massachusetts: law "to protect the sepulchres of the dead," makes unauthorized disinterment or *possession* of a dead body punishable by $1,000 fine and imprisonment for a year

1819   New York: makes grave robbing a felony, with penalty of five years in prison

1820   Maine: passes an anti-grave-robbing law modeled on Massachusetts statute

1831   Massachusetts: first American anatomy act, applies only to Boston

1832   Great Britain (the Warburton Act)

1833   Connecticut

1834   Connecticut act repealed; New Hampshire

1842   New Hampshire act repealed

1844   Michigan: provides bodies of criminals who die in prison to medical societies and proposed University of Michigan medical department; but in 1846 abolishes the death penalty (in some accounts the MI law is said to be similar to MA 1831 law)

1846   Ohio: makes exhumation for "dissection or any surgical or anatomical experiment, . . . without consent of the near relatives," punishable by up to $1,000 or six months in jail or both

1854   New York: "Bone Bill," limited to cities over 30,000 (of which there are six)

1867   Pennsylvania: Armstrong Act (aka "Ghastly Act"), limited to Philadelphia and Pittsburgh

1869   New Hampshire; Maine: give medical schools the bodies of convicts who die unclaimed; also provide that a person can bequest body to advance anatomical science if relatives do not object (precedent breaker), but abolishes capital punishment in 1876

1870   Vermont: assigns bodies of executed criminals to medical schools for dissection

1871   Connecticut

1872   Minnesota, California

1879   Indiana, Ohio, Michigan, Iowa

Continued on next page.

TABLE 4.2. CONTINUED

1882	Pennsylvania: extends anatomy act to entire state
1884	Vermont, Virginia
1885	Illinois
1889	California: revises anatomy act to exempt the bodies of Union Army and Navy veterans
1890	Maryland
1901	California: exempts bodies of widows of veterans and men honorably discharged from the U.S. armed forces; burials provided, not to exceed $50
1902	District of Columbia: passed by U.S. Congress
1927	California
1944	Louisiana
1947	Tennessee

their advantages over rural schools: they had more bodies to dissect and were close to large hospitals, where students could receive instruction that at least gestured at the French or British model of clinical medicine.[68] Location within New York City, the largest city in the United States, with a population of over 200,000 in the 1830s and growing rapidly, was undoubtedly a competitive edge. Both P&S and UNY were among the most prestigious colleges in the country. As part of their pitch for students, the catalogues of UNY and P&S featured prominently the claim that "anatomical material" was abundant and legally obtained. In fact, both schools continued to get their bodies illegally from Potter's Field and other sources.

So did many other schools. James Silk Buckingham, a British traveler in America in the late 1830s, remarked that it was "common practice in New York, to ship off the bodies of dead negroes, male and female, for various ports, but especially the south, to the medical students, for dissection; . . . to elude suspicion, these dead bodies were put up in salt and brine, and packed in the same kind of casks as those in which salted provisions are exported."[69] The prodigious availability of cadavers, many of them black, but increasingly Irish and German, was a source of pride to New York City medical schools. "[I]t is a fact of notoriety," the 1841 catalogue of UNY boasted, "that a considerable part of the supply required in the dissecting-rooms of Philadelphia has . . . been obtained from New-York; and a number of other medical schools in the country are mainly dependent on [New York City], even for . . . the illustration of their anatomical lectures."[70]

Anatomy professors from outside the city expended fairly large sums of money, anywhere from $10 to $30 per body. Even W. E. Horner, professor of anatomy at the haughty University of Pennsylvania, was forced to import bodies from New York.[71] At Harvard, J. C. Warren's hopes that his perennial shortage of cadavers would cease with the passage of the Massachusetts Anatomy Act of 1831, were thwarted when the superintendent of the House of Industry refused to implement the law. Warren looked again to New York, contacting several professors at P&S and UNY.[72] As his agent, he hired Dr. Cyrus Weeks, a former student who supplemented his income by acting as a procurer of bodies.[73]

The business did not run smoothly. The entry of new schools and new agents complicated matters. In November 1843, Samuel Parkman, demonstrator of anatomy at Harvard, advised Warren—who had traveled to New York to make "inquiries into the mode of obtaining subjects"—to negotiate with the firm of Millet & Brown, at 280½ Broadway. They had sent Parkman a letter offering to supply bodies to Harvard for $20 apiece, $5 less than Weeks's price. Parkman wrote Warren that he now believed that Weeks had been cheating them.[74] Two weeks later, Warren received a letter from Weeks, marked "Private," in which the agent complained that

> In consequence of some of your people having been too communicative to two foreign interlopers named Millet & Brown[,] one an Englishman & the other a Philadelphian[,] we have had considerable trouble . . . and to add to the difficulty the New School [UNY] notwithstanding their professions of penitence last winter are again . . . endeavoring to prevent any goods going out of the city. . . . Their noses will soon be upon the grindstone of repentance never to be relieved by the party who served you last winter.[75]

The net effect of the rivalries among schools and body snatchers was "difficulties" for all parties. Warren noted in his journal that P&S and UNY were "in violent opposition & many improprieties are the consequence."[76] By January 1844, a New York medical professor wrote Warren that even P&S and UNY were "badly supplied," but allowed that if he was "in want" one or two subjects might be obtained.[77]

The situation became further complicated when UNY recklessly directed the attention of the public to the burgeoning export of bodies from the city. According to UNY's 1846 catalogue, "Schools of Medicine, in almost all parts of the country, have mainly drawn their supplies," from New York City's "large surplus of *materiel* . . . thus instituting a traffic most dangerous to the interests of Practical Anatomy." But UNY went further, delivering a threat: "The attention of the municipal authorities has been drawn to the subject, and hereafter, it is understood, the *trade* will be at an end," thereby locking in UNY's advantage over schools located outside the city.

However, UNY's understanding with the authorities quickly collapsed when the faculty of upstate Geneva Medical College printed and circulated a sharply worded rebuke addressed to "the Medical Profession of the City of New-York" and Mayor Abraham Mickle. The Genevans sarcastically pointed out that, if UNY's assertions were true, then the mayor and members of the city council were "parties to the procurement of the dead bodies of the poor of [the] city, for the purpose of dissection in the University of New-York"—probably true, but certainly impolitic for UNY to advertise. And in alleging "that Medical Schools abroad depend exclusively" on the illegal disinterment and exportation of bodies from New York City, UNY was impugning not merely the honor of the medical college at Geneva, but also the honor of the profession—here again the allegation was at least partly true (outside schools also had local and regional sources, and Baltimore also supplied cadavers), but not prudent to advertise. With an eye toward maximizing UNY's embarrassment, the Geneva faculty pointedly reminded its rival that "the laws of this State protect alike the dead bodies of the poor as well as the rich, therefore the Professors of the University of New-York have no more right to them than those of any other Institution, or individual, in or out of State, and are subject to the same penalties for their infringement"—a statement that stands as perhaps the sole public expression of funerary egalitarianism on the part of any group within the antebellum medical professoriate with regard to provision of cadavers.[78]

UNY responded with some quick backpedaling. Without giving full satisfaction to the Genevans, the faculty apologized to the mayor and disavowed any statements that could be taken to imply that Geneva was deficient "in the supply of *material* for dissection."[79] There the matter rested. With UNY chastened, the traffic in bodies resumed and, apart from an 1847 altercation over the alleged sale of bodies at Bellevue Hospital by the resident physician, for the next few years there were no major controversies concerning anatomy in New York City (though there were plenty elsewhere).[80]

THE BONE BILL

> [T]his prohibition against the only means of acquiring [medical] knowledge . . . is made not at the request of the emigrant . . . ; but all this is done merely for
> *political effect.*
>
> E. R. PEASLEE, *The Moral Character of the Medical Profession: An Address Introductory . . . in the New York Medical College, Session of 1852–53* (New York, 1852), 11

> [S]ome politician whispers to me, "The intelligent part of the community understands perfectly your professional necessity; and these penal enactments [against

bodysnatching] are a dead letter—intended merely as an offering to popular prejudice. You doctors should set about overcoming that prejudice, and we statesmen will quickly remove such inconsistencies from the statute-book. If it was our affair, we could persuade the people that it is pleasant to be dissected, just as we so often persuade them that it is profitable for them that we should put our hands into their pockets."

J. W. DRAPER, *An Appeal to the People of the State of New-York, to Legalise the Dissection of the Dead* (1853)[81]

This brings us up to the 1850s. Medical education was continuing its rapid expansion; the curriculum was continuing to become more anatomical; and competition among schools remained fierce. New York City was continuing to grow with extraordinary rapidity, the population exceeding 500,000 persons, largely from an influx of German and Irish immigrants, and its burial grounds were still being plundered to supply the city's and the nation's dissecting rooms, by one estimate a yield of 600 to 700 bodies a year.[82] Some difficulties in the flow of bodies, however, persisted. E. R. Peaslee, a medical professor, reminded his incoming class of a "well known" fact, that during the winter of 1851–1852 "more than 600 young men in the medical schools of this city . . . had their anatomical studies arrested for weeks in succession," due to an interruption of supplies that could only delicately be "alluded to."[83]

Given such hardships, a new effort commenced to push a remedial measure through the state legislature in Albany, largely at the prompting of Whig party members. The 1851 model, "An Act to Promote Medical Enquiry and Instruction," introduced in the assembly by Franklin Tuthill (Whig-Suffolk), a physician-legislator, went nowhere, as did the 1852 model, retitled "An Act to Promote Medical Enquiry and Instruction and for the Better Protection of Burying Grounds and Cemeteries." In 1853, after debate and negotiation, the bill attracted support from members of both parties and nearly passed, but was narrowly defeated at the end of the session.

In the fall 1853 elections, the Whigs won control of both houses of the state legislature, despite the fact that the party was disintegrating at the national level (in 1856 the Republican party would pick up the Northern pieces). At the state level, both major parties were fissured by the temperance agitation, the free-soil/slave-soil controversy, and the byzantine machinations of state politics—the Democrats had Barnburner and Hunker factions; the Whigs had Dries, Wets, Compromisers (on the extension of slavery), and Free Soilers; and there were also third-party Free Soilers—but observers linked the fortune of the anatomy bill to the Whig victory. The difference on anatomy was most pronounced within the New

York City delegation. There the party system was based on rival coalitions that had a distinctive class character. Wealthy voters divided evenly between the two parties, but the middle classes and small master craftsmen preferred the Whigs, whose rhetoric typically invoked moral discipline, sobriety, and progress, a Protestant and reformist individualism. The philanthropic-minded portion of the middle and upper classes generally voted Whig, but both parties competed for the more numerous working-class vote. Workers tied to trade with the South went with the Democrats; those with upward aspirations, and a more mutualist, less antagonistic social ideology went with the Whigs. After the Loco Foco revolt of 1837–1838, Democrats stepped up rhetorical appeals to "the common man," gesturing in the direction of working men, egalitarianism, and a more open economy (while doing nothing for organized labor). Finally, the Irish, previously only a bugaboo for nativist voters, began to become an electoral force, generally voting Democratic.[84]

The supporters of anatomy legislation—the 1854 model was titled an "Act to Promote Medical Science and Protect Burial Grounds," but usually referred to as the "Bone Bill"—were energized by the new Whig legislative majority. County medical societies and the chartered medical colleges sent petitions, expressions of support, and lobbyists. UNY dispatched Martyn Paine, professor of the institutes and practice of physic; P&S sent Willard Parker and Bellevue sent James R. Woods, their professors of surgery. John W. Draper, professor of chemistry and president of the medical faculty of UNY, wrote "An Appeal to the People of the State of New-York to Legalise the Dissection of the Dead," which circulated throughout the state in pamphlets, newspapers, and medical journals. The bill's supporters and the Whig press were well informed on the legislative history of anatomy acts in Massachusetts, New York, and Great Britain in the 1820s and 1830s, and recycled the standard arguments, along with some new themes and variations.[85]

The act, they argued, would put a finish to grave robbery and commerce in bodies, remove the taint of association between ghoulish body snatchers and respectable anatomists, provide the state's medical colleges with a regular and cheap supply of bodies, and end the threat of mob violence against medical schools. (A riot of volunteer firemen against the Eclectic Medical College of Rome, New York, took place just prior to the final vote on the act, but seems to have had little impact on the bill's progress.) As a result, surgeons and physicians would be better trained; medical science would advance more rapidly. Poor people, J. W. Draper argued, would especially benefit through a reduction in their high rates of mortality and morbidity: "The knowledge . . . gathered in the dissecting-room will produce its results in the railroad shanty; it will be felt among that wandering population which fringes the advance of civilization; . . . even here at home, it will find its way into those sinks of destitution and vice which your hospitals can never reach." (13) Still another set of arguments related to the economic health of the state, whose medical schools would attract students and prosper, while the medical schools of other states, which lacked anatomy acts, would wither and die. Thus the battle was waged simultaneously on moral and economic grounds.

Advocates of the bill disparaged the opponents of dissection as barbarous, ignorant, and superstitious. F. A. Conkling, a wealthy New York City merchant who was the bill's floor manager, began an hour-long oration on the Assembly floor by invoking the "great example" of Jeremy Bentham, whose "skeleton still occupies the arm-chair in which he was accustomed to sit when living, where it was placed in honor of his superiority to one of the groundless prejudices of his age."[86] The "feeling of repugnance" for dissection, Conkling continued, "is entertained most strongly by heathen nations." Funerary sentiment, however noble, is illogical. In the absence of spirit, the body is "but the material tenement of man, from which the spirit has fled. . . . It is a piece of inanimate clay, that cannot . . . be preserved from instant decay" and therefore should be used to benefit mankind or disposed of in such a way as to mitigate its deleterious effects.[87] Better to follow the example of the city authorities of New Orleans who, during a yellow fever outbreak, decreed the cremation of "a vast multitude of human bodies . . . , lest the atmosphere be rendered still more pestilential by their effluvia." (4–5)

Finally, like Southwood Smith, Conkling inveighed against the "remorseless vampires in human shape, bearing the name of 'resurrectionists,' . . . who grow rich by this atrocious iniquity." Their "nefarious trade" was not directed toward the provision of local anatomists, but "to supply the wants of other medical schools," a "demand [that] has received a new impetus of late, from the greater facilities for safe and rapid conveyance furnished by railroads." The anatomy act then would end "the traffic in human bodies," sever the "involuntary connection" between the medical profession and these "miscreants" (10), who threatened even "the strongest vault or tomb," the resting places of the respectable classes (although few middle- and upper-class graves were plundered). Again the argument turned on an appeal to class interest. The condemnation of "traffic" signaled not so much a critique of capitalist practice as a desire to regulate or eliminate the bottom end of the market, the distasteful entrepreneurial activities that enterprising members of the lower classes engaged in.[88]

In another floor speech supporting the bill, Assemblyman Rollin Germain (Whig-Erie), took the appeal to class interest a step further:

> The supply of bodies which this bill may furnish will be mainly from those . . . brought to wretchedness by improvidence or crime. Having either afflicted

the community by their misdeeds, and burdened the State by their punishment; or having been supported by public alms—by offering up their bodies,
to the advancement of a humane science, they will make some returns to
those whom they have burdened by their wants, or injured by their crimes.[89]

The poor, lumped together with criminals by their common impositions
on the public purse, owed a debt to society. Anatomy legislation was a
form of retributive justice.

The debate on the Bone Bill was lengthy and vociferous, and the popular press reported and commented on it in detail, printing transcripts of
speeches, floor debates, texts of petitions, and editorial appraisals of the
merits of the arguments and the bill's progress. The willingness of propo-
nents to publicly campaign for the bill represented a departure from past
practice. Up until 1853, they had operated on the assumption that the
anatomy question had to be handled quietly. It was risky to openly crusade for such a measure, the *Times* editorialized, "the superstition of its
opponents would then be sure to take alarm and bring out all their
forces."[90] Given the public's riotous response to grave robbery and the
stigma attached to dissection, politicians shied away from expending any
political capital on the question. In 1854, by contrast, there was no shortage of advocates willing to join the battle for public opinion.

Lining up against the measure were egalitarian Free Soilers and fellow-
traveling upstate Whigs, Democrats from the Finger Lakes and the Cat-
skills, and, most vocally, New York City Democrats whose districts had
substantial numbers of immigrants. Petitions, resolutions, and editorials
denouncing "the obnoxious dissection bill" came from *Freeman's Journal*
(a popular Irish newspaper); the Germania Society and some German
language papers; the Irish Emigrant Society; and Tammany Hall, which
was beginning to reach out to the Irish vote.[91] Although the Whig leadership was based in New York City and strong in Brooklyn, the New York
Common Council and Brooklyn Board of Supervisors both passed resolutions calling for the bill's defeat.[92]

Downstate opposition was fervent. Assemblyman Peter Dawson (12th
District–NYC), a Tammany Hall Democrat, proclaimed that "ninety-nine
hundredths" of his constituents despised the measure. The Irish Emigrant Society's "Remonstrance" conceded that Irish immigrants were often "poor and helpless," but were not generally criminals; "their remains"
should not be "subjected to the fate of felons." The Irish, the society
pleaded, were "distinguished by their adherence to the rites of decent
sepulture": "any violation of the remains of the dead are abhorent [*sic*] to
their feelings."[93] As the debate in Albany heated up, the Hibernian Burial
Society marched in the New York City St. Patrick's Day parade, carrying a
"green silk banner, fringed with gold, on it reading, beneath a deathbed

scene:—WE PROTECT THE SICK AND BURY THE DEAD."[94] (But, the Irish opposition was hobbled by the absence of Archbishop John Hughes, who spent most of the winter and spring in Cuba and the American South to restore his health; he returned in mid-April, after the bill had passed.)[95] Patrick Maguire (Democrat-NYC) denounced the bill as anti-Christian: believers deserved a decent burial. "The raw and bloody bones bill" treated "the bodies of men of no greater import than the bodies of dogs": "I believe in the resurrection of the dead. Man dies not though his ashes may mingle with mother earth."[96]

Objectors also came from upstate, especially the Finger Lakes and western New York, the region dubbed the "Burned-Over District" for its waves of religious revivals and susceptibility to new prophets and new cults. Whig Assemblyman Joseph Cook of Genesee fulminated against the bill in language that blended theology with class analysis. According to the "Holy Writ . . . God made man in his own image: . . . We may pass a bill to permit the immolation of this sacred image upon the altar of science, yet . . . a higher law . . . will hold us responsible for granting so questionable a license to a class of men . . . who laugh at the jest and top off the bowl, while before them quivers the flesh of inanimate humanity." The anatomist revels in carnality and deliberately profanes the dead bodies of the poor. "Is poverty a sin—misfortune a crime? Is it not enough that the recipient of these drank life's bitter cup while living, without subject his dead body to insult and sacrilege, and the heartless jeers of those knights of the dissecting-knife who are besieging this House in behalf of the bill?" The utilitarian detachment that would permit "insult," "sacrilege," and "heartless jeers" is "a cold philosophy that would brutalize the finest feelings and defile the image of God."[97]

At every turn, the bill's opponents contested the anatomist's claim of moral superiority over the agents who procured his bodies for dissection. "If they are remorseless vampyrs who steal a dead body for dissection," Assemblyman Benjamin Joy, an upstate Free Soiler, wondered, "what will those be who take bodies for dissection under the law?"[98] The poorhouse "had horrors enough now, without adding the further dread to it of a legalized dissection after death." The humane thing would be to dissect "the bodies of all who die rich," so that nothing be added "to the sufferings of the poor." Better yet, as Cook, Joy, Maguire, and J. E. Willis, an upstate Democrat and a former blacksmith suggested, physicians should be required to contribute their own bodies to the dissection tables.[99]

In short, opponents condemned the bill as the ghoulish and illegitimate exercise of class privilege. Anatomical dissection served as a metaphor for class relations: the poor were meat, preyed upon and eaten by the upwardly aspiring professorial elite. The figures of the anatomist and the body snatcher were incorporated into a parable of capitalism, which turned everything, even the dead, into a commodity traded on the market. The bill's object, Patrick Maguire jeered, "is to obtain dead human bodies for mere purposes of speculation, to be made merchandise of. New York will then truly be made a commercial city, where the dead cannot escape the rapacity of speculators."[100] And in a certain way, both sides agreed. Supporters of the bill also denounced the market in bodies, but in their discourse the traffickers were the enterprising lower-class "wretches . . . who prowl about . . . grave yards like hyenas and ghouls," not the noble and disinterested medical profession.[101]

THE DIVIDED SOUL OF THE BOURGEOISIE

> A bill introduced into one of our Legislatures to give the
> bodies of paupers to surgeons, was probably to get rid of
> the expense of burying them. . . . Oh! there is no
> boundary to human selfishness.
>
> REV. SAMUEL HAYES ELLIOT, 1858[102]

Thus the debate over the Bone Bill and anatomical dissection encoded a critical discourse of social identity and the market. This was not merely a matter of the poor and their representatives versus the bourgeoisie: the middle- and upper-classes of the state were not united in favor of the bill. Although the progress of medical science was precious to the bourgeoisie (which defined itself in opposition to the insensibility, inertia, and ignorance of "the million"), humanitarian sentiment demanded a show of empathy with the sufferings of the poor.

This critique of the market and the performance of humanitarian empathy was a mark of bourgeois cultivation that was obsessively staged in sentimental poetry, fiction, melodrama, and reformist rhetoric. It was an especially favored theme in sentimental death narratives. *New England's Chattels: or, Life in the Northern Poor-house*, an 1858 novel by Congregationalist minister Samuel Hayes Elliot, is structured around a morally redemptive series of deaths in the poorhouse, in which each pauper's demise is an imitation of Christ. Elliot's principal target was the rural practice of auctioning off the poor (which he regarded as another kind of body trade), but he also condemned the Bone Bill. At the end of the book, reform triumphs and a new humanitarian poorhouse system is instituted. When one of the worthy inmates, the widow Prescott, dies, she receives a beautiful funeral:

> Every one of the paupers who was able went to her grave and saw her buried. . . . They could not avoid thinking it was a handsome thing to be decently buried; to see a good many people at your grave—i.e., at your companion's grave; to be thought a human being worthy of a burial notice, and

perhaps a marble slab in memory of one, as at least belonging to the great race—the HUMAN people. (473)

For Elliot, those who treated the dead of their fellow humans without "reverence," as a commodity, suffered from a fatal lack of empathy, the very trait that distinguished the "human" from the "inhuman." The supporters of anatomy legislation thus could also be conscripted to serve as the Other against which bourgeois social identity defined itself.

This logic helps to explain why some highly respectable prohibitionists, moral reformers, and antislavery Whigs opposed the Bone Bill. *Harper's Monthly*, a house organ for bourgeois reform, ran a lengthy editorial denouncing the bill: "An increasing irreverence for the *body* may well characterize a time when men's *souls* are everywhere bought and sold for political offices, and the highest weal or woes of the most important nation on earth is staked on measures having no purer motive than the party advantage they may give . . . to this or that clique of spoil-hunting factionists."[103] The dead body, like the "human" body (antislavery), the female body (antiprostitution), and the political body of the nation, should be sequestered from any calculus of advantage or disadvantage.[104] The dead human body, that is, contains an implicit critique of "the claim of science, and the claim of the mart," the utilitarian calculus and the commercial calculus that underly capitalist economics and political culture, and that violate customary funerary practice:

> The human body, on the departure of the spirit from it, has never been regarded in the same light as other matter. . . . It has a deeper ground. The body is not like a picture, a book, a garment, or any thing else that once *belonged* to the deceased and which recalls him to our remembrance. It is something more than a belonging, a property, an association. (691)

The possession of such "deep" sentiments defines the transcendental moral self that is signified in the term "human." "Science may prove" that the dead body consists of

> nothing . . . but carbon, and oxygen, and lime, and phosphorus, and azote [nitrogen]; . . . but all this can never eradicate the sentiment we are considering. It enters too deeply into our laws of thinking, our laws of speech, our most interior moral and religious emotions. . . . Scripture and nature both protest against the wrong it would inflict upon . . . [all] that is most pure, most tender, and most precious in our humanity. (690)

It was a mistake then to assume that dissection "does no hurt to the dead." Anatomy, the *Harper's* editorialist argued, does "an immense injury to the living," to society as a whole: it "breaks up the sympathies which unite us with the dead" and "make life serious, rational, and religious." Anatomy "must produce a state of mind at war [with] feeling," a callous indifference to the "continued identity of being" that links the living and the dead (691)—the linchpin of Adam Smith's *Theory of Moral Sentiment*. All the more objectionable, then, the respectable classes' willful insensitivity to the sufferings of the poor:

> The poor think more of death—they have more to remind them of it—than their wealthy brethren; and . . . are ever more alarmed at the thought of sepulchral violation than those "who fare sumptuously every day" . . . Every truly sensitive mind must feel more pain at the thought of the poor Lazarus being dragged from his grave, than of the rich Dives being subjected to the same treatment. (692)

IN the end, despite the outcry, the Bone Bill passed, by one vote more than the necessary two-thirds majority. With slight modifications—a requirement that the remains of the dissected be interred in a wooden coffin; the omission of the word "almshouse," so that technically the unclaimed body of a rich person dying at home might be taken for dissection—the Governor signed the bill into law, on 3 April 1854. The contest was over in New York, but would continue in other states for another 40 years.

Over the next few decades, the Bone Bill did help New York's medical schools get the bodies they needed, but in other respects it was poorly enforced. Waiting periods were sometimes ignored, and next of kin haphazardly notified. The covert taking of bodies by professional and student body snatchers diminished markedly. However, as long as other states lacked similar legislation, commerce in bodies continued, albeit at a lower level. In the 1870s and 1880s, as the number of medical schools and medical students continued to multiply across the nation, anatomy scandals proliferated, including in New York State.[105] But, as other states successively adopted anatomy acts, a new, legal system of cadaver provision slowly came into being. By 1900, the process was complete, except in the South, where most states lacked anatomy acts and bodies were requisitioned from state prison systems where large numbers of prisoners—inmates were disproportionately black—labored under terrible conditions that produced high mortality rates.

However, if the debate was finished, this did not mean that the anxieties of the poor were laid to rest. In postbellum America, a decent burial became even more of an imperative for working-class people. From the 1850s to the 1890s, philanthropic institutions that provided burials for the poor proliferated. The compelling existential necessity of such a burial served to bind working men and women to religious institutions and charities. The Catholic church made a particular point of offering spaces in its cemeteries for indigent parishioners.[106] Always at risk of destitution through the vagaries of the economic cycle, incapacitating sickness, and accident, working men and women built up a vast web of fraternal, religious, and ethnic burial societies; for the destitute there were also informal neighborhood collections. From the mid-1870s onward, there was a great expansion of cheap commercial death insurance for the poor. The Prudential and Metropolitan insurance companies became corporate giants through their cultivation of the mass market in penny death insurance policies.[107] We cannot attribute the demand for such policies solely to the fear of dissection—burial in Potter's Field was the primary fear—but dissection served as the cautionary worst-case scenario.[108]

The new funerary economy then enforced a kind of discipline on the poor, something like the Christian afterlife: the good burial was a reward and the bad burial (or no burial at all) a punishment. Anatomy laws drew a moral boundary between the respectable working poor and those below, a depth into which the working classes lived in perennial terror of falling: the limbo of the unclaimed.

"Indebted to the Dissecting Knife"

ALTERNATIVE MEDICINE AND ANATOMICAL
CONSENSUS IN ANTEBELLUM AMERICA

IN NOVEMBER 1851 the body of a sixteen-year-old girl was discovered missing from a grave in Ohio City, a village about 150 miles west of Cleveland. Several months later, a newspaper reported that "mangled remains" were found discarded in a cesspool adjacent to a Cleveland medical school. Suspecting the worst, the girl's bereaved father and a group of sympathizers hurried to the school and, "with axe in hand," gathered a large crowd. After a battle with medical students and police in front of the college, a delegation from the mob was permitted to search the premises. A local medical journal printed an account of the ensuing riot:

> [The delegation] proceeded to the dissecting room, where . . . several bodies were found. They also found several limbs, hands, feet, &c. One of the father's friends seized a hand, and swore that that was the hand of his daughter, and of this he was perfectly positive, from some marks upon it. A physician present . . . declared it to be the hand of a man. . . . A foot was also discovered, which the friend and a ringleader of the mob declared was the girl's foot. The committee then descended the stairs, and the father took the hand, and, swinging it around, said, "This is my daughter's hand." The mob then became perfectly furious. . . . The windows (nearly sixty) were broken out; the beds and furniture of students destroyed; the chemical apparatus, collection of minerals, museum, valuable anatomical models, &c., broken up and thrown out of the windows and carried away. For an hour or more the mob had entire possession of the building, and did not retire until they had finished their work. Before leaving, they set fire to the building.[1]

The anonymous author of the account (probably a member of the college faculty) denounced the assemblage as "the veriest looking scoundrels that have thus far cheated the penitentiary out of its due." The school's dean, concurred: the riot was nothing but "the aimless fury" of "a mob . . . of Germans, Irish, . . . drunken Americans . . . and idle boys."[2] But, as historians of the crowd have amply demonstrated in similar instances, the episode did have a social logic, a cultural poetics that was played out in every aspect of the riot, especially in the physician's comment about the sex of the hand. For the respectable person, the hand of a "genteel," bourgeois woman should be easily distinguishable from that of a man by virtue of its "delicacy." If the crowd cannot discern the difference then it has demonstrated its brutish insensibility, its lack of "humanity." If, however, there *is* no discernable difference then this proves the coarse indelicacy, the vulgarity, of the woman to whom it once belonged. Bourgeois identity is signified through the highly developed performance of the feminine; the lack of such a distinction is fatally damaging to one's social standing. For the crowd, the defense of family honor, especially the honor of a female family member, was an imperative affirmation of social being, of inclusion in the moral community.

The reports of the riot connected performances of social distinction to the spirit/matter dichotomy. The superiority of spirit over matter was encoded in the disciplined bodies and language of the bourgeois physicians, and in their command over the dead but powerfully evocative bodies of anatomical subjects. On the other side, the mob continually signified its affiliation with the body: it brandished dismembered limbs of the body and reveled in the dissected flesh. According to one account, the rioters threw "blood remnants of mortality . . . helter-skelter out of the windows[,] on to the side-walks, the crowd below, or wherever else they might land. . . . [One] full length skeleton was lashed to a barber's pole," as if an effigy, "and all sorts of fiendish demonstrations made."[3] The mob asserted the moral superiority of body over spirit, alternately mocking and assaulting the social and cultural pretensions of the anatomist, the professional privilege that affirmed itself by dishonoring the dead bodies of people who worked with their hands. The riot was a carnivalesque leveling: stripped of protective social wrapping, the anatomist was a butcher, fatally contaminated by matter.

Up until 1852, such riots were not unusual. The Cleveland riot is notable for being the last major American anatomy riot. But also for another reason: the college in question was an alternative medical institution, a homeopathic college. To historians of American medicine, this has not seemed remarkable. In the nineteenth century, they tell us, anatomy riots and scandals afflicted schools of every medical sect and faction.[4] Regulars, homeopaths, neo-Thomsonians, and eclectics alike emphasized the importance of anatomical dissection in the education of physicians, using the same anatomy textbooks, making the same gestures and claims in the anatomical theater, and performing the same rituals at the dissecting table.

But if antebellum alternative medical sects were trying to differentiate themselves from the regulars, as they surely were, why embrace anatomical dissection?[5] Anatomy was in most places illegal or only quasilegal. It was difficult and expensive to do, requiring a medical library and anatomical theater; dissecting rooms; anatomical objects to be manufactured or bought, and museums to be maintained; storage and waste disposal areas for anatomical material; and, above all, a steady supply of cadavers, supplied by the exertions of medical students or paid bodysnatchers and corrupted Potter's Field officials. Anatomy also incited the fury of the crowd. Why didn't homeopathic, botanic, and eclectic colleges place themselves on the side of anatomy's critics, both the crowd and more genteel objectors? And how did homeopaths and botanics get around the fact that Samuel Hahnemann (1755–1843), the founder of homeopathy, and Samuel Thomson (1769–1843), the founder of sectarian botanical medicine, were distinctly averse to anatomy?

THE BOTANICAL CRITIQUE OF ANATOMY

[A] college diplomatic doctor is a privileged character.

SAMUEL THOMSON (1843)[6]

To answer these questions it will be necessary to look at what botanics and homeopaths had to say about dissection. Samuel Thomson himself initially had nothing to say: his major works, all written in the 1810s and 1820s, make no mention whatsoever of anatomy; his critique of "learned medicine" was conducted along other lines.[7] Thomson denounced medical orthodoxy as an antidemocratic cabal whose "diplomaed" members aped the effeminate foppery of European elites ("[t]he doctor comes with great perfume") and stifled upstart, socially inferior, competitors.[8] Just as the Roman Catholic priesthood concealed knowledge of scripture in Latin, the regulars, he warned, concealed "the knowledge and use of Medicine, "in a dead language." Although logically this might include the greco-latinate nomenclature that designated body parts in anatomical discourse, his main target was the "unnatural" and "poisonous" metallic drugs, prescribed in a cultish vocabulary and symbols indecipherable to the public. In contrast, Thomson advocated the use of steam and herbs (primarily lobelia and cayenne) by lay healers.[9] His "plain and simple" theory of the body—"formed from the four elements," earth, water, air, and fire—lacked any explicit reference to anatomy, although it implicitly opposed the knowledge claims of the "learned physicians."

However, as anatomy ascended to an increasingly privileged position in the regular medical curriculum, Thomson felt obliged to confront it. In 1836, he revised *Learned Quackery Exposed* to include a two-page critique entitled, "Study of Anatomy; or the Skeleton in Its Natural Dress." One "view of the skeleton, . . . the study of a live anatomy," he complained, "has scarcely entered the mind of the anatomist."[10] The regular physician's understanding of the *living* body derives from a course of study of

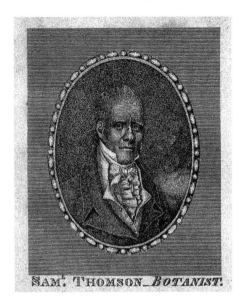

SAM. THOMSON__BOTANIST.

Figure 5.1. Samuel Thomson (1769–1843). Engraving. *The New Guide to Health; or Botanic Family Physician.* . . . (Boston, 1835), frontispiece. Courtesy of the Library of the College of Physicians of Philadelphia.

texts and the dissection of the *dead*. The regular interposes himself between the patient and the patient's body, claims jurisdiction over the body. In contrast, true healing ability comes from an unmediated understanding of the body, from self-contemplation, something everyone can do:

> When I studied the live anatomy of my own body, I observed when I was mowing, or making hay, and the sun came the nearest being directly over my head, . . . I had the most heat, most life, most sensation, and most ambition. Here was my college; here was my book open; here was the God of nature, my president and instructer [*sic*]; here I graduated; here I got my diploma. Here I come before the world to prove the facts and instruct others in the true principles of anatomy of human life, and how to restore the decaying spark of life in suffering humanity.[11]

Thomson's knowledge comes direct from "the book of nature," from God, not anatomy books or the examination of cadavers. His revelation occurs, significantly, while he performs manual labor. His "president and instructer" is God, not hubristic medical professors who are members of the social class that does no manual labor and who look down on work and workers. Knowledge of the body properly belongs to the divinity (and, by extension, believers), not a medical priesthood. In effect, Thomson renarrates the Protestant critique of Catholicism, with the human body substituted for scripture. Anatomical dissection is symptomatic of larger social ills: anatomy is linked to scholasticism, popery, and the ancien régime of Europe. Life in a nonhierarchical society, Thomson insists, requires that knowledge of the body be "plain and simple" self-knowledge. The problem is not anatomy per se, but rather anatomy's exclusionary epistemology and the social hierarchy that is erected around it. Anatomy competes with a "commonsensical," "natural" knowledge of the body.

Except for "The Skeleton in Its Natural Dress," Thomson did not bother with anatomy, but other botanics did. An ephemeral and anonymously edited monthly journal, the 1823 *Medical Reformer*, published out of New York City, devoted much of its second issue to the subject, condemning "the fashion" that "represent[s] a knowledge of anatomy as the almost exclusive foundation of pathology and therapeutics" and judges "the practical skill of the physician by the extent of his anatomical information."[12] Anatomy, the *Reformer* asserts, confers no real medical knowledge; no therapeutic advances follow from its progress. "[T]he learned doctors . . . wait for the sick to die to know what caused their death"; then the physicians rush to dissect the find the cause of death. But this confers no practical benefit. Doctors may understand the course and location of the disease better, but still do not know how to cure it: "They are called learned men. . . . It is said they understand anatomy, and know the name of every part of a man. All this they may know, and yet not know how to cure a sick man." A knowledge of anatomy is a "philosophical" display of learning that diverts the physician from the practical task of treating patients. Moreover, the dead body cannot be used to give an accurate account of the living body: after death the body undergoes a transformation into something that is qualitatively different. Given these limitations, only "a general knowledge of the structure of the animal body . . . is requisite to form the most able physician."[13] (Such criticisms of anatomy were not distinctively botanical: orthodox physicians who felt threatened by the Parisian school made similar arguments. Regular doctors could not deny that anatomy was the foundation of medicine, but they condemned the enthusiasm for pathological and comparative anatomy, arguing that medicine was more an "art" than a science.)[14]

The *Reformer*'s critique is a response to the emergent institutionalization and professionalization of contemporary medicine: "There are about twelve hundred students attending lectures in the different medical colleges in the United States. What a blessing would it be to society had their parents trained them up to agriculture instead of . . . the idle speculation, and dogmas of medical schools."[15] In such institutions, the medical professoriate used anatomy to forge medical authority and identity. In contrast, the *Reformer* argues, botanical physicians "cannot be indebted to the dissecting knife."[16] The botanic relies on easily obtained local herbs and on practical experience, which can be gained by ordinary people.

Botanical healing is an indigenous approach to medicine that fosters egalitarian social relations, unlike European medicine with its hierarachical and social distinctions.[17]

Anatomy is hubristic at its core, the *Reformer* contends. The dissector arrogantly seeks to uncover what God keeps hidden. The anatomist conceives of the body as a machine and aspires to be the machine's operator. But this expansion of medical agency is morally corrupt, because a spiritual and holistic "principle of life" operates the "animal body"—the "powers of the mechanist" are reserved for God (and derivatively the individual soul): "we can neither change, remove, or restore a part, we cannot even interfere with its action, without influencing the whole system."[18] This divine holistic principle elevates the human "animal body" to a privileged status. In dividing the body into functional parts, anatomy reduces the human body to the status of a material thing, a mechanism.

Going further, the *Reformer* offers a final social and aesthetic indictment of anatomy, reprinted from an unidentified "Medical Newspaper":

> A gentleman . . . visited a chamber in Market-street . . . and [was] much surprised. . . . Human bodies, sacrilegiously stolen at midnight from the grave, in various stages of putrefaction, and exhibiting various operations of the dissecting knife, filled the atmosphere of the room, with the most nauseous exhalations. On one end of a table lay a body, dismembered of its limbs; on another, the head, robbed of its contents, was placed as if to gaze in mockery at the mutilated trunk, which it had once surmounted. Arms, legs, feet, ears, heart, liver, and lights of human beings . . . of all sizes, from six inches to six feet . . . , male and female, were scattered in profusion and disorder about the room. Here was a bowl containing the brains of some new-laid corpse, and there a tub filled with "guts and garbage," while on a slow consuming fire, were laid the parts for which there was no further use, frying in their own fat and marrow. The furniture was besmeared with blood and filth . . . without regard to decency and cleanliness. The slaughter-houses . . . where cattle and sheep are butchered by hundreds, are perfumed palaces compared with this school of anatomy! The gentleman who communicated these particulars and requests their publication, has left his name, which is at the service of any one who may doubt the correctness of the representation.[19]

Through its association with the proliferating corruptions of the dead body (odors, repulsive mess, violation of funerary custom), anatomy implicates its practitioners, and offends and endangers the respectable public. Far from being a constitutive performance of genteel medical science, anatomy has affinities with the abattoir. It brutalizes its participants and society at large.

This critique of anatomy has a different social origin than the critique offered by the Cleveland rioters, and a different social meaning. The tone is literary, in the genre of mannered correspondence. The instigator of the piece, several times identified as a "gentleman," is so delicately re- fined—so disembodied—that he "communicates these particulars" through the pen of a third party, rather than directly. In effect, the article inverts the logic deployed by the medical reporter of the Cleveland riot. The chaos of the dissecting room, the "profusion and disorder" of disaggre- gated bodies is laid at the foot of the anatomist and contrasts with the delicacy of the offended gentleman. Where he is abstracted to the degree that the name of this "individual" can only be supplied on request, the bodies of the dead are very present, very concrete, with invasive smells and scenes so repulsively powerful that they excite involuntary loathing, even nausea. Absent the anatomy rioters, the dissecting room itself has a carnivalesque quality that works to subvert the rule of spirit over matter; the anatomist demotes the human body to the level of butchered and cooked animal meat. The dissecting room scene is a riot of carnality. The anatomist is "soiled with trade," imbued with the taint of bodily corrup- tion, in contrast to the literary sensibility of the gentleman and his pen- man, who signify their class affiliation by gestures that link them to a morally pure disembodied spirit.[20]

THE ANATOMICAL CRITIQUE
OF BOTANICAL MEDICINE

But this particular critique of anatomy did not originate with the botanics and was far from their usual style and concerns. Thomson and friends were never known for excessive gentility and the Thomsonian system re- quired only a modicum of literacy from its practitioners. Thomsonians regarded themselves as plain-speaking democrats, and identified with the agrarian, antimonopoly politics of the Jacksonian Democratic party. The regulars, they complained over and over again, were trying to monopolize medical practice and introduce the hierarchical structures of ancien ré- gime Europe into American medicine and society. Much of the Thomson- ian medical politics of the 1820s and 1830s, therefore, was taken up with lobbying state legislatures to deprive regular medical colleges and soci- eties of the exclusive power to license practitioners.

Here it bears repeating that the colleges were selling anatomy and ana- tomical dissection. Anatomy legitimated medicine as "scientific." Anatom- ical knowledge served to distinguish the medically educated from the ig- norant; and anatomical credentials were necessary to achieve status within the profession, and with the public. The orthodox supporters of medical licensure scorned the Thomsonians on anatomical grounds. An 1828 New York State Assembly subcommittee reported that it was "a mat- ter of notoriety, that the botanic or Thomsonian practitioners are almost universally ignorant of the anatomy of the human system, and of its condition in disease." The botanics' "only claim to professional knowledge" was by virtue of "patents" that Thomson issued for a fee. Such arguments assume that true knowledge is privileged above "traffic" that soils the hands of those who conduct "trade" in patents and that illegitimately markets healing authority to unrefined "individuals of the most limited mental attainments, and of the lowest capacities." In contrast, the legitimate physician should dwell in a disinterested, protected genteel space, sequestered from the sordid compulsions of the market economy.[21]

In the 1830s and 1840s, the regulars beat the anatomical drum: anatomical medicine is learned medicine; nonanatomical medicine is ignorance and quackery. We have studied and dissected: we know the body; they do not. Such arguments had force: as critics denounced them, botanics and homeopaths conceded the point, reconciling themselves to and even embracing the anatomical body. In the 1830s, Thomsonians and eclectics (another medical sect that adopted many Thomsonian ideas and assimilated many Thomsonian practitioners) began to adopt the orthodox model of formal medical education—much against the wishes of Samuel Thomson, establishing colleges that granted degrees certifying medical competence. These schools included, even emphasized, the teaching of anatomy and anatomical dissection; no medical college could claim legitimacy if it did not promise to provide such instruction.[22] Thus, the first fully operative eclectic medical school, the Worthington Reformed Medical College of Columbus, Ohio, which opened its doors in the fall of 1839, advertised its intention to offer anatomical instruction, and its professor of anatomy, T. V. Morrow, renounced any links to Thomsonianism. Morrow agreed with the critics of botanic medicine that possession of anatomical knowledge marked physicians as persons of liberal culture and strong character—in other words, anatomy was linked to bourgeois professional identity.[23] His attempt to make good on his claims proved his undoing. A few weeks after opening, a "resurrection" riot forced the closing of the college.

Wooster Beach (1794–1868), often regarded as the founder of the eclectic sect, was more ambivalent, or perhaps confused, on the subject of anatomy. His enormously popular 1836 compendium *The American Practice of Medicine* relied on John Wesley's century-old pronouncement that "neither the knowledge of astrology, astronomy, natural philosophy, nor even anatomy itself, is . . . necessary to the quick and effectual cure of most diseases incident to human bodies," and Beach went to some lengths to deny that anatomy was "a foundation of the healing art": "I treated complaints quite as successfully before I studied anatomy as afterward; indeed it is almost proverbial, that a great anatomist is a poor practitioner."[24] Yet Beach also proclaimed that "All classes should possess a general knowledge of anatomy, physiology and the practice of medicine, both as a matter of interesting information and practical utility" (xv), while stipulating that this could "be acquired without those disgusting and revolting scenes which are exhibited in the lecture and dissecting rooms of our medical colleges": "Plates, wax preparations, &c., are sufficient . . . , for all practical purposes, anatomy needs not many lectures, descriptions, nor minute dissections" (738).

But in the 1840s Beach came fully to terms with anatomy, even publishing in 1847 *A Treatise on Anatomy, Physiology, and Health, Designed for Students, Schools, and Popular Use.* The same year, he purchased a large collection of anatomical specimens, both wax and natural, and opened the New York Anatomical Gallery and Academy of Natural, Medical and Moral Science, a popular anatomical museum (for more on such museums, see chapter 9 below).[25] But he never purged or revised the antianatomical sections of *The American Practice of Medicine,* which continued to be published into the 1860s.

Eclecticism, as its name implies, exhibited a spongelike capacity to absorb contradictory theories and practices, including spiritualism, hydropathy, Thomsonianism, mesmerism, electrotherapy, phrenology, eugenics, "natural bonesetting" (a British folkhealing tradition, discussed below), and so forth. Although Beach and some other eclectics may have initially hesitated, anatomy and anatomical dissection quickly achieved high status within eclectic discourse: claims of anatomical competence authorized eclectic practitioners to adopt or reject various theories and therapies in the name of disinterested medical science. From the 1850s on, eclectics wholeheartedly endorsed anatomy.

THE THOMSONIAN ADOPTION OF ANATOMY

Thomsonians could not renounce Thomson, but they also came to embrace anatomy, a transition facilitated by the fact that some influential botanics were converts from regular medicine. Dr. Thomas Hersey, twice president of the U.S. Botanic Convention and editor of the *Thomsonian Recorder* (the first avowedly Thomsonian journal), by his own account had been an orthodox surgeon "of the old school" for forty years before adopting the Thomsonian system. Hersey's training and experience predisposed him to retain his anatomical commitments.[26] Under his editorship, the *Thomsonian Recorder*'s first two volumes (1832–1834) reprinted portions of William Paley's pietistic and deeply conservative *Natural Theology* (under the title, "Anatomical") and a lecture by John Abernethy, an eminent British anatomist. But the journal's stance toward anatomy was not sharply defined. Hersey also published "Logical Deductions from Anatomical Facts," by Wilson Thomson (one of Samuel Thomson's five

sons), a wary effort to appropriate anatomy while retaining a critique of
the "specious developement [*sic*] of the mechanical or anatomical structure of the human frame."[27] Tellingly, although Wilson Thomson distanced himself from anatomy, only deploying it "for useful illustrations
. . . of certain principles inherent in the living animal body, without attempting any thing like a vain parade of scientific ingenuity," he assigned
anatomical knowledge the status of a "fact" determined by that ultimate
authority, "the anatomist." His use of anatomy, however, was deliberately
unsophisticated, a translation of anatomy into the commonsensical idiom
of Thomsonianism and deployed only insofar as it buttressed and ampli-
fied Thomsonian doctrine.

In a later lecture (1834), also published in the *Thomsonian Recorder*,
Wilson Thomson elaborated upon his objections to anatomy. Like the
elder Thomson's "Living Anatomy," these were not religious in the sense
that dissection was described as a desecration of the dead body, but were
articulated within a religious narrative, "the reformers" versus "Popery."
This was the Whiggish history of anatomy stood on its head. In Wilson
Thomson's view, medical science and superstition are structural and ideological kin; both are obscurantist: "Why did the Bishops of Rome perform
the service of the church in Latin? Because they wished to keep the people in ignorance, while they made a gain of them and established their
own infallibility. And why have physicians concealed the healing art under
the same language? . . . [F]or the same purpose." The regulars complain
"How can these men [Thomsonians] cure the sick, who never studied
anatomy and chemistry? They know nothing about the human system."
But this, Wilson Thomson argued, was medically irrelevant: "the study of
anatomy is little more than the study of foreign names and technicalities":

> [R]eason and a close examination of ourselves will teach us more useful anat-
> omy than any system now in use in the schools of science. . . . While I feel
> friendly to learning, and wish it to flourish in our country, and every branch
> of science to be pursued with avidity . . . , yet I wish it to be distinctly under-
> stood that a good classical education is one thing, and the secret by which
> the sick is to be cured, another.[28]

Anatomy cannot coexist with American national identity. Anatomical terminology is "foreign" and elitist. The nation's progress requires that science flourish here (a conventional trope of patriotic rhetoric), but that
science must be skeptical, pragmatic, democratic, and anti-institutional.

In contrast, Thomas Hersey made fairly sophisticated and extensive use
of anatomy, and abstained from any criticism. The second edition of Hersey's *Midwife's Practical Directory* (1838), dedicated to the "Thomsonian
brethren" and the "numerous intelligent Thomsonian sisterhood," contains chapters on menstruation, gestation, the female organs of genera-

tion, prenatal development, and the process of conception, and featured eleven engraved plates illustrating female sexual anatomy and the stages of pregnancy, one of them a tinted foldout that showed a fetus in the womb. Hersey responded to the botanical critique of anatomical medicine's social pretensions by working to democratize anatomy, to spread anatomical knowledge beyond the boundaries of the regular profession, to midwives and the public. Thus, in a sharp, but unavowed, departure from Samuel and Wilson Thomson, Hersey championed the acquisition of anatomical knowledge as a key objective of oppositional medical politics.

At the same time, Hersey linked the acquisition of anatomical knowledge to a gentrifying self-improvement in language: "by becoming familiarly acquainted with a delicate mode of conveying ideas on such matters," readers could render "useful instruction to others, and extend a salutary influence in correcting the taste and improving the habits of conversation in those circles where occasional hints on these subjects appear to be indispensable." This too was not previously a Thomsonian concern. Anatomy provided a vocabulary and a "site" in which the body, and especially the sexual body, could be textualized, articulated as respectable discourse—the body domesticated.[29]

Thomas Hersey and Wilson Thomson coexisted within the pages of the *Thomsonian Recorder*. They engaged in no debate on anatomy; rather, the two men addressed their shared audience separately and without reference to Paley and Abernethy, or each other. This incoherence was customary in the popular medical journals that flourished in the 1830s. Like other contemporary periodicals, editors had space to fill: a good portion of their pages were taken up by articles reprinted from other periodicals, or by unpaid correspondents. Incompatible voices cohabited, even in a journal ostensibly published "under the direction of Dr. Sam. Thomson."[30]

Still, it was no coincidence that anatomical articles were increasingly encountered in the pages of irregular publications, given the growing importance of anatomy in orthodox discourse and practice, and the enthusiasm for anatomy among the laity (an interest cultivated by contemporary middle-class reformers like William A. Alcott and Sylvester Graham, discussed in chapter 6 below).[31] In adopting anatomy, Thomsonianism took a bourgeoisifying turn and shed its distinctive social character. In the late 1830s, one begins to see the change, especially in urban locales. For example, the *Boston Thomsonian Manual* of 1 December 1837 devoted its first three pages to an article entitled "On the Structure of the Human Body." By mid-1838, almost every issue of the journal, renamed the *Boston Thomsonian Manual and Lady's Companion*, led off with three or more pages on "anatomy and physiology."[32] As Thomsonianism began to fracture, and anatomy increasingly found an audience among the laity, the Thomsonian stand against anatomy eroded. Nathaniel S. Magoon of Boston, who credited himself as the "successor to Samuel Thomson" in his *Thomsonian Almanac for 1844*, repeated Thomson's stand on the superiority of "the study of living bodies" over an anatomy based on the dissection of the dead. But in an item titled "Necessary Science" Magoon provided a virtual compendium of contemporary arguments for the teaching of anatomy in elementary and secondary schools. A knowledge of anatomy would beget in children "a sense of self confidence and respect" and help them "more than a thousand sermons" to keep "to a line of habitually virtuous action." Anatomy would have a inherently disciplinary effect. Children "would at once see and feel the importance of doing exactly as they are required to do by the soundest system of ethics":

> The miss and young lady would scarcely dare to corset themselves a single hour! They would know that in that short time an adhesion might take place to obstruct circulation between the most delicate and important viscera in the human body, and be followed by slow, lingering disease, fearful pains, and certain death. [Anatomical knowledge] would do more to promote habits of temperance . . . [and] to induce the rationality of feeling and judgment than any thing else ever devised. . . . Let schools and academies teem with instruction on this subject.[33]

This new Thomsonian interest in anatomy extended beyond the schooling of children. *The Philadelphia Botanic Sentinel*, while deploring "the fact that many professional Thomsonians are induced, from the opinions of others, to attend 'scientific' (so-called) lectures, before they become properly informed as to Thomsonian remedies," argued that "Anatomy is an accomplishment which every practitioner should acquire."[34] The proliferation of anatomical articles in botanical journals of all factions suggests that the Thomsonian public, increasingly interested in adopting aspects of bourgeois identity, found anatomy useful, even compelling. And, as the addition of *Lady's Companion* to the title of the *Thomsonian Manual* evidences, the sect's growing audience of women fostered the process of gentrification. The plain-spoken masculinist style of Thomson and sons increasingly gave way to more mannered prose.

By the mid-1850s the botanical assimilation of anatomy was institutionalized in ways that Thomson would have found inconceivable. The neo-Thomsonian *Journal of Medical Reform* (*JMR*) reported on new developments in physiology and pathological anatomy, and favorably reviewed texts written by orthodox medical professors. The newly established Metropolitan Medical College of New York City advertised that it offered "Anatomical and Hospital privileges . . . never before . . . enjoyed by Reformers" and an anatomy teacher "as scientific and thorough as any Anatomist of Allopathic Colleges." As in orthodox schools, the enthusiasm for anatomy was driven largely by student demand: "we think the *most* 'anxious' student will be fully satisfied with the completeness of the Ana-

tomical Instruction."[35] Again, the tone was genteel and the zeal for anatomy linked to the democratization of medical science and the profession.
Gone was Thomson's condemnation of orthodox medicine as effeminate,
aristocratic medical science; botanical medicine shed its masculinist coloring. The *JMR* supported the opening of medicine to women (Metropolitan Medical College was a coeducational school), and published
Lydia Fowler's "Suggestions to Female Medical Students," which stressed
the importance of "an *intimate* knowledge of anatomy" for women entering medical schools.[36]

HOMEOPATHY'S ANATOMY

A parallel story obtains in the case of homeopathy. Samuel Hahnemann,
the sect's founder, argued that the body was opaque, a black box, and
condemned anatomy as a hubristic effort to tear the veil that God placed
over the body. He denied the usefulness of anatomy in the understanding
and cure of disease. In *The Organon of Medicine* (1810), *Lesser Writings*
(New York, 1852), and other works—all of which had scriptural status
within homeopathy—Hahnemann made many negative pronouncements
on anatomy and physiology: "we [cannot] witness what is passing in the
interior of our bodies . . . these processes remain concealed from us,
[even] as they lie open to the sight of the Omniscience."[37] Hahnemann
doubted the very possibility of anatomy. The anatomist might claim that
dissections provided him with the equivalent of "a mental eye" that enabled him "to penetrate through flesh and bone into that hidden essential nature of things," but that "pretension" was nothing more than
"boastful charlatanry and mendacious delusion."[38] Anatomy had no useful
role in determining the origins of disease. Hahnemann derided the anatomist who "took upon him[self] to explain the functions of the living
body; and, by his knowledge of . . . the internal parts, to elucidate even
the phenomena of disease."[39] The action of disease on the body was subject to its own unique and specific laws, an "immaterial, vital principle."
The homeopath therefore worked on spirit, not gross matter:

> The materials of the mechanical workman . . . have physical and chemical
> properties, and can only be fitfully and fully employed by one who is well
> acquainted with these properties. But it is quite otherwise with the treatment
> of objects whose essential nature consists in vital operations . . . the living
> human frame. . . . The matter on which we [homeopaths] work is not to be
> regarded and treated according to physical and chemical laws like the metals
> of the metallurgist, the wood of the turner, or the cloth and colors of the
> dyer.[40]

The effect of such a critique was to brand orthodox medicine and the
anatomical conception of the body as "materialism" (a code word for

atheism), but also as "coarse," tainted by the materiality of manual labor, manual laborers, and the material world. The orthodox physician (and especially the anatomist), unlike the homeopath, must get his hands dirty.

What this suggests is that the homeopathic adoption of anatomy—the transformation of homeopathy into a fraternity of dissectors—represents a disjunction between discourse and performance. In homeopathic discourse, medicine should be a science of the immaterial: this is what gave homeopathy its distinctive appeal. Thus the contradiction at the heart of American homeopathy: initiation into the mysteries of anatomical dissection and certification of anatomical training on actual bodies served as a credential to practice a technology of the ethereal self.

If homeopaths claimed a shared epistemological affinity with the regulars, based on anatomical dissection and derivative texts then this obscured the differences between the two sects. Dan King, a searing critic of homeopathy, charged that the "veneration [of homeopaths] for Hahnemann is entirely hollow and hypocritical, since they . . . practically deny all his principles."[41] Disagreements between homeopath and allopath were relegated to the therapeutic arena. And there the homeopathic critique of "rational" medicine converged with the increasingly scientific orientation of the New England (European-trained and -influenced) medical elite.[42] Thus Constantine Hering, an eminent disciple of Hahnemann, claimed that the "wonderful discoveries in Pathological Anatomy" were easily incorporated into the homeopathic canon as "a valuable addition to our knowledge." Far from refuting homeopathy, scientific medicine deprived the *orthodox* materia medica of its rationale, and so left the regulars with only a futile therapeutic nihilism.[43]

Hering overstated the case: materialism and immaterialism were not so easily squared. Although anatomical dissection was invariably a requirement of formal homeopathic education, as late as the 1860s some homeopathic colleges resisted pathological anatomy.[44] Nevertheless, the move to identify homeopathy with anatomy and physiology succeeded to the extent that, by the turn of the century, the homeopathic profession (although not lay practitioners) could without much difficulty be absorbed into the regular profession.

By the 1860s, homeopathy had achieved a level of respectability never achieved by the botanics. From the very beginning, there were crucial differences in the cultural and social position of the botanics and homeopaths. Thomson knew manual labor; Hahnemann was an upper-class German physician, patronized by the aristocracy. In America, homeopathy presented itself as an exotic European cultural innovation. Rather than offering a critique of medicine as science, it claimed to offer a superior, more empiricist, medical science. It extended the Baconian inductive method to therapeutics via the technique of "provings." Hahnemann was "the Bacon of Medicine" and claimed his *Organon of Medicine* (1810) as a descendant of Bacon's *Novum Organum*.[45] In homeopathic renditions of the sect's history, homeopathy was set securely in the scientific Grand Tradition.

This identification with science was consistent with homeopathy's social character. Mid-nineteenth-century homeopathy, observers typically noted, attracted as patients "the refined, the learned, and the wealthy"—and disproportionately women.[46] D. White, a homeopathic practitioner, argued that homeopathic patients came from among "the most enlightened classes . . . the reading and thinking portions of mankind. . . . [T]he illiterate and unintelligent portion of the community cannot appreciate [homeopathy's] doctrines. . . . , while on the other hand the more intelligent admire the beauty and symetry [*sic*] of all that is really scientific."[47] The doctrine of "infinitesimal doses" (the progressive attenuation of potent substances, with powerful but subtle therapeutic effect) was aesthetically appealing to those who cultivated a rarefied sensibility. On their bodies, a princess-and-the-pea effect seemed plausible. A healing system that did not puke, blister, and bleed, that worked on immaterial spirit, fit comfortably with the aestheticizing requirements of bourgeois identity: a scrupulously clean body, pleasantly arranged appearance, moderate disposition, beautiful surroundings, and a cultural poetics that privileged the abstract and disinterested spirit over the desirous, disorderly body. Thus, in contrast to the Thomsonians, homeopaths more often than not abstained from a critique of class distinction and were not much interested in constructing an antielitist and anti-European American national identity. Although some homeopaths (mainly lay practitioners or female physicians) did participate in the movement to democratize medicine and disseminate anatomical knowledge, this was never the dominant tendency within homeopathy.

Because Hahnemann, unlike Thomson, endorsed the idea of scientific medicine—and because a large number of homeopaths had originally been trained as orthodox physicians in orthodox medical colleges—homeopaths were well positioned to drop their founder's objections to anatomy. Homeopaths assimilated surgery into their practice—and incorporated anatomical instruction, including dissection, into their college curriculum.[48]

DISSECTING THE BODY ELECTRIC: ALTERNATIVE MEDICINE, ENTREPRENEURSHIP AND THE ANATOMICAL CONSENSUS

By the 1840s, the connection between anatomical expertise and healing authority had been firmly established throughout the spectrum of medical belief, among both the laity and professionals. Anatomy had the status of a legitimating, foundational discourse. "So great and universal has the prevalent delusion upon the subject of dissection become," complained Samuel Dickson, English founder of yet another alternative medical sect (Chrono-Thermalism), "that almost everybody, from the peer to the peasant, shares in it."[49] Patients sought out anatomically trained healers. Medical practitioners, high and low, sought to advertise their anatomical credentials. Even Vair Clirehugh, a British haircutter and wigmaker relocated to lower Manhattan, made claims of anatomical expertise. To tout a remedy "to prevent Baldness and Grey Hair, . . . restore the Hair where it has fallen off, and . . . eradicate Scurf and Dandriff" [sic] he wrote a small pamphlet entitled "Clirehugh's Anatomy of the Skin":

> According to the researches which I have made, the skin consists of three distinct layers, the outer of which is called the *epidermis* or cuticle, . . . popularly known as scarf skin; it is a dense impermeable envolope [sic], adhereing [sic] by its inner surface to the rete muscosum. . . . The *Dermis or true Skin* in which the hair is rooted, is the innermost layer and the thickest part of the skin, is of a white color, and possesses great strength. . . . It rests upon the adipose and cellular tissue formed by numerous threads closely interwoven together, besides an extensive system of arteries, veins, and nerves. . . . [V]iewed through a microscope, it is found to be studded with little eminences, . . . named papillae, . . . [which] contain branches of nerves of exquisite sensibility.

Clirehugh boasted of having studied with "the most celebrated Physiologists in London and in Edinburgh," where he "dissected the different layers of the skin," and "examined the nerves, vessels and bulbs, connected with both skin and hair."[50] The invocation of anatomical science was meant to bolster Clirehugh's claims, and clinch the argument in favor of his baldness cure. Whether such claims were effective with the public is unknown, but, whatever the case, the authority of London and Edinburgh could not be denied. Anatomy was a cultural gold standard.

Within the regular medical profession, there were, of course, still debates over which kind of anatomy was to be privileged, the dangers of specialization, and the political, social, medical, and empirical conclusions to be drawn from the anatomical body, but anatomy's high status was a settled issue among entrants at every level. Physicians established their credentials within the profession through the intensity and competence of their commitment to anatomical medicine. And in professional performance even the humblest practitioners cited this filiation, displaying in their offices wired skeletons, anatomical preparations, anatomical diagrams, and diplomas with anatomical iconography. Such were the icons that signified healing authority, and if irregulars wanted to make

equivalent claims, then they had to wield the same signs, to place themselves inside the anatomical consensus.

And so they did. Homeopathic, eclectic, and neo-Thomsonian schools
all advertised their identification with anatomy, their commitment to provide anatomical instruction, including the dissection of cadavers. The critique of anatomy, if present at the origin of the sects, no longer served to
define sectarian difference. There was, instead, a competition to wield the
signs of anatomical authority, and this contest had a destabilizing potential. It was hard to stage anatomy: the growing prestige and progress of
the Parisian school, with its emphasis on pre- and postmortem examination, meant that medical legitimacy increasingly depended on a knowledge of a growing number of difficult texts, possession of ever larger
numbers of cadavers—in most cases from illegal sources—and examination of ever larger numbers of living bodies, which required access to
hospital patients. Such strenuous demands, in turn, created counterin-
centives to place limitations on the commitment to anatomy. Complacent
authorities, impecunious, undereducated, or lazy medical students, and
insecure rural physicians alike felt threatened by the rising anatomical
ante—not to mention a populace that recurrently mobilized to protect its
dead from the depredations of medical grave robbery. At the same time,
such limitations in turn provided opportunities for enterprising critics to
take the regular profession and local medical establishments to task for
failing to adequately teach anatomy to medical students, keep pace with
the latest scientific advances, and disseminate anatomical knowledge
among "the million." In making such charges, reformers, unorthodox
healers, and popular lecturers could rhetorically assert their own anatomical competence and commitment, articulate their own anatomical visions, and cultivate their own audiences.

This fissure was avidly exploited by electrotherapeutic, mesmeric, and
phrenological practitioners whose relationship to orthodoxy was often
nebulous. To stake out the contours of the emergent anatomical consensus in 1840s America—and the entrepreneurial niches it opened up—
it will next be instructive to look at two men who operated near its
boundaries: Andrew Jackson Davis, the magnetized "seer of Poughkeepsie"; and Henry Hall Sherwood, "a regularly educated" but heterodox
physician, magnetizer, astrologer, and journalist.[51]

Henry Hall Sherwood (b. 1796; fl. 1840s) was a minor contributor to
the demimonde of spiritualism, phrenology, Swedenborgianism, and mesmerism that flourished in America in the late 1830s and 1840s. Between
1836 and 1847, Sherwood developed a thriving practice in electromagnetic medicine and authored a flurry of books, with titles like *The Motive
Power of Organic Life, and Magnetic Phenomena of Terrestrial and Planetary
Motions, with the Application of the Ever-Active and All-Pervading Agency of*

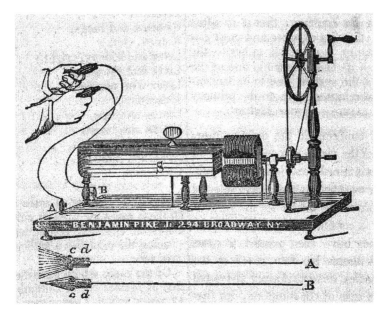

Figure 5.2. "Rotary and vibrating" electromagnetic machine. Henry
Hall Sherwood, *Manual for Magnetizing with the Rotary and Vibrating
Magnetic Machine in the Duodynamic Treatment of Diseases* (6th ed.,
New York, 1845), 26. Courtesy of the National Library of Medicine.

Magnetism, to the Nature, Symptoms, and Treatment of Chronic Diseases.[52] His
therapy, like chiropractic, attempted to regulate the flow of electromagnetic force from the brain to the organs and extremities, with a corollary
emphasis on the disposition of the spine.

In the 1830s and 1840s, electricity and magnetism inspired widespread
enthusiasm. Following from Galvani's famous experiments on frogs, the
electric researches of Alessandro Volta, Michael Faraday, and others, and
the healing wonders attributed to Anton Mesmer (whose theories were
popularized in America through lecture tours by Charles Poyen and Robert Collyer), electromagnetism could plausibly be identified with the *élan
vital*, the force that animated the living body, and possibly the inorganic
universe as well. The vogue for animal magnetism and medical electricity
was, if anything, heightened by the invention of electromagnetic telegraphic devices in the late 1830s and 1840s. The construction of telegraph lines in Great Britain, and Samuel F. B. Morse's celebrated 1844
demonstration of the telegraph, followed by the rapid proliferation of
lines between major cities, palpably demonstrated the power of electricity
and provided a model of information transmission that seemed analogous or identical to that of the human nervous system. Orson Fowler, the

phrenologist, wrote that "Magnetism, or electricity, or galvanism . . . is now generally conceded to be the grand instrumentality of life in all its forms."[53] Electricity was an exemplary transformative technology; electromagnetic healers and therapies multiplied; the body pulsed with electric force. This was the cultural moment in which Walt Whitman wrote "I Sing the Body Electric" (published, not coincidentally, by the phrenological publishing house of Fowlers & Wells). An anonymous 1843 pamphleteer estimated that twenty or thirty mesmeric lecturers were busily crisscrossing New England, speaking to audiences that sometimes numbered in the thousands, and that the Boston area had over 200 practitioners engaged in some kind of "magnetic healing" or "patho-mesmerism."[54]

It was also the moment in which Whitman resolved to "Read the latest and best anatomical works / talk with physicians / study the anatomical plates."[55] And, like Whitman, Sherwood's passion for electricity and animal magnetism was connected to a passion for anatomy and physiology. In the mid-1840s, Sherwood edited a medical journal called the *New-York Dissector*.[56] Modeled on *The Lancet*, the *Dissector*'s title signaled its critical project: to cut to the bone, pare away the unessential and the false, and reveal inner truth.[57] The dissector locates, names, and extirpates the pathological element, the source of bodily corruption. There is menace in the keen blade. The anatomist metaphorically kills his subject, reduces it to its component parts, takes power over it and augments his own—the dissector as castrator. Sherwood favored a "cutting tone," but, more than that, he deployed anatomical discourse to legitimate his own efforts and delegitimate competing healers.

The regulars were Sherwood's principal targets, but he also went after magnetizing rivals, many of whom also used anatomy to authorize themselves. One such healer was Andrew Jackson Davis, the eighteen-year-old "seer of Poughkeepsie," who made his debut in 1844. A barely literate shoe-maker's apprentice, Davis claimed that, while he was mesmerized, he possessed a knowledge of anatomy and physiology, "without ever having gone through the labor of study." "The human system seemed utterly transparent to him," William Fishbough marveled, "and to our utter astonishment he employed the technical terms of anatomy, physiology, and *materia medica*, as familiarly as household words!"[58] Placed in a trance by his magnetizer, he would diagnose and prescribe for patients, and, according to reports, cured them instantly. The Reverend Gibson Smith, who witnessed the mesmeric examination of a young woman, testified that Davis described her condition "perfectly, . . . pointing out the seat of her disease and pain, designating the different organs by their technical or scientific names, and locating every part of the system which he had occasion to name."[59] This clairvoyant power to gaze into the body was a kind of postmortem dissection, but on the living.

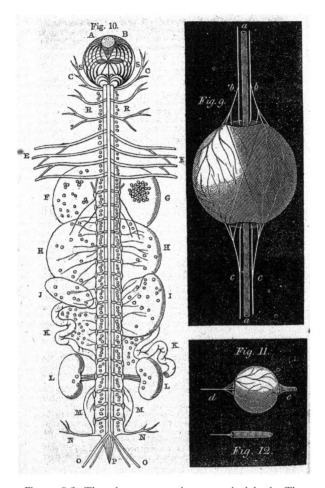

Figure 5.3. The electromagnetic anatomical body. The diagram is Sherwood's revision of a plate taken from an anatomical textbook; Sherwood has added an electromagnetic globe at the head of the spinal column; the whole thing appears to be effervescing. Henry Hall Sherwood, *Electro-Galvanic Symptoms, and Electro-Magnetic Remedies, in Chronic Diseases of the Class Hypertrophy, or Chronic Enlargements of the Organs and Limbs, including All Forms of Scrofula, with Illustrative Diagrams and Cases* (New York, 1837), 18. Courtesy of the Library of the College of Physicians of Philadelphia.

In 1847, Davis visited New York City, where, in a trance state, he treated clients and delivered a series of lectures. Sherwood immediately responded by itemizing Davis's numerous anatomical errors, and denounced him as a quack.[60] But the Seer, already consolidating his reputation, held fast to his anatomical claims and rhetoric. His *Great Harmonia*, published in 1850, mingled mesmerism, Swedenborgian cosmology, anatomical and physiological jargon, and health advice. *The Harbinger of Health*, published in 1861, carried the anatomical motif further, with chapters on the "Pathological Offices of the Sympathetic Ganglia" and "A Pneumo-Gastrical Discovery," which Davis claimed to have made "by means of clairvoyant examinations of the human body." *The Harbinger of Health* remained in print for more than fifty years.[61]

Sherwood and Davis shared common interests: a fascination with electromagnetic forces, a fascination with anatomy. But condemnation of Davis and other healers as quacks served to bolster the credibility of Sherwood's own healing practice—treatments with "magnetic" pills and plasters, and electromagnetic stimulation with "rotary magnetic" and "duodynamic" machines—all of which made reference to new scientific knowledge and technology.[62] So did Sherwood's enthusiastic advocacy of pathological anatomy. He advertised this filiation by reprinting the texts of celebrated European pathologists and physiologists, and mingling their writings beside, and within, his own. He also bound in or copied finely detailed plates from authoritative anatomical texts to illustrate his own writings. *The Motive Power of Organic Life* is a pastiche of writings by Sherwood and writings and illustatrations taken from the works of elite European anatomists.

He claimed the right to keep such company by virtue of original contributions to medical science. In an article entitled "Anatomy and Physiology," Sherwood claimed that, as far back as the 1810s, he had "ascertained by the magnetic symptoms, and by post-mortem examinations, that there was a direct connexion between the ganglions of the spinal nerves, and the serous surfaces of the organs, as well as with the muscles." The rhetoric of scientific prose, the stance of disinterested observation, the latinate terminology, diagrammatic illustrations, and verification via autopsy, all served to link magnetic medicine with pathological anatomy, the most sophisticated and most prestigious medical discourse of the 1840s. Magnetic medicine, Sherwood insisted, should use the same language, procedures, and standards of proof, as the most advanced scientific investigations:

> The intermediate ganglions are no doubt connected with the different viscera, and a physician of this city has . . . has been trying to determine these connections by the action of the magnetic machines. . . . No opportunity has, however, occurred to test their correctness by post-mortem examinations, and

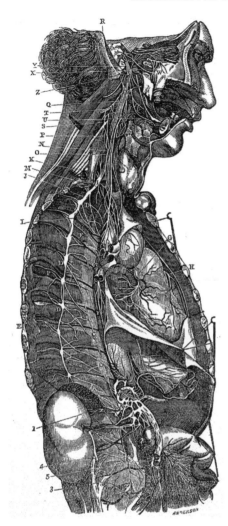

Figure 5.4. "The ganglions of the organs of the body, connected with the great sympathetic nerve, reduced from Manec's grand plate. . . ." Sherwood, *The Motive Power of Organic Life and the Symptoms and Treatment of Chronic Diseases* (New York, 1844), plate between pp. 64 and 65. Courtesy of the Library of the College of Physicians of Philadelphia. The same plate appears in works by Calvin Cutter, Mary Gove, and other popular anatomists.

we would now suggest to physicians who are . . . using the magnetic machines, the importance of these scientific investigations, and of ascertaining, and publishing, as soon as possible, the true connections of these ganglions with the viscera. . . . This is a fine field for investigation and for distinction, and we hope that the enterprising young men of the profession will not fail to enter upon it.[63]

While not as emphatic as Horace Greeley's call to "Go West young man," this last counsel suggests that in the 1840s anatomy presented an analogous set of opportunities: like the West, the anatomical body was a large and poorly defended territory, potentially a prime chunk of real estate if only you could figure out how to exploit some corner of it. It could be capitalized on by a variety of hands, at a variety of levels: wholesale, retail, or for individual consumption; it could be either master craftsmanship or shoddy work. Sherwood was closer to the shoddy end of the spectrum, though not so far as Davis, but even so anatomy was a discursive resource that helped make credible his magnetic theories and therapies.

Davis and Sherwood both directed their syntheses of anatomy and magnetism to a public eager for new scientific technologies of self-making and self-regulation. But what precisely was the promise of anatomical self-making, as Sherwood retailed it? To which particular segment of the public were his efforts directed? The market for popular anatomy (discussed at length in the next chapter) consisted of that large number of people who wished to acquire some version of bourgeois identity. For them, anatomy acted as a template, disciplining and distancing the body by overlaying it with a textual form. Inscribed with borders and place names, the body was rendered into a rational, legible, manageable, and aesthetically ordered self. Anatomy and physiology provided a secular morality—what Andrew Jackson Davis termed "physiological virtue"—enforced by scientific law. The rule of a systematic, abstemious reason over the impulsive, desirous "animal economy" produced a temperance body. Contemporary moral reform literature increasingly made use of physiological arguments.[64]

The acquisition of such a body gave the promise that, with new scientific discoveries, the human body, and human society, would undergo physiological improvement corresponding to the moral progress promised by evangelical Protestantism. At the same time, in adopting the anatomical body, aspirants to bourgeois status signified in their very embodiment an affiliation with a progressive and sophisticated learned tradition that made powerful epistemological claims, one that, above all, was distinct from the coarse, carnal embodiments of their undisciplined social inferiors, those who were without anatomical knowledge or who actively objected to it, the anatomy rioters (about whom Sherwood had nothing to say)—and also distinct in its materiality, lucidity, and improvability from the voluptuary or ethereal bodies of the aristocracy and its upper-middle-class emulators.

But, as any reading of *Leaves of Grass* and the numerous popular anatomy books of the period demonstrates, the anatomical body had the discursive potential to support an extravagant materialist-vitalist synthesis that far exceeded its disciplinary agenda. Alongside aesthetics, morality, rationality, and technological innovation, anatomy promised a radical expansion of human agency that was also a part of bourgeois identity. The telegraph seemed to be an especially paradigmatic example of the coming transformation of self and society. A New Hampshire homeopathist enthused that

> Telegraphs . . . will vibrate all over the world, even as the nerves of the human body ramify every root and branch of the living man. Another progressive philosopher . . . claims that even the *telegraph* will soon be surpassed, and all mankind be brought into immediate *mental* communication with each other on psychological principles. . . . [O]ur people have come to regard "all things possible," even with man, which the human intellect is capable of conceiving.[65]

In the writings of Sherwood and his contemporaries, the body electric is extravagantly productive: "[The] structure, arrangement, and order of the different parts of the human body . . . are recognized by every anatomist of the present age, and now present to our view a galvanic battery altogether superior to any ever made by man."[66] The "animal economy" explodes with competing and complementary transactions, radiates electromagnetic forces. The body flows and overflows with blood and sera; grows thickets of veins and nerves; pulses with excitations and exhaustion; ingests, processes, and excretes outside material—a constant churning of spirit with matter, matter with spirit. If anatomy carved the body into bounded regions and subjected it to a physiological jurisprudence, the

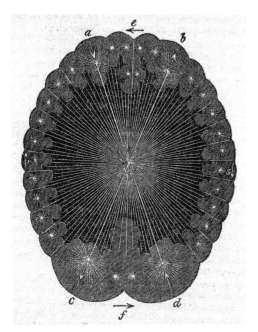

Figure 5.5. Radiant heart, with magnetic diagram underneath. Sherwood, *The Motive Power of Organic Life and the Symptoms and Treatment of Chronic Diseases* (New York, 1844), 231. Courtesy of the Library of the College of Physicians of Philadelphia.

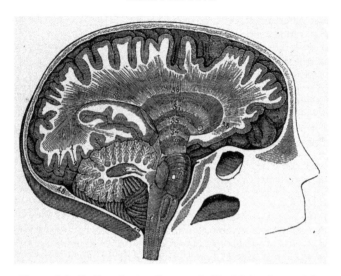

Figure 5.6. Radiant brain. Sherwood, *The Motive Power of Organic Life and the Symptoms and Treatment of Chronic Diseases* (New York, 1844), plate between pp. 50 and 51. Courtesy of the Library of the College of Physicians of Philadelphia.

anatomical body could also be unstable, an inebriate body where boundaries and forces proliferated. This generative anatomy was in some ways a return of the repressed "enchanted" body that disciplinary anatomy had originally defined itself in opposition to.

The proliferating body was appealing for other reasons as well. It modeled the social experiences of its public: the feverish boom-bust economy of early industrial capitalism; the insatiable expansion of the nation-state across the North American continent; the jostling competition of political parties; the emotional upheavals of religious revival; class antagonism and insurrection; the incitements of the consumer culture of the 1840s; and the transformative power and danger of industrial technology. If harnessed, this anatomical/magnetic body had millennial implications, but the prospects were not altogether comforting. The alternative healers and popular anatomists of the period, especially marginal operators like Sherwood, characteristically oscillated between arousing and allaying the anxieties of their public, a state of suspension that readers and patients found in some ways pleasurable, at any rate compelling.

In producing the body as the "real," a thing of nature exempt from the vagaries of political and social strife, anatomy naturalized contingent social orders, ideological regimes, and historical experiences. This, it should be emphasized, did not merely ratify the status quo. If the ana-

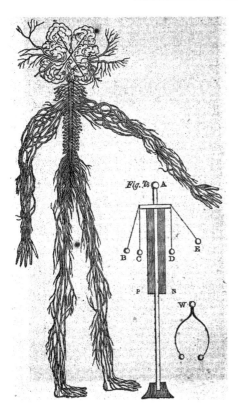

Figure 5.7. Nervous/electromagnetic man. Henry Hall Sherwood, *Electro-Galvanic Symptoms, and Electro-Magnetic Remedies, in Chronic Diseases of the Class Hypertrophy, or Chronic Enlargements of the Organs and Limbs, including All Forms of Scrofula, with Illustrative Diagrams and Cases* (New York, 1837), 23. Courtesy of the Library of the College of Physicians of Philadelphia. Similar or identical illustrations of nervous, arterial, and venous man (minus the magnetic apparatus) appear in works by Frederick Hollick, Wooster Beach, Edward Bliss Foote, S. G. Goodrich, Catharine Beecher, T. S. Lambert, and other popular anatomists.

tomical body increasingly became a prerequisite of a hegemonizing bourgeois identity, that identity was no fixed thing. There were ongoing contests over who was to be eligible for such an identity, and over the agendas to which it would be linked. Such questions keenly interested the large segment of the population that was on the cusp of bourgeois identity. This was the public to whom Sherwood appealed when he criticized the regular medical profession as "aristocratic," when he championed anatomy as a democratic alternative practice. The medical politics complemented the entrepreneurship: Sherwood was in the business of retailing the bourgeois self to people who were only a thin stratum above the anatomy rioters, and maybe not even that.

His anatomy, however, was derivative. Although he was a surgeon, he had no highly specialized training by any recognized authority, and did not regularly perform dissections or provide anatomical training to others. And this defined the limits of his cultural authority: Sherwood transmitted anatomical knowledge via articles reprinted from (mostly foreign) medical journals; he identified with anatomy and assimilated its

language into his magnetic healing practice. He did not produce anatomical knowledge like the Europeans he admired. Despite his extravagant
claims, he had to defer to Flourens, Magendie, Bell, Bichat, and Broussais. Not that Sherwood ever adopted any sort of deferential tone: in the
pages of the *Dissector*, he posed as a visionary prophet of medical electricity and magnetism, a stance asserted more by rhetoric than real erudition.

"Different From All Book Knowledge": Waterman Sweet's "Natural Anatomy"

Electrotherapists, spirit healers, homeopaths, and Thomsonians embraced the anatomical consensus. Who (if anyone) remained to dissent?
In the fall of 1837, F. H. Hamilton, then a 25-year-old professor of anatomy and surgery at a small medical school in Auburn, New York, touched
on this topic in his introductory address:

> the importance of anatomy is at the present time conceded by most, if not by
> all—the poor and affluent—the learned and unlearned. . . . Even the super-
> stitious old woman who . . . mutters an ill-omened curse at the . . . unholy
> student of the charnel house . . . , will when in her ague of fear she shatters
> her brittle bones, seek for the same unsanctified man to adjust the several
> parts, and restore her limbs to nature's comely proportions. Indeed . . . nei-
> ther *Sweet* with his instinctive . . . faculty of adjustment . . . nor *Thompson* [*sic*]
> with the mysterious power of pepper and steam, can arrange a dislocated or
> fractured limb, or perform any surgical operation, unless they possess both
> anatomical knowledge and professional skill.[67]

Hamilton, like other ambitious young medical men, sought to advance
within the medical professoriate by riding the anatomical wave (Auburn
was a good place to begin because the state prison there provided a
cheap and quasilegal supply of cadavers; Hamilton was the prison surgeon). He too made common cause with French pathological anatomy
and physiology, insisting (more rigorously and credibly than Sherwood)
on the importance of "*actual dissection* alone."[68]

The success of that position, and his competence in asserting it, can be
measured by the trajectory of his subsequent career: Hamilton ascended
from his position at the state penitentiary to professorships at Fairfield,
Geneva, Burlington, Buffalo, Brooklyn, and finally, in the postbellum era,
the prestigious chair of surgery at Bellevue Medical College in New York
City. His 1837 lecture features a number of arguments relevant to our
discussion. First, from a position of newly minted authority within the
orthodox profession, Hamilton condemns those regular physicians who
still resist pathological anatomy and disparage the Parisian emphasis on
dissection, but argues that even so there is essentially a consensus on the

value of anatomy. At the same time, Hamilton points to three representative figures who stand outside the consensus: "the superstitious old woman" who opposes the medical desecration of bodies, but nevertheless resorts to an anatomically trained surgeon when in need; Samuel Thomson (whose followers were already adapting anatomy to their needs); and Waterman Sweet, a "natural bone-Setter." (Elsewhere, in Hamilton alludes to a class of uneducated persons—anatomy rioters—who conceive of death as a kind of sleep, and regard the "dissector [as] a rude and unnatural wretch," who amuses himself by "violating the sanctity of the grave, and disturbing by wanton slaughter the repose of the dead.")[69]

Bonesetters specialized in the setting of broken bones, replacement of dislocated joints, relief of spinal and musculo-skeletal pain, and treatment of "lameness." The art was a European folkhealing tradition that combined physical manipulation, tying of splints, and applications of herbal plasters and dressings.[70] Introduced into North America from Wales by James Sweet, when he settled in Rhode Island in the early seventeenth century, the "hereditary faculty" passed through at least seven generations of Sweet men, most of them farmers, artisans, and sailors. Bonesetting was the family sideline.[71]

In the nineteenth century, the art's most well-known practitioner was Waterman Sweet (b. 1796, fl. 1829–1843). A notice, printed in an 1830 Rhode Island newspaper, gives an indication of the nature of his practice: "Waterman Sweet, Bone setter, hopes to meet the applause of all who may be under the necessity of employing him. He may be found at the Market Cellar, where he has a lot of good butter for sale, fit for table use."[72] Sometime thereafter, Sweet moved from Providence to upstate New York, not far from Schenectady, and "left the plough" to become a full-time itinerant healer, "called from Canada to New-Orleans."[73]

Hamilton, the anatomist, positioned himself with respect to bonesetting. How did Sweet, the bonesetter, position himself with respect to anatomy? The testimonials published by Sweet make it plain that typically his "employers" (patients) had first been treated by anatomically trained physicians and surgeons. They came to him only after regular physicians and surgeons failed to cure their ills.[74] Given the vast number of untreatable conditions in the late 1820s, anatomical medicine was not so hegemonic that it could afford to ignore folkhealers like Sweet, who may have been more effective in treating dislocations and chronic conditions than the regulars.[75] Usher Parsons, professor of anatomy at Brown University, in a lecture to the (nonmedical) upperclassmen, denounced bonesetting as "a burlesque on common sense, . . . a term implying that some persons come into the world, possessed of a particular knowledge of the joints, more perfect . . . than can possibly be acquired by repeated and close examination of them, in a dissecting-room."[76] Other regular physicians of Providence followed suit, condemning Sweet as "an impostor and a quack."[77]

Under siege, Sweet began styling himself a "natural anatomist," a practitioner of "one of the most complicated sciences known to man," in two pamphlets: *An Essay on the Science of Bone Setting* (1829) and *Views of Anatomy and Practice of Natural Bonesetting, by a Mechanical Process, Different from All Book Knowledge* (1843). His claims of "eminence in the sciences of intuitive and self taught surgery and anatomy" (5) were in keeping with common usage of the time which was already beginning to identify the word "science" with the Baconian program, while retaining older constructions like "science of theology" and "science of law."[78] The bonesetter did not derive his healing authority from Baconianism or any textual canon: his repeated invocation of "science" was a counterclaim against physicians who did refer back to those sources. Bonesetting, Sweet argued, "like other sciences," is progressive and empirical, and does not derive from the study of books: "the practice of about forty years . . . and cases of almost every description that have come under my inspection, like all other sciences, is continually adding to my faculty . . . " (6). Similarly, he used "profession" to mean any skilled occupation, such as carpentry ("the profession" always refers to regular medicine), implying that skilled crafts are equivalent to the "learned professions" of law, theology, medicine.

Bonesetting was self-avowedly an oral healing tradition. Although textual evidence reveals Sweet's familiarity with Samuel Thomson's work, Sweet boasted that no book had ever influenced him, "nor have I ever discovered one idea in all I ever read . . . respecting the science of Bone-Setting. . . . " (1843, 19).[79] Yet in writing and publishing his "few illiterate lines," Sweet turned bonesetting into "book knowledge," if only for the purpose of contesting the hegemony of the printed word. Given the language and rhetorical strategy of Sweet's 1829 essay, a mannered retort to the "malevolence, satire and ridicule of the 'learned doctors'" of Providence (1829, 5), it is likely that he had assistance in writing. Against formal "unnatural" medical education and book learning, Sweet claimed to possess have an "intuitive predilection," "taste," "talent," "faculty," or "natural" knowledge conferred at birth by "a Superior Being"; Sweet could heal where educated physicians failed.[80] But he also claimed to "worship . . . at the shrine of the muses," and love "the wild and sublime" (1829, 6–7). His argument about natural versus book knowledge was thus linked to a notion of original genius derived from romanticism.

The bulk of the 1829 essay seeks to authorize natural practices like bonesetting through lengthy quotations from two works: a 1565 letter by "Count La Sallee [*sic*] . . . to the Academy Des Arts at Paris"; and a letter by the Moravian missionary John Zimmerman who, in 1620 made a voyage to Patagonia. Both European travelers described natives who had mastered "the art of surgery" and whose medicine was superior to that of "civilized nations," even though they were "unacquainted with any of the sciences." In both cases, the nonliterate Indians insisted that true healing power derived from God, not texts. Thus Sweet cites textual authority, in the genre of the learned essay, in a printed pamphlet, to argue the superiority of "natural," orally transmitted, or divinely revealed knowledge.

Sweet's 1843 pamphlet, in rough prose that must be his alone, goes further and (repetitively) confronts the sources of formal anatomical knowledge, in "the great cities, where the most flourishing institutions are in operation . . . where . . . all knowledge . . . of anatomy [has been] . . . acquired, from . . . books of thousands of years [old], as well as of more recent date . . . [where] they have been dissecting and wireing dry bones together, and attending lectures for a number of years." (1843, 42–43) Sweet saw "little useful knowledge" there. Physicians still fail to cure lameness or relieve pain, and even make things worse, because they have wrong "views of the anatomy of living forms"—an echo of Samuel Thomson's short antianatomy essay of 1836.

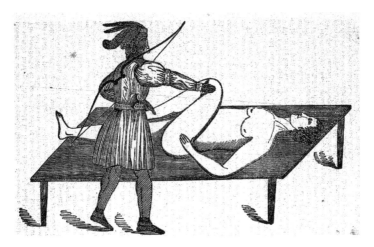

Figure 5.8. "Representation of the SWEET or lever principle of reducing Dislocations," Wooster Beach, *The American Practice Condensed* (New York, 1860), 551; rpt. from *The American Practice of Medicine . . .* (New York, 1833), 2 (pl. 11). Courtesy of the National Library of Medicine. In the 1830s and 1840s, some botanical healers called themselves "Indian doctors" and claimed their knowledge of herbs and "natural" healing methods came from study with Native American healers. Sweet, while not an "Indian doctor," claimed to practice a natural healing tradition. Here, the "natural bonesetter" is represented as an Indian.

As we have seen, by the 1840s the anatomical consensus had grown formidable, gathering unto itself even the critics of regular medicine. Perhaps for this reason, in his 1843 essay, Sweet felt compelled to provide an alternative vision of "the formation of the Anatomy of the human body," "easy to be understood . . . so that the smallest and most illiterate in community can comprehend it: . . . [A] duty was enjoined on me to . . . make known my views of the . . . intricate formations of the bones and situation of the compact frame, together with the compactness and unitedness of the bones or joints; and also of the whole human system which may be said to be composed of the four elements of fire, water, earth, and air." (1843, v) Sweet's "intuitive knowledge" of the body revives the Aristotelian theory of the four elements, again likely via Samuel Thomson.

But Sweet cannot fulfill his promise to provide a "science" of the body. The lack of a descriptive vocabulary confines him to a meager litany of parts, with only the most sketchy explanation of their connection: "The structure of the human Anatomy is erect, standing upright, composed of a head, neck and shoulders, two arms, two hands, four fingers on each hand and one thumb; one body extending from the neck to the hip joints, where the sockets receive the heads of the thigh bones," and so on (1843, 23). Exhausted, in the scant space of seven pages, Sweet drops his inventory and renews the attack on anatomical medicine:

> A child of common sense . . . will tell you your joints are out of place; a lady will say the same, as soon as she looks at it; a farmer or mechanic, or any man in different occupations; if a regular built Doctor should happen to know, it would be no strange thing or trick at all, because every body has an idea that Doctors must and do know, they have studied it for years from books, attended lectures, and many have dissected dead bodies to get information; . . . they have boiled up the dead bodies and wired them together; they have hung them up in their offices and if properly put together and set up, what specimen would that be of a person whose joints are out of place. (1843, 26–27)

I have quoted Sweet at length because, except for the anatomy rioters, it is difficult to document the response of "plain and illiterate" people to anatomical representations, practices, and claims. But Sweet's dilemma is telling. To oppose anatomy, he had to repackage bonesetting as a "natural anatomy"—and advertise it in the form of a published essay, thus undermining his own critique of literate medicine.

The paradox serves to remind us that many Americans in this period felt ambivalent about bourgeois culture and identity, and hence anatomy, even as they increasingly resorted to anatomically legitimated healers. But by mid-century anatomy and the anatomical body were ascendant. In an 1854 critique of the medical monopolization of anatomical knowledge,

Frederick Hollick, a popular lecturer on anatomical topics and a "neuro-pathic" (electromagnetic) physician, lauded "first rate *bone-setters*, who . . . , without any special . . . instruction, . . . are far superior to most medical men":

> Let the human skeleton be studied in all our schools . . . and there would be natural bone-setters everywhere, ready and able to give relief in any emergency. . . . The old idea that such knowledge is *exceedingly difficult* to obtain is not true,—give the right instruction and it is easy. . . . [T]he *knowledge* would always be at hand when wanted; while the medical man is *not* always there, nor always competent when he is.[81]

Thus, in the late 1820s in some places, and nearly everywhere by the 1850s, you could stand outside the anatomical consensus, but you could not ignore it, and it would not ignore you. In the twentieth century, later generations of the Sweet family carried on their healing tradition as conventionally trained orthopedic surgeons. Natural bonesetting was consigned to the antiquarian past. Today, osteopaths and chiropractors, Sweet's spiritual descendants, carry on something akin to bonesetting but translated into anatomical terms.[82] Both sects accord dissection a privileged place in their scholastic curriculum, much like the regulars did in the mid-nineteenth century.

6

"The House I Live In"

POPULAR ANATOMY AND

EMBODIED SOCIAL IDENTITY IN

ANTEBELLUM AMERICA

> "Philosophy," exclaimed Dupaty, on seeing the magnifi-
> cent anatomical museum at Florence, "Philosophy has
> been . . . wrong not to descend more deeply into physi-
> cal man; *there* it is that the moral man lies concealed."
>
> ANONYMOUS REVIEWER, *Annals of Phrenology*, 1835[1]

IN AN ENTRY dated 27 January 1860, Samuel Edgerly, a young merchant's
clerk, confided to his diary that "after wishing for a long time," he had
finally managed "to see the inside of a 'dissecting' room," at the College of
Physicians and Surgeons.[2] Edgerly, who had arrived in New York City a few
months earlier, worked as the "white-collared" employee of a respectable
firm. He had no particular interest in medicine: other entries in his diary
show him attending church; taking his leisure in a parklike cemetery; going
to the circus; perusing books and periodicals in a reading room set up for
the moral instruction of young people; "thrashing" wheat and picking
cherries on an excursion to the countryside; hearing a lecture by Wendell
Phillips on Toussaint L'Ouverture; and enjoying the antics of Wood's Min-
strels. Clerks like Edgerly formed a sizeable audience for an array of entertainments, diversions, and self-improving activities. Some of these were
anatomical in nature. Middle-class men and women crowded into popular
anatomical museums, heard lectures by "popular anatomists," and purchased anatomical books and pamphlets. In the antebellum period, anatomy overflowed the boundaries of professional medical discourse and performance, and became important to the American middle class.

We will explore Edgerly's dissecting-room visit in more detail at the end
of this chapter, but first it is necessary to ask: How did the lively popular
anatomical discourse that flourished in the antebellum era come into
being? Who developed it and toward what ends? Who was its audience?
What ideological duels were conducted on its terrain?

As we have seen, physicians defined themselves professionally and socially in opposition not just to lower-class healers and anatomy rioters, but

also to the body. In the rituals of the anatomical theater and the anatomy room, ambitious young men learned to dissect, and to regard that operation as a paradigm for the broader mastery of instrumental reason over the body, the lower classes, the savage races, the material world, women, animals. Such mastery was not just an isolated part of professional identity, but (at least potentially) part of two larger projects: the making of the bourgeois self and the making of bourgeois society. Anatomy provided a discursive vocabulary of bourgeois identity—and the opportunity for medical professionals to take on an expanded role in the making of that identity. In reading the body as anatomical text, anatomy opened up the interior of the private body and made it public domain, to be surveyed and regulated by the profession and by the reasoning mind. The "intellectual faculties," argued C. B. Coventry, dean of the Geneva Medical College in the early 1840s, should discipline human "physical wants and moral sentiments": "If men were left to the unrestrained and unguided influence of these impulses it would not only lead them into excesses inconsistent with their own welfare, but to trample on the rights of others and the general interests of community."[3] Ignorance of the "animal economy" affects society as well as the individual. Coventry called on Geneva's graduating class to exercise their professional authority beyond the sickroom, to offer their services as guardians of public health and morality, but also to transmit anatomical knowledge to the people so that every person could acquire a self-regulating "internal monitor."

In taking on this enlarged mission, Coventry conceded that the Thomsonian critique of regular medicine was in some respects justified. The profession had built up its mystique by jealously protecting a body of secret knowledge, but this worked against the formation of a cultivated public that would respect and defer to its claims. Coventry therefore urged the Geneva graduates "to improve every opportunity of giving popular lectures on Anatomy, Physiology and Hygiene," and saw a ready market for such undertakings: "There are few places where an audience could not be collected to listen to a lecture on those interesting subjects."[4] Such lectures would help the public to appreciate the importance of anatomy and the ways in which regular medicine was grounded in anatomical science (as Thomsonian medicine was not). As a secondary benefit, it would also bolster public support for legislation benefitting the regulars, including anatomy laws modeled on those passed in Massachusetts and Great Britain.

"THE DOMESTIC SCIENCE *PAR EXCELLENCE*": POPULAR ANATOMY'S EARLY BEGINNINGS

In the 1830s and 1840s all this seemed very new, but the makings of a popular anatomy had been percolating for decades. At the opening of the nineteenth century, Thomas Beddoes, an English physician and chemist, wrote a multivolume health manual, *Hygëia*, which called for "popular anatomical lectures." Like other medical writers of the period, Beddoes worried that "middling and affluent" men and women, made prosperous by Britain's burgeoning capitalist economy, were impairing their health through gross overindulgence. Anatomical lectures, he expected, would awaken them to "the mischiefs arising from systematic irregularity" and the "innumerable ordinary errors of individual conduct" to which they were prone. Although he anticipated that higher authorities and the public would oppose allowing women to learn about the interior of the body, Beddoes predicted that "physiology" would eventually "come to be considered . . . the domestic science *par excellence.*"[5]

Hygëia was prescient but failed to attract a lasting readership. In the high tide of anti-Jacobin reaction that swept Britain, Beddoes's participation in the circle of radical scientists grouped around Joseph Priestley, and his avowed sympathy for revolutionary France, made for a difficult reception.[6] More significant for our purposes was the roughly simultaneous appearance of William Paley's *Natural Theology* (1802), which did attract a large readership and quickly attained canonical status. Paley, an Anglican archdeacon, presented anatomical descriptions "without plates or figures, or technical language," with the aim of fostering a pietistic appreciation of the "human frame" and "nature." In providing "evidences of the existence and attributes of the Deity," whose creation was providential, immutable, and perfect, Paley sought to link the English political and social hierarchy with a divinely ordained natural order, and dismantle the links between science and revolution, science and materialism (i.e., atheism).[7] The many editions of *Natural Theology*—some of them with plates and lengthy footnotes with "technical language"—became a touchstone for writers and lecturers, even radical egalitarians like Walt Whitman, who favorably reviewed a new American edition in 1847.[8] Paleyite arguments sprouted in sermons, religious tracts, verse, and political oratory. More importantly, in the 1830s, 1840s and 1850s, natural theology became a staple of American pedagogy.[9]

The public could also learn about anatomy through lectures. From 1816 to 1820, Alexander Ramsay, a well-regarded Scottish anatomist, delivered "Lectures on the Anatomical Structure of Man" to lay audiences of men and women in New York, Montreal, Concord, Boston, Charleston, and elsewhere (he dedicated one of his pamphlets "to the ladies of Boston"). As part of the course, he dissected an unspecified member of "the ape species." Ramsay sounded many of Paley's themes—design as evidence of God's existence, the moral value of anatomical knowledge in instilling an appreciation of the divine creation, opposition to materialist interpretations of the physical body—and enthused over the potential

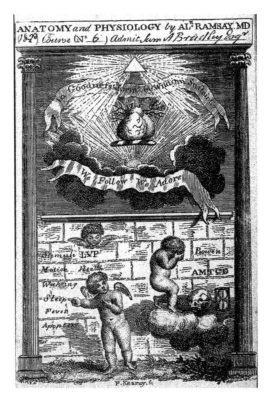

Figure 6.1. Ticket to Alexander Ramsay's lectures on anatomy and physiology, 1820. Courtesy of the New York Academy of Medicine Library.

uses of anatomical knowledge "as the basis of the conduct of the nursery in rearing the child, and schools in cultivating the mind."[10] Admission to his 1818 series of lectures in Montreal was set at a dollar per lecture, not cheap in an era when a skilled journeyman might earn $10–$30 a week and a day laborer $1 per day or less.[11] Another well-regarded Scottish anatomist, Granville Sharp Pattison, delivered a similar "popular course of lectures on General Anatomy and Physiology, as Illustrative of the Natural History of Man" in Philadelphia in 1819. Pattison charged a $10 tuition fee for the entire series.[12]

Colleges were also venues for anatomical lectures to the laity. In the mid-1820s, Usher Parsons, a Brown University anatomy professor, lectured to the upperclassmen on "The Importance of the Sciences of Anatomy and Physiology as a Branch of General Education." Parsons argued that such instruction would profit students practically, morally, socially,

and intellectually: they could call "things by their right name" when discussing problems with their physician; they could avoid displays of "palpable ignorance on such subjects" that would "diminish" their "respectability"; they would learn the limitations of their bodies and so avoid
injuries; and they would be protected from becoming the gullible prey of
natural bonesetters like Waterman Sweet (who was then residing in Providence). Parsons predicted that such lectures would make the public more
appreciative of anatomical science, less averse "to touching animal substances, especially the human body, while in a state of putrescence," and
therefore more supportive of an act to supply the colleges with the bodies
of indigents.[13] John Collins Warren offered similar lectures to the senior
class at Harvard in the 1810s, 1820s, and 1830s. In 1814, when Warren
declined to offer a lecture, the president of Harvard personally requested
that he change his mind, saying that the "present senior class . . . feel
much chagrin & disappointment at the information that the anatomical
professors will not . . . give them any dissections."[14]

The popular lectures discussed above were delivered by skilled anatomists, and often included actual dissections of a human or animal. While
aiming to gratify public "curiosity" about the body's interior and the work
of the dissector, they addressed the social and moral concerns of audience members: "cultivating the mind," fostering piety, and promoting an
understanding of the disease-producing consequences of unchecked desire.[15] The anatomically conscious person, upon learning how immoral
behavior affected the liver, brain, stomach, heart, skin, etc., and how
bodily dysfunction could affect one's moral and intellectual status, would
exercise greater control over bodily desires. Such lectures also provided
audience members with the opportunity to covertly respond to their own
sexual desires and anxieties within the idiom of anatomy.

At the same time, public lecturing furthered the goals of the lecturer.
They advertised his erudition as an anatomist and physician, and helped
to attract patients and students; earned public acclaim and raised money
through ticket sales; served as a forum to link anatomy to Christian morality and gentility; publicly repudiated sinister associations with atheism,
revolutionism, necrophilia, and cannibalism; helped the lecturer make
and solidify connections to local elites and their networks; and enhanced
the cultural authority of both the speaker and the profession. Such lectures were especially valuable for Ramsay and Pattison, controversialists
who had left behind enemies in Scotland and were trying to make fresh
starts in America.[16]

Early nineteenth-century audiences were obviously attracted to the subject of sexual anatomy, but public discussion of such topics could be dangerous to the lecturer's social standing. Parsons and Warren, solidly embedded in local networks, declined to pursue it. Pattison and Ramsay,

transient foreigners, proceeded cautiously, arguing that anatomical knowledge served to confirm and further Christian sexual discipline, although perhaps protesting too much. (Women and minors, Ramsay complained, were wrongly excluded from his lectures on the reproductive system.)[17]

The Emergence of Popular Anatomy: Discursive Sources

Up until the early 1830s, the American audience for anatomico-physiological discourse was small and fairly elite. But by the 1850s lectures, pamphlets, home manuals, and newspaper and magazine articles on anatomy and physiology, illustrated by engravings and lithographs, were being produced in large numbers, for an avid mass audience. This anatomical industry was made possible by converging technological, infrastructural, and social developments: the invention of the steam press and other new print technologies, the spectacular growth of old and new cities and towns, and the emergence of new markets opened up by successive transportation revolutions in road and canal building, steamboats, and rail.[18] In the mid-1820s and 1830s, there was an explosion of cheaply produced newspapers, magazines, and books, many of them devoted to health and medicine. When popular lecturers preached the gospel of anatomy and physiology, their audiences, principally composed of the emergent middle class, were primed to receive them.

Anatomy traveled to socially and culturally distant places. Jeffries Wyman, a young Harvard-trained anatomist teaching in Virginia in the mid-1840s, wrote his sister a teasing letter reporting "the scientific acquirements" displayed by some "Richmond ladies" over a game of cards: "one of them . . . gave me a good description of some of the bones, of muscles of the eye & shewed her proficiency in various ways. I asked some tough questions in anatomy—Can *you* answer a question which she answered correctly—has the 12th rib a tubercle? Let us see whether the science of the North or South is the strongest."[19]

Agitation for the passage of state anatomy acts also helped to foster public awareness of anatomy. The Massachusetts Medical Society's 1829 *Address to the Community* argued that "[i]f dissection shall ever become a legalized pursuit" (as it did in 1831), then anatomical

> knowledge . . . must be spread through the community: . . . [P]opular lectures upon Anatomy . . . [must be] as common as those upon Astronomy, and other branches of natural science. . . . Let Anatomy no longer be viewed with horror, but . . . form a part of the education of every well-informed man, and . . . the standard of knowledge will be raised. Physicians must be better informed, because the public is better informed. The . . . weakness, igno-

rance, and prejudice of mankind will not so readily afford stepping-stones to employment for the incompetent and unprincipled [healer].

The logic was circular: the passage of an anatomy act will stimulate public interest in anatomy; a knowledgeable public will demand the increasing anatomization of the medical profession, reject quackery, and (again) support anatomy legislation. But the idea that anatomy should "form a part of the education of every well-informed man" resonated beyond the immediate question.[20] The same arguments were recycled, sometimes verbatim, in later anatomy act debates in other states.

Perhaps the greatest contributor to anatomy's popularity was the phrenology movement that took America by storm in the 1830s and 1840s. After Johann Gaspar Spurzheim's lecture tour of 1832, George Combe's tour of 1838–1840, and Robert H. Collyer's tour of 1839, phrenological societies formed in nearly every major city. Lesser-known phrenological and "phreno-mesmerist" lecturers crisscrossed the country, giving public readings of the skulls of eminent personages and local townspeople before large and enthusiastic audiences.[21] George Combe's bestselling *The Constitution of Man Considered in Relation to External Objects*, printed in Boston in 1829 and reprinted in numerous editions for the next seven decades, came close to achieving scriptural authority in many circles.[22]

The excitement over phrenology stemmed from its claim to be a scientific technology of self-making, a claim that overlapped anatomy and physiology. In the mid-1830s, Dr. Amariah Brigham, who was then America's most prominent phrenologist, insisted that "of course," the study of anatomy and physiology was to be "strenuously recommended . . . as that on which all plans of education ought to be founded."[23] In fact, phrenologists claimed to derive their doctrine from anatomy: the craniological dissections of Gall, Spurzheim, Combe, and later exponents. Roger Cooter, one of the leading historians of phrenology, argues that Combe's success in popularizing phrenology was accomplished through the attenuation of its anatomical content; Combe made phrenology less technically demanding, more "user friendly." But anatomical dissection is at stage center of phrenology's founding drama: Combe avowed that his conversion experience occurred after witnessing a dissection of the brain performed by Spurzheim, which inspired Combe to perform his own dissections.[24] Combean phrenology gave a place of epistemological privilege to the act of anatomical dissection and located personal identity in the brain. Its credo was "brain is the organ of mind." Phrenologists presented their science as a subset of anatomico-physiological science: Nelson Sizer, a far-ranging phrenological lecturer, asserted that the science did not lie in the reading of bumps, but rather in the assessment of the "radial distance from the *medulla oblongata*, or capital of the spinal marrow, to the surface of the brain."[25] Critics were quick to seize on phrenology's link to anatomy. An anonymous editorialist in a Methodist newspaper lambasted phrenology as an "ignoble doctrine, born of the dissecting knife and a lump of medulla." Phrenology converted the "beautiful region of mental philosophy . . . into a barren *Golgotha*, or place of sculls":

> Yes! This . . . carnal philosophy . . . is to supplant the lofty faith of antiquity, and the sublime philosophy of the Bible, and to sit in judgment on the Infinite. . . . ! These powers, those thoughts, are the products of little lumps of flesh, measuring each an inch in diameter, weighing, altogether, about two pounds avoirdupois. Behold here the true nature and the full dimensions of the human soul![26]

In its first wave in America, many anatomically minded physicians embraced phrenology; many phrenologists discoursed on anatomy and physiology. The phrenological publishing house of Fowlers & Wells issued many popular anatomy books and pamphlets. Yet phrenology and anatomy were not entirely compatible. Popular anatomists were free to pick and choose what they liked from Combean doctrine, but what they did choose they found compelling. In an editorial entitled "Books on Anatomy and Physiology," William A. Alcott instructed his readers to "Reject, if you choose, [Combe's] Phrenology, for that is not . . . necessary to the right understanding of his remarks and arguments; but study the rest [of Combe's writings] with great care."[27] Alcott was referring to Combe's emphasis on self-formation and reformation, and his belief in physiological "laws of organization" which rewarded moral behavior with good health and punished immoral behavior with disease. These were to become sustaining themes of American popular anatomy—with or without reference to the phrenological belief in mental faculties and moral characteristics that corresponded to regions of the brain and topography of the skull. At the same time, phrenology's influence on popular anatomy was practical as well as ideological: Anatomical proselytizers copied phrenological practices and forms: the public lecture/demonstration, the popular journal, and the society of interested lay enthusiasts.

ANATOMICAL DOMESTICITY: WILLIAM A. ALCOTT'S *THE HOUSE I LIVE IN*

The vogue for phrenology heralded the emergence of a new and larger audience for scientific discourses of self-making. It was this market that William A. Alcott, Jerome Van Crowninshield Smith, and George Hayward sought to exploit in the early 1830s, with low-cost books that offered selections of anatomical illustrations.[28] Illustration gave the anatomical body the status of "fact": seeing (the inside of the body) is believing. Before

1832, home manuals and school books sometimes included a cursory paragraph or two on anatomy, but almost never pictures—anatomical illustrations could be found only in expensive and inaccessible medical texts. After 1832 came a deluge of cheap and easily accessible anatomical picture books and textbooks, many of them using the same illustrations, recycling the engravings presented in these pioneering works.[29]

Imagine then the impact on contemporary readers who saw, for the first time, maps and inventories of the physical body. The fact of graphic representation dematerialized the body, made it textual. The self was reconceptualized as an aggregate of anatomical parts and zones, organized around a locus of agency, the brain and nervous system, which operates through muscular and cerebral action on the external natural world. If anatomical templates could be imprinted on the "impressionable" minds of readers, then the voice of the rationalizing, moralizing agent—the disembodied author—would produce a population of anatomically conscious individuals devoted to continually rehearsing the inventorying operation on their own bodies. Implicitly, the body would take up a double existence, as both the originator and object of discourse, as flesh and text.

William Andrus Alcott (1798–1859), the son of a Connecticut farmer (and cousin of Bronson Alcott), was the true pioneer in the field.[30] His improbably titled autobiography, *Forty Years in the Wilderness of Pills and Powders*, informs us that he grew up in "extreme indigence." "Nearly as poor as John Bunyan and his wife," his parents owned not much more than "a looking-glass, an old iron kettle, an axe and a hoe." In 1822, at age 24, he began a course of self-instruction in medicine, carrying to his father's house "an old dirty skeleton," a small eighteenth-century anatomy book, and also a "more extended British work on anatomy and physiology," all borrowed from his family physician.[31] After a brief apprenticeship with another local doctor, he entered Yale Medical College in 1825 (a year after the anatomy riot there). Upon graduation, he became a practicing physician, schoolteacher, and farmer. (About this time, he and his cousin Bronson jointly decided to change the family name from "Alcox," which carried a distasteful association with male genitals and roosters, to the more refined "Alcott.") Four years later, he helped start a school near Hartford that operated along reformist pedagogical principles. In 1832, he moved to Boston to become an editor of the *Annals of Education*, a monthly magazine devoted to educational reform; he also edited the *Juvenile Rambler*, the first American weekly magazine for children, and, slightly later, *Parley's Magazine*, another magazine for children. Over the next three decades, while remaining a practicing physician, he wrote or edited over a hundred books, journals, pamphlets, and Sunday School tracts, gave public lectures on Christian and medical themes, and worked tire-

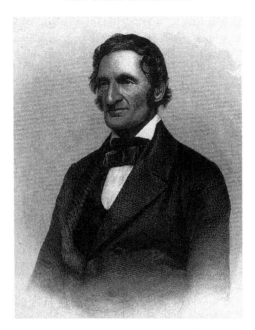

Figure 6.2. Frontispiece portrait. William A. Alcott, *Forty Years in the Wilderness of Pills and Powders* (Boston, 1859). Courtesy of the Library of the College of Physicians of Philadelphia.

lessly to promote hygienic principles, both in the school curriculum and in the architectural design of schools. (He is said to have visited over 20,000 schoolhouses.) He also advocated a distinctive medical politics. Like his close associate Sylvester Graham (the inventor of the graham cracker), Alcott criticized regular medicine and its predilection for metallic-based medicines and bleeding. He enthusiastically endorsed vegetarianism, teetotal temperance, personal cleanliness, and sexual restraint.[32]

Alcott introduced anatomy to his youth readers in the November 1832 issue of *Juvenile Rambler*, an unillustrated dialogue on "The Human Hand. Bones, Muscles, Tendons, &c" between "Mr. Williams" and a boy named "Thomas." Thereafter, the *Juvenile Rambler* featured a piece on anatomy and physiology in almost every number.[33] These early dialogues had a strong natural theological component. The anatomy mainly involved the recitation of an inventory of parts: "Now how many [finger bones] have you? Nineteen."

In the spring of 1833, Alcott abandoned the dialogue form and began an illustrated series in the form of letters written to "a young friend George," using wood engravings copied from eighteenth-century anatomy books and more modern sources. The mixture of descriptive anatomy and physiology, medical advice, and moral and religious exhortation was entitled "The House I Live In." Further installments followed in the *Juvenile Rambler* in the spring of 1833 and *Parley's Magazine* in 1834.[34] "[T]he solicitations of parents and teachers," and "an increasing conviction of the absolute necessity of something of the kind," induced Alcott to prepare it as a book "for families and schools." Part one appeared in 1834; the full volume came out in 1836 and remained in print long thereafter.[35]

The House I Live In is remarkable for the insistence with which it identifies the self with the anatomical body, and its determination to link anatomical embodiment, domesticity, hygienic reform, and Christian morality. As in Paley's *Natural Theology*, readers are exhorted to meditate upon the divine architecture of their own bodies, "a machine so ingeniously constructed, that . . . an inspired writer exclaimed, 'I am fearfully and wonderfully made?' [Psalms 139:14]."[36] But the mystery of embodied life, so evident in the psalms, is transmuted here. The chaotic body must be subjected to medical management:

> Our minds . . . are the tenants of bodies so constructed as to be continually liable to waste, as well as to become disordered; and yet we are neither taught

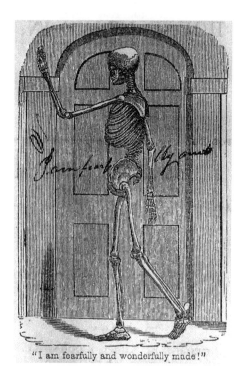

Figure 6.3. "The Frame of the House I Live In," William A. Alcott, *The House I Live In . . .* (5th ed., Boston, 1839), frontispiece. Courtesy of the American Antiquarian Society.

"I am fearfully and wonderfully made!"

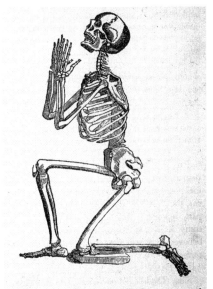

ANATOMY.—The study of the nature and structure of the bones, and nothing but the bones, is called *osteology*; that of the muscles,

Figure 6.4. Praying skeleton, *The House I Live In* . . . (2d ed. enl., Boston, 1837), 107. Courtesy of the National Library of Medicine. The figure, copied from William Cheselden, *Osteographia* (London, 1733), pl. 36, also appears in J. V. C. Smith, *Class Book of Anatomy* (2d. ed., Boston, 1836), 48, and Mary Gove, "Lectures to Ladies on Anatomy and Physiology," *Graham Journal of Health and Longevity* 2.2 (1838): 325.

the way to keep them in order nor to prevent them from premature decay. These bodies act also on our minds in a wonderful manner; for if anything in the body is wrong, it affects either our thoughts or feelings, or both.

The body must become rationalized, made into a morally and logically ordered home to its inhabiting "mind and heart" (v–vi).

The incorporation of anatomy and physiology into the school curriculum therefore has a compelling goal: the moral transformation of the public. Alcott prophetically predicts that soon "a knowledge of the physical nature of man will be generally taught to every individual of the whole race as arithmetic and geography now are; and will be as universally taught in our schools." But the habit of regarding the body with disgust, especially the dead body, stands in the way: "Many connect with the thoughts of studying the human frame, the idea of skeletons, dead bodies, knives, dissections, disinterments, and violent deaths. No wonder the mind should revolt at so horrible a picture! No wonder that Anatomy and Physiology . . . should be neglected and despised, as if these things are inseparable from it!" (vii) Alcott treads cautiously here, acknowledging the disturbing connection between anatomical dissection and the desecration of the dead. The production of anatomical knowledge, and the training of physicians, requires dissection, but dissemination of that knowledge to the public does not:

Much may be learned with the aid of nothing but a book and a few good engravings; and in fact without either of these. The body itself may be studied; that is always at hand. And if dissections are even made, portions of birds or quadrupeds may be obtained, which will partly answer the purpose. The heart, for example, of most . . . common domestic animals, nearly resembles the heart of man. . . . All good citizens disapprove of every form of disrespect for the bodies of the dead; and, above all, the barbarous practice of robbing graves. (vi–vii)

This is a tricky business. The distasteful facts must be evaded, but not to the point of denying the body altogether. The self must be divided, but the parts must also be reconciled. Against the ancient Christian preoccupation with spirit, Alcott argues for an embodied, worldly Christianity: "Man . . . has a body as well as a mind" (vii). Alcott asks his readers to identify that body with the anatomical illustrations.

At the same time he asks his reader to identify that body with the extended metaphor signaled in the title. The first chapter of *The House I Live In* is devoted to a discussion of dwellings, an architectural history of civilization that goes from "brute animals" who "build themselves houses," to ancient and primitive humans who live in huts and tents, to Euro-Americans who live in "improved" houses made of brick and stone, and, finally, that marvel of the 1830s, the "modern" wooden-frame house. What distinguishes contemporary Western humanity from beavers, bees, and savages is "improvement": no animal or savage "builds its house one

Figure 6.5. "Huts, or Wigwams," *The House I Live In* . . . (2d ed. enl., Boston, 1837), 13. Courtesy of the National Library of Medicine.

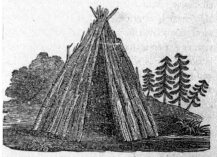

BEFORE describing "the house I live in," it will be necessary to give a short account of other houses.

HUTS, OR WIGWAMS.

Among what we call savage nations, buildings are very simple in their construction, and rude in their appearance. They are often nothing

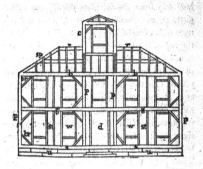

INTRODUCTION. 21

then they set up other upright sticks upon them, and frame them into the sills at the bottom, and fasten them together with beams, studs, braces, &c., in such a manner that they cannot fall down; and this they call the *frame*.

Here is a view of the front or fore side of the frame of a wooden dwelling house. The engraver has marked it with letters, so that I can describe it to you without difficulty. As you look upon the front part of it, you can of course see only one of the sills.

Figure 6.6. "Account of Framed Houses," *The House I Live In* . . . (2d ed. enl., Boston, 1837), 21. Courtesy of the Library of the College of Physicians of Philadelphia.

jot better now, than it did 5000 years ago." The chapters that follow develop the metaphorical connection between the body and house: "The Frame-work of the House: The Thigh Bone. The Leg. The Knee Pan . . ."; "The Material of the Frame: Structure of Bones. Shape of Bones . . ."; "Furniture of the House, and Its Uses . . ."; etc.

The analogy connects anatomical discourse to the contemporary obsession with house building, furnishing, and renovation.[37] As Richard Bushman has shown in *The Refinement of America*, "In the first four decades of the nineteenth century, white frame houses with green shutters," featuring parlors with finished and upholstered furniture, knick-knacks, framed engravings, rugs, bookcases, and picket-fenced lawns and gardens, "came to characterize New England townscapes and to appear nearly as commonly in other sections of the country." The creation of such homes was linked to the emergence of a large class of persons who "had the desire and the means to bring their houses up to a modest standard of respectable gentility."[38] Alcott's body is a well-designed middle-class house:

"The house I live in" is a curious building. . . . Not that it is the largest, or the oldest, or the most beautiful, or the most costly; or that it has the greatest

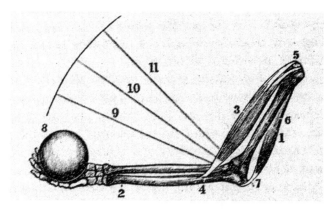

Figure 6.7. Technical description of the shoulder and
elbow joints. *The House I Live In* . . .(2d ed. enl., Boston, 1837),
90. Courtesy of the National Library of Medicine.

number of rooms or occupants, or the most fashionable furniture. But it is
one of the most wonderful buildings in the world, on account of the skill and
wisdom of the great Master Workman who planned it. (25)

The extended metaphor detaches the body from its associations with
death, desire (especially sexual desire), mess, and smell, in the same way
that the respectable home segregates its beautified parlors, bedrooms,
porches, and fenced gardens from odorous, chaotic, and ugly areas for
labor and waste. The separation, in both cases, serves to stake out boundaries between civilization, work, and unruly nature.

In making the body over into a house, the self is compartmentalized,
aestheticized, and domesticated. But the metaphor only extends in certain directions. "The house I live in" is not a node of communal life, not
part of a village, city, or neighborhood. It is abstracted from any social
context, sealed off from other selves. The effect is to forestall the emergence of a collective identity. The body is unsituated; it exists in relation
to nothing except God—and his interlocutor, the physiological advisor.

Sermons on diet, cleanliness, dress, and the prevention of disease are
threaded throughout the text. There are also many technical descriptions
of the body, both written and illustrated: "The lower portion of the arm is
made up of two bones; one larger, called the *ulna*, and another smaller,
called the *radius*. The upper end of the smaller bone, *d*, is a little rounded
and lies against a smaller hollow in the other at *g*, to which it is tied by
cords, called ligaments, particularly by one which goes round it like a
band" (90–91). The inventorying, mapping, and labeling of body parts
create a geography of the body, a terrain to be surveyed and controlled by
a disembodied moral will.

The prose throughout is in the first and second person, a textual strategy designed to encourage reader identification with the narrator's voice,
to help persuade the reader to assimilate the anatomical body and make
it the basis of his or her own self-identity. In adopting this anatomical
persona, the reader is distanced from sensation, desire, and death, which
then become merely formal properties of the body that the "I" inhabits.
The body is simultaneously self and other, a stance that gives Alcott lee-
way to speculate about the location and identity of the self within the
body:

> One of the chambers in the interior of the brain was supposed by the philos-
> opher Descartes to be the particular residence of the spiritual inhabitant.
> Now I will not stop to say . . . how it may be with *all other* spiritual inhabitants
> of houses of clay, but for myself I can assure the reader with certainty that I
> do not exclusively reside there. I live in all the parts of the brain, spinal
> marrow, and nervous system; though I will not deny that the brain is my more
> special residence. (191)

The "I," the spiritual tenant of the house, inhabits the body. The body
acts on the "I" by affecting "thoughts or feelings" when it needs to alert
the "I" that "anything in the body is wrong" (v). Subjectivity is split between spirit and body (which is objectified but still possesses agency). At
the same time the voice that speaks in the text emanates from two locations: the inhabiting soul (or mind, but not brain), and the anatomist
who operates from a subject position above and outside. Thus the Alcot-
tian self anticipates the Freudian tripartite arrangement: id (body)–ego
(mind)–superego (anatomist).

The body is subordinate to the mind, but exerts a reciprocal moral
force. If neglected or overindulged, it produces mental distress. In effect,
there is a constitutional structure of checks and balances: body and soul
continually monitor and regulate each other. The body is a complicated
mechanism ("the builders of machines have sometimes made joints in
their machinery very much like the shoulder joint," 93).

The House I Live In also sounds some of the themes of Benthamite utilitarianism. Separation between mind and body raises the possibility that
the dead body can be a material resource, to be exploited for the moral
and medical benefit of both individuals and society. In ancient Israel,
people believed it to be "wrong to use the dead body for any such purpose." But in modern times people have come to "think it quite right to
dissect . . . dead human bodies, if by so doing they can learn . . . to cure
or prevent diseases of the living. Not very often to be sure; and only the
bodies of criminals, such as have no friends, relatives, &c." (108–09).
Dead bodies, Alcott suggests, can also be put to other productive uses,
such as the making of "a very excellent manure." After the Napoleonic

Wars, the bones of "thousands of men . . . left dead" on the battlefields of Europe, were "ground up by means of steam-engines and other powerful machinery, and used as manure. . . . [I]n 1832, a million . . . bushels of bones of men and horses, were brought . . . to England, and used by the farmers of Yorkshire, Nottinghamshire, and the neighboring counties" (111).

MISSIONARY ANATOMY:
MARKING THE BODY AS "HUMAN"

The House I Live In, "that little juvenile anatomy," was explicitly designed to help children acquire an anatomical conception of self. Alcott and other reformers regarded childhood as the period in which the people were most malleable and educable. But, as the titles of his other works suggest—*The Young Man's Guide* (1834); *The Young Wife* (1837); *The Young Mother* (1836); *The Young Husband* (1840); *The Young Woman's Book of Health* (1850); *The Physiology of Marriage* (1855)—Alcott also catered to an adult audience and wrote about physiological laws that governed gender relations, sexual reproduction, bodily functions, and erotic pleasure (though not very explicitly). A millenialist and a believer in human perfectibility, Alcott's popular writings drew vitality, and even urgency, from the desire of a large segment of the population to acquire an identity that conflated Christianity, "civilization," and, crucially, "humanity": "The time has come when anatomy, physiology and hygiene must be taught, or man must cease to be *man*."[39] In *The House I Live In* and other works, anatomical boundaries mark the individual as a civilized human and function as signposts of a Christian disciplinary regime: the "LAWS which obtain in the habitation of an immortal spirit."[40]

This "science of human life" articulates a kind of universalism. A dedicated abolitionist on moral grounds, Alcott argued that science confirms the unity of the human race.[41] Skin color, anatomists had proven, is only a superficial difference:

> [S]pread over the true skin . . . on a thin gauze-like membrane, and under the outside membrane . . . is a soft pulpy or jelly-like substance, containing the color. In the African, this pulpy substance is black; in the native American or Indian, it is red . . . ; in the Asiatic, it is yellow, and in the European, white. . . . Some [people] suppose that the whole mass of our bodies is darker or lighter, according to the indication of our faces; others suppose the color is in the blood. . . . But we see none of these are right[;] . . . the skin . . . is alike in the whole human race, . . . it would form leather of the same color in all; and . . . the color might be removed, though not without much pain, leaving one individual as white and as dark as another.[42]

Alcott's anatomy also minimized gender difference, but in a different way. *The House I Live In* abstains from any discussion or illustration of sexual dimorphism, makes no mention of the typical difference in facial hair, hips, breasts, height, or musculature. The masculine is universalized: "man" is used interchangeably with "human" and "the race." The text does include a discussion of "the evils of tight lacing," but this only reinforces the universalist premises of Alcott's anatomy: corsetry exerts a harmful effect on "human chests," "the human frame," "our health" by imposing sexual difference on the body. The illustration of the deforming effects of tight lacing is the book's only reference to sexual dimorphism.[43]

The rest of the engravings represent an idealized "human" anatomy: there is nothing to show gender, race, age, pathology, or any specific identifying sign. Vesalius and other early modern anatomists often posed their cadavers in the graveyard, dissecting room, or other scenes, and showed the faces of their subjects. These older anatomical illustrations can be read for signs of the cadaver's social identity—generally the subject is a prostitute, criminal, or indigent—and also for moral instruction: "all is vanity," "the wages of sin are death" (and anatomical presentation), and so on. In contrast, *The House I Live In* erases the body's particularity. There are no poses, no faces, no backgrounds. The bodies and body parts are abstracted from any real or imagined context, with two exceptions that refer back to the older iconographic tradition: a skeleton standing in the doorway of a house (the frontispiece, which illustrates the title of the book); and a praying skeleton (copied from an eighteenth-century text), which begins the section on anatomy.[44]

This universalism has expansive, colonizing aims. The identification of

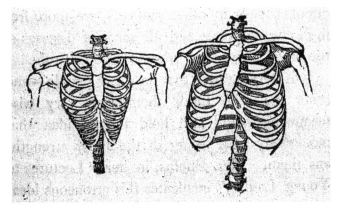

Figure 6.8. The pathological effects of tightlacing. *The House I Live In* . . . (2d ed. enl., Boston 1837), 238. Courtesy of the Library of the College of Physicians of Philadelphia.

the self as human and anatomical is a crucial step in a civilizing process that brings every aspect of life under a medico-moral regime. The anatomical human will carefully regulate food intake; abstain from tobacco, alcohol, coffee, and tea; bathe regularly and in cold water; go to sleep early and on a regular schedule; avoid "immoderate" sweating; engage in sex only in marriage and then not more than once a month; avoid inhaling fetid air and drafts; wear loose-fitting and modest clothes; etc. Submission to such medical discipline offers the prospect of moral equality for those who enter into it—and the prospect of a larger social transformation. In subsequent works, Alcott adopts a prophetic voice: "[I]f . . . we obey all the laws of life from first to last . . . , what . . . is to hinder an organ, naturally imperfect, from becoming, in process of time, comparatively perfect? . . . [I]f the individual, in view of the perpetual renovation of his system, can do much for its improvement, in his own life time, how much can be done in a series of generations for the improvement and elevation of the human race?"[45] The sum total of individual "improvement and elevation" will result in the gradual redemption of original sin, the abolition of morally disfiguring hereditary/congenital disease—the incremental perfection of humanity. Anatomy ushers in the millennium.

The underlying assumption, derived from Combean phrenology, is that Christian morality and laws of health are mutually supportive, or identical. Given the status of "physiological law," morality takes on a higher epistemological status, is made over into a scientific fact or principle. Like Newtonian laws of physics, physiological law is no longer open to debate or interpretation. But unlike the "law of gravity," which leaves no room for the play of free will and requires no moral decision about whether it will be obeyed, physiological law operates in a juridical fashion. It can be violated, but such violations incur certain punishment: disease and death. Compliance can be assured only if people become conscious of their anatomical makeup, learn the laws that govern the specific regions of their bodies, and are persuaded to refrain from activities that endanger their physiological and moral health.

Thus, and here is the heretical aspect of Alcott's teaching, Christianity is not sufficient: "teachers of christianity, science and morals" must ponder "whether men at the present—even civilized men—can ever be made what they should be, without a knowledge of anatomy and physiology."[46] Moral redemption requires that people have scientific knowledge of the body: "It is the office of physiology, in the light and under the sanction of christianity, to redeem man's physical frame from the curse under which sin, in all ages, has brought it."[47] As John M. Keagy, one of Alcott's close allies, put it: "Three fourths of the vice that entails wretchedness on the human family, is . . . physiological vice. . . . I know of scores of pious persons, who, for the want of physiological knowledge, cannot be the perfect men and women they desire to be."[48] Keagy, a Philadelphia physician and a one-time "burning and shining light" in the Methodist Church, contended that such knowledge was indispensable even if a "high degree of moral excellence associated with the practice of religious principles" is also present.[49] Ezra Stiles Ely, a prominent Presbyterian philanthropist and theologian, preached that "no education should be deemed *biblical*, in which the student have not been introduced to an acquaintance with the general principles of jurisprudence, anatomy and physiology." Alcott approved and went further: "We . . . insist that the Bible cannot be thoroughly understood otherwise."[50] In marked contrast to Waterman Sweet, who praised the Indians for having a natural, intuitive understanding of the body, and Samuel Thomson, who believed that an apprehension of the divinity of the body was accessible to Christian believers without anatomical study, Alcott and friends argued that the anatomical body was an indispensable commentary on and adjunct to biblical texts.

If so, then the extension of Christianity depends on the teaching of anatomy. Here, Alcott cited the precedent of the "Indian Apostle" John Eliot who, in the seventeenth century, was said to have instructed the natives of New England in anatomy in an effort to free them "from a blind and superstitious obedience to their powaws or sorcerors."[51] Anatomical instruction had an intrinsically "civilizing" effect, crucial in dispelling a barbaric attachment to animistic belief. Beliefs in a body, and a world, full of magic and spirits could not survive the adoption of an anatomical persona.[52]

The connection between medicine and Christianity was therefore more than just a fulfillment of the requirements of Christian medical charity, it had to become a part of missionary practice. Thus, an 1838 issue of *Graham's Journal* lauded Dr. G. R. Judd, a medical missionary, for producing an anatomy manual in the Hawaiian language for his seminary students.[53] A few years later, in 1843, Mrs. Stella Kneeland Bennett, a Baptist missionary, translated *The House I Live In* into Burmese. It remained in print in successive Burmese editions until at least 1884.[54]

This was not merely a perfunctory gesture. The lady missionaries in Burma took great pains to ensure that anatomy and physiology were taught thoroughly and scientifically. They purchased animal organs at the local market, to be exhibited and dissected in classroom demonstrations, and undertook a laborious second translation of Calvin Cutter's *Anatomy, Physiology and Hygiene* in the Karen language, after rejecting the first version as inadequate. They even commissioned an agent to procure additional illustrations, so that the human body could be represented more precisely.[55] Only a course in anatomy, including dissection, could persuasively demonstrate that spirits did not reside within, and show the moral and scientific logic that governed the "untenanted" body.

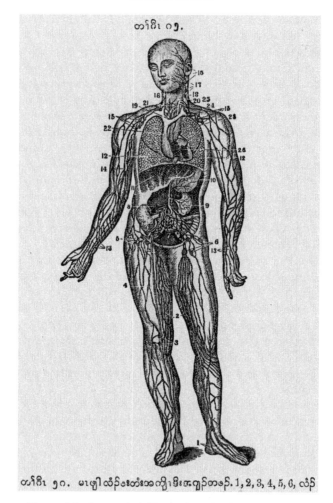

Figure 6.9. Anatomical illustration. Calvin Cutter, *Anatomy, Physiology and Hygiene (in Sgau Karen)*, trans. and adapt. Mrs. J. G. Binney (Rangoon, 1872). Courtesy of the American Antiquarian Society.

Such missionary efforts were compelling to antebellum New Englanders because they referred back to their own recent histories. In his autobiography, Alcott describes the "rude and uncultivated" Connecticut village of his childhood as a place where "the majority . . . knew something of the dream-book and of palmistry, and of the influence of the moon," a place full of magical beliefs, where troubles were betokened by the howling of a dog, the blossoming of a flower out of due season, or the beginning of journey or a job of work on Tuesday or Friday. Many . . . knew how to tell fortunes in connection with a cup of tea. . . . [M]ore . . . could tell under what planet a person was born, and perchance, could predict thereby the future events of his life.[56]

In this cultural context, the study of anatomy and physiology expedited the passage of a segment of the population from the unrefined uneducated yeomanry into a "more rational and elevated" bourgeois order. This new identity required the adoption of a body governed by natural and moral law rather than unaccountable and arbitrary forces. In the work of medical missionaries then, the experience of contemporary New Englanders, who had only recently acquired their own anatomico-physiological conception of self, was dramatized and incorporated into a sentimental narrative of evangelical and social progress.

But, if anatomy was as potent as Alcott and other physiological evangelicals made out, there was a lurking danger. When violations of moral laws were automatically punishable by disease, what need was there for the Bible and its interpreters, for the church? Physiological morality raised anatomical texts over scripture, earthly medical authority over God, and body over soul as the privileged object of divine agency. No wonder then that Keagy was purged from organized Methodism. In the 1850s and later decades, the natural theological element in popular anatomy became increasingly attenuated, eventually reduced to an obligatory trope. Popular anatomists, while never daring to endorse atheism, became more secular—and began paying more attention to sexual topics.

Anatomy's New Destiny: The Popular Audience

After the appearance of *The House I Live In*, popular anatomy gathered momentum, especially in New England, New York, Philadelphia, and other northeastern cities and towns. Inspired by the example of the Boston Phrenological Society, in 1836 Alcott helped to found the Boston Physiological Society, which in turn became a model for similar organizations.[57] The BPS held monthly meetings and sponsored public lectures on anatomy and physiology. In 1836–1837, Alcott, Jerome Van Crowninshield Smith, a professor of anatomy and pioneer medical journalist, and Sylvester Graham, the popular "physiological" advisor, all made appearances there. Graham was particularly active in the 1830s, giving popular lectures in many northern cities.[58] An advocate of the strict monitoring and reform of bodily functions (eating, drinking, and sex), Graham developed his "physiology," a system of rules of diet and hygiene, after encountering the works of Xavier Bichat and François Broussais during a sojourn as the agent of a temperance society in Philadelphia.[59] His books and lectures initially contained little in the way of anatomy, but as time wore on the anatomical element expanded. By 1838 and 1839, *Graham's Journal* was regularly printing anatomical lectures and engravings, and reporting on efforts to spread the anatomical gospel.

In the late 1830s and even more in the 1840s, a cadre of anatomical lecturers and writers sprang up to meet the growing demand for anatomical instruction.[60] Some were obscure, like Paul W. Allen of Springfield, Massachusetts, who advertised lectures to "Ladies and Gentlemen" on "Popular Anatomy & Physiology . . . and its application to the Laws of Health," illustrated by "anatomical paintings" in an 1843 issue of the *Botanico-Medical Investigator* (a Thomsonian newspaper). Others were well known. The *Botanico-Medical Investigator* printed and endorsed Horace Mann's celebrated report advocating the teaching of "physical education," a term that encompassed instruction in anatomy and physiology, as well as physical exercise.[61]

As early as 1837, Alcott noted happily that courses in anatomy and physiology were increasingly taught in private academies, at both the secondary and collegiate levels.[62] Educational reformers harped on the importance of such teaching. "Why should Physiology be introduced into Common Schools?" asked T. S. Lambert, a popular anatomical lecturer and author. His answer was that "the moral and physical health of the community would be benefited beyond computation":

> [T]he increased profits of every farmer would more than pay all the educational expenses of his family. . . . [O]ur young ladies would be more beautiful, graceful, and healthful than now, and at less expense; our boys would be more easily governed, our young men more expert as laborers, tradesmen, or scholars; the middle-aged and advanced in life would be still better and more efficient members of society; our homes would be more happy.

"[A] correct view of physiological principles," Lambert rhapsodized, will not only lead to the "increased docility" of young students, but also build up in them "a laudable enthusiasm in all their pursuits; . . . their delight will be to please their instructor, their parents, and their mates." As "children . . . learn the character of [anatomical] objects in a scientific manner" and learn "to give complete, thorough, and direct descriptions" of body parts, they would develop mental discipline and a rationale for productive behavior. A knowledge of anatomy and physiology would profoundly alter students, families, and communities.[63]

The push to incorporate anatomy into the public school curriculum was wildly successful. In New York State, where only two common schools taught anatomy in 1840, fifty taught it by 1850, and 258 by 1885.[64] The movement to require such studies—by the mid-1880s nearly every state

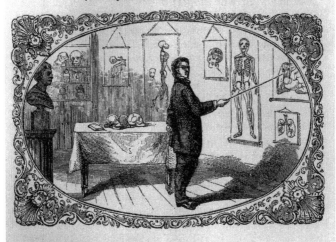

PART I.

FIRST DIVISION OF HUMAN PHYSIOLOGY AND HEALTH.*

(This subject is continued in the Fifth Reader.)

LESSON I.

THE FRAME-WORK OF THE HUMAN BODY.

1. ALL persons know how important it is that the frame-work of a house, such as the walls, the posts, the beams, the braces, and the rafters, should be made of strong materials, and be well put together. If there should be any thing wrong

Figure 6.10. Schoolbook lesson on "physiology" (actually anatomy). Marcius Willson, *The Fourth Reader* . . . (New York, 1861), 15. Courtesy of the American Antiquarian Society. Like many mid-century textbooks, Willson borrowed liberally from Alcott's *The House I Live In.*

outside the South had such a requirement—may perhaps be regarded as an instance of professional empire building, or as a bourgeois program to institute social control over the working and middle classes. But the reprinting of Mann's manifesto in irregular and ephemeral publications like the *Botanico-Medical Investigator* suggests that in this instance supply arose to meet demand. A growing number of people looked to anatomy as a resource in the making of some version of the bourgeois self and wanted anatomically trained physicians and teachers to advise and oversee that self. They avidly sought anatomical instruction for themselves and their children.

Physicians, high, low, and middling, were glad to cater to this enthusiasm, in a variety of forums and genres. In the first four decades of the nineteenth century, books on medicine for the general public circulated widely, usually with the words "domestic medicine" or "family physician" in the title. These manuals for home treatment of common illnesses usually omitted anatomy or included, a meager paragraph or two, and never had anatomical illustrations. But in the mid-1840s the genre was revised to include anatomy. Calvin Cutter's *The Physiological Family Physician* discussed "common diseases . . . in connexion with anatomy and physiology," using over 100 engravings, "making the work one of popular anatomy." Cutter, a Massachusetts physician, also produced well-illustrated textbooks in "anatomy, physiology, and hygiene" for elementary and secondary school classes. These were fabulously successful, going into multiple stereotyped and revised editions, and were translated into Tamil, Arabic, Japanese, Russian, and other languages.[65] By 1850, anatomical lecturers plied the lecture circuit and a small industry was devoted to the production and distribution of popular books with anatomical illustrations and explanations.

The medical establishment for the most part endorsed these developments, but not unreservedly. An editorial in the *Boston Medical and Surgical Journal* complained that "a mad system of itinerating with a manakin [*sic*] has been much in vogue":

> People love to have their marvellousness excited by looking on while muscle after muscle is detached, dry as a ribbon—and a promiscuous assembly of men, women, and children, imagine that the exhibiter who picks the artificial model of humanity to pieces so easily, must be a prodigiously learned professor of exceedingly profound sciences. This racing over the country from village to village, and exhibiting the mysteries of animal organization with a manakin, is falsely called popular anatomy. The truth is, it is a superficial show of superficial things, and far too often by very superficial persons in pursuit of pence.[66]

Clearly some elite physicians feared that popular anatomy debased the coinage of medical knowledge, but the medical brahminate also participated in efforts to instruct the laity. Zabdiel Boylston Adams, the son of a well-born Boston physician, remembered Sunday school in the late 1830s as the site of boyhood anatomy lessons. His teacher, Dr. Samuel Parkman,

> used to gather together the boys . . . at his home in West St., and pass the Sunday morning hour in instructing us in anatomy. I remember his beautiful french models and cast of the eye and ear, and dissections, human and of the lower animals, to illustrate the lessons. . . . I can still recall with pleasure the

hours when I listened . . . to his explanation of the wonders of God as shown in the mechanism of sight and hearing.[67]

John Collins Warren, Parkman's colleague at Harvard, delivered an anatomy lecture to a crowd of "50 ladies and gentlemen" at a party in 1839; he also invited a group of "ladies" to view the school's anatomical museum.[68] A few years later he delivered a lecture to the Massachusetts legislature on the anatomico-physiological effects of alcohol, exhibiting "magnified views" of "the drunkard's stomach."[69]

Women formed a sizeable constituency for anatomical and physiological instruction: they made up almost one-quarter of the American Physiological Society.[70] Contemporary doctrines of domestic individualism assigned women a crucial moral role in the formation of the bourgeois self, as mothers and wives, as teachers, cooks, clothiers, and home decorators. For middle- and upper-class women searching for modern means of improving self and society, anatomy had an undeniable appeal. It also served as a wedge through which they could expand their scope of action. Long debarred from the dissecting room, women moved to become consumers and transmitters of anatomical knowledge in their own right. In the late 1830s, Mary Gove, a protegé of Graham, began lecturing to hundreds of women, "among the most intelligent of the city," reportedly causing a "sensation." Gove went on to a career as an anatomico-physiological speaker, writer and reformer.[71] Other women followed—Harriot K. Hunt, Pauline S. Wright, Lydia Fowler, Jane Thompson—and the late 1830s and 1840s saw the formation of organizations like the Boston Ladies Physiological Society, where audiences of middle-class women could hear anatomical lectures.[72]

No longer coded masculine, anatomical discourse was even dispensed in Catharine Beecher's enormously popular manual for women, *A Treatise on Domestic Economy* (1841). Beecher, the daughter of a prominent Congregationalist preacher and sister of Harriet Beecher Stowe, included a chapter "on the care of health" with engravings of skeletons, vertebrae, arm muscles, spine and central nervous system, the brain and nerves, spinal curvature, heart, lungs, etc., "sanctioned by the highest authorities" (presumably earthly and male). Beecher refrained from including illustrations of the female breasts and the organs below the waist, but within those limits claimed anatomical knowledge for women. The illustrations (mainly copied from J. V. C. Smith's *Class Book of Anatomy*, George Hayward's *Outlines of Human Physiology*, and *The House I Live In*) were linked to technical discussions of erect posture, hygiene, and the prevention of deformity and disease. Anatomical knowledge had become necessary to the rationalization of the household.[73]

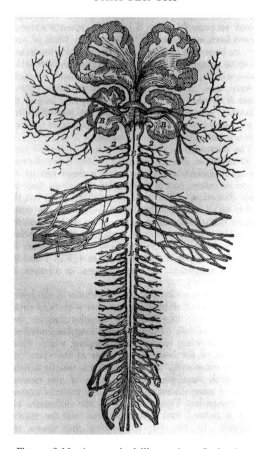

Figure 6.11. Anatomical illustration. Catharine
Beecher, *A Treatise on Domestic Economy* (2d ed.,
Boston, 1843), 79. Courtesy of the American
Antiquarian Society. The plate is copied from
J. V. C. Smith, *The Class Book of Anatomy* . . . (2d
ed., Boston, 1836). Popular anatomical illustrations were often aestheticized representations
of the body's interior, suggesting the interior
order and symmetry of the body. The brain cut
open here looks something like a flower or
ornamental lettuce.

   In the domestic ideology of the period, the home was woman's domain, the place where children were nurtured and "the future of the
race" determined. Accommodation with male authority, medical and otherwise, was fairly easy where transmission of anatomical knowledge was
from woman to child, from woman to woman, within the home—and

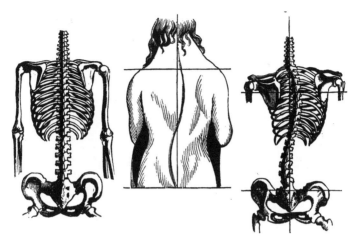

Figure 6.12. Anatomical illustration. Catherine Beecher, *A Treatise on Domestic Economy* (2d ed., Boston, 1843), 81. Popular anatomical texts often contained discussions of proper posture. Courtesy of the American Antiquarian Society.

where the taboo on discussion of sex and sexual anatomy was respected. Beecher's *Treatise on Domestic Economy* and Jane Taylor's physiological primers (which borrowed liberally from Alcott) were never a threat in this respect. They were writings intended for use in the home and school and omitted any discussion of sexual anatomy.[74] Mary Gove initially did likewise, but later (as Mary Gove Nichols) she crossed the line and presented adult readers with discussions of sexual anatomy and physiology, attacked the institution of marriage, and even presumed to address an audience that included men.[75] Elizabeth Blackwell, though never as radical, dared to challenge the male monopoly on knowledge of the body by becoming a physician herself—and by dissecting. She was followed by a cohort of middle-class women. The popular anatomy movement of the 1830s, 1840s, and 1850s was the indispensable prerequisite to the emergence of the first cadre of formally trained women doctors.[76]

"Adapted to Popular Comprehension": The Anatomical Careers of John Wieting and Frederick Hollick

From the early 1830s to the 1870s, anatomy expanded its audience: demographically, to men, women, and children; socially, to the upper and middle classes, and upwardly aspiring skilled workers and farmers; and geographically, from its base in Boston, New York, and Philadelphia to

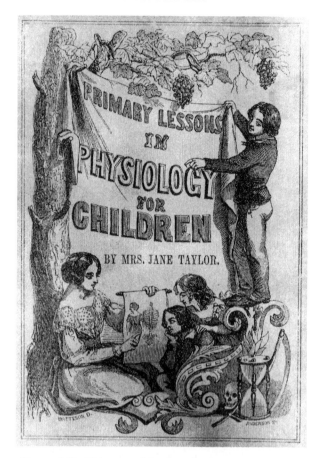

Figure 6.13. Title page. Mrs. Jane Taylor, *Primary Lessons
in Physiology for Children* (New York, 1858). Courtesy of
the American Antiquarian Society.

the rural hinterlands, the Midwest and, to a lesser degree, the South. By
the end of the 1840s, the market had grown large enough to support, and
in several cases make wealthy, an enterprising new generation of anatomical lecturers.[77] For contemporaries, the two most significant figures were
John M. Wieting and Frederick C. Hollick.

Born in Springfield, Otsego County, in upstate New York, in 1817, John
M. Wieting fit the contemporary definition of a "self-made man." At age
fourteen, when his father's business failed, he was forced to take a job
teaching elementary school. At age eighteen he assisted in the survey of
the New York and Erie Railroad. At age twenty, he moved to Syracuse,
New York, and for the next six years worked as an engineer on the con-

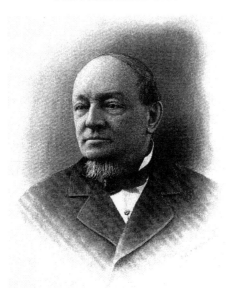

Figure 6.14. John M. Wieting (1817–87).
M. E. Wieting, *Prominent Incidents in the Life
of John M. Wieting* . . . (New York, 1889),
frontispiece. Courtesy of the Library of the
College of Physicians of Philadelphia.

struction of the Syracuse and Utica Railroad, and as a street grader. In his
mid-twenties, he became interested in "the natural laws governing the
world and man" and apprenticed himself to a local doctor. In late 1842 or
early 1843, he attended a course of popular lectures on "Physiology," delivered by Austin Flint, an ambitious young medical professor from New
York City. Seizing the main chance, Wieting made Flint an offer for his
"lecturing apparatus," his anatomical charts, and a papier-maché anatomical "manikin." Flint accepted, and Wieting, who had to borrow money to
finance the purchase, embarked on a career as a lecturer.[78]

He began by touring small towns and villages in upstate New York.
Over the next twenty years he perfected and polished his performance,
"increasing his apparatus by judicious purchases, until he possessed the
largest and most complete apparatus for lecturing on these subjects ever
owned in this country." His tours were extensive and frequent, including
over a hundred lectures in Boston. According to a biography written by
his wife, he was "brilliant, entertaining, and instructive," the first man to
render "physiology and the laws of life and health . . . attractive and
agreeable to the masses." At 12½ cents a lecture, with the first lecture
free, the admission price was affordable to almost anyone. An 1850 newspaper described the enthusiasm that surrounded his appearance:

Dr. Wieting has created a perfect furore of excitement in Boston upon one of the most scientific of all scientific subjects—anatomy. His lectures at the Tremont Temple are attended by upwards of two thousand ladies and gentlemen every night. Not a single seat in that vast hall . . . is unoccupied; . . . the aisles are filled with people seated on benches or stools, or standing. . . . We have been there several nights three quarters of hour before the commencement of the lecture, and found upwards of a thousand persons already in the front seats. Such an immense rush was never caused in Boston by any lecturer on a scientific subject.

A Wieting lecture was a "brilliantly illuminated" anatomical spectacle. His elaborately printed handbill boasted of

SIX SPLENDID FRENCH MANIKINS, LIFE-SIZE.
TWELVE BEAUTIFUL FRENCH SKELETONS,
VARYING IN SIZE FROM AN INCH AND HALF TO SIX FEET IN HEIGHT:

The Manikin, which seems only to want the breath of life to make it a thinking, walking, human being, is the greatest, most wonderful and curious piece of mechanism of the age in which we live; was made by that distinguished anatomist, Dr. Auzoux, of Paris; is the result of nearly thirty years of labor, and the admiration of the literary and scientific men of this country and Europe; is constructed so that it can be taken apart in such a way as to exhibit not only the Form, Size, Location, and attachments, but the actual color and appearance of every essential organ in the constitution; exhibiting
OVER 1,700 PARTS OF THE HUMAN BODY, ETC., ETC.
THE MANIKINS AND SKELETONS WILL STAND ERECT. . . .
THE PROPER STUDY OF MANKIND IS MAN. . . .

The lecture circuit was arduous, but lucrative. In 1862, at age forty-five, Wieting retired from the field, having acquired enough capital to become one of the leading men of Syracuse, the builder of its first opera house and theater. Upon his death in 1887, an obituary rated him the top money earner of all the public lecturers of his day, ahead of Mark Twain and Henry Ward Beecher. His fame notwithstanding, we know surprisingly little about Wieting's lectures, his tour itineraries, and his audiences. Unlike other anatomical lecturers, whose earnings partly derived from the sale of medicines, mail-order medical consultations, and books and pamphlets, no published work of his survives.

We can compensate for this gap in the historical record by turning to Wieting's contemporary, Frederick C. Hollick (b. 1818, fl. 1843–1870). In his late teens and early twenties Hollick was an Owenite social missionary and phrenological lecturer. He came to the United States from England around 1842, having somehow acquired the title of "Dr." Within a couple of years, he was doing a good business as an electro-therapeutic practitioner and popular lecturer.

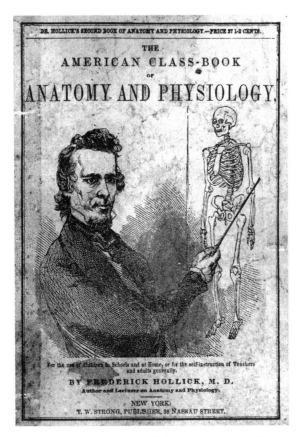

Figure 6.15. Frederick C. Hollick lecturing. F. C. Hollick, *The American Class-Book of Anatomy and Physiology* (New York, 1853), cover illustration. Courtesy of the American Antiquarian Society.

He also pulled in a good income through the sale of mail-order remedies, aphrodisiacs, and books and pamphlets on medical topics.[79] Hollick was quick to seize the production and marketing opportunities presented by new print technologies, the extension of the U.S. Mail and lowering of postal rates, and the decreasing distribution costs resulting from the extension of canals and railroad and steam lines.[80] His profusely and sometimes colorfully illustrated books sold extremely well. *The Origin of Life* went through ten stereotyped editions its first year (1845–1846), *The Diseases of Woman* fifty-three editions between 1847 and 1855, *The Matron's Manual of Midwifery* 100 editions between 1840 and 1853, and *The Marriage Guide* over 500 editions between 1850 and 1877. We don't know how large each edition was—at least 2,000 books, probably closer to 5,000, with stereotype editions running closer to 10,000—but clearly a mass readership appreciated Hollick's work. In the late 1840s he boasted of sales "so great that it has scarcely been possible to print [books] fast enough, particularly the *Outlines of Anatomy*."[81]

Outlines of Anatomy and Physiology for Popular Use featured a striking "dissected plate of the human organization," with successively overlaid pages of colored lithographs, cut to shape, that "opened up" so that readers could perform a "dissection" just by removing the flaps. *Outlines* was designed as a pedagogical aid "like our Primary School *Geographies*, simple

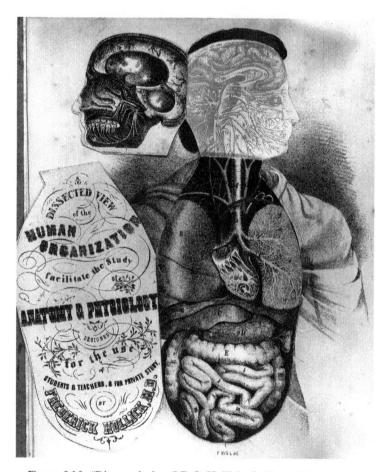

Figure 6.16. "Dissected plate." F. C. Hollick, *Outlines of Anatomy and Physiology* (Philadelphia, 1847). Courtesy of the American Antiquarian Society.

yet complete": "everything [is] represented . . . so that the young pupil may be taught by the *eye*, as in studying Geography by a *map*" (x–xi). Hollick urged teachers, parents, and children to make "museums of anatomical objects" and provided detailed instructions for making a cast of the air passages of a sheep's lungs (98–99).

Like Wieting, Hollick also appeared on stage alongside anatomical manikins, skeletons, and charts. Between 1844 and 1852, Hollick gave "courses of lectures" for runs of up to four weeks on "The Origins of Life," "Physiology," "The Physical Man," etc., to separate audiences of men and women in New York City (his home base), Hartford, Philadelphia, Baltimore, Washington (with John Quincy Adams and other congressmen in attendance), Richmond, Boston, Worcester, Pittsburgh, Cincinnati, Louisville, St. Louis, New Orleans, and on a riverboat between the latter two cities. His venues were generally large auditoriums (he also appeared at Barnum's). Crowds in many places were in the thousands.[82] A newspaper account of Hollick's lectures in Boston in the early months of 1848 at Washingtonian Hall and Tremont Temple (where Wieting was acclaimed) gives an indication of his reception. The halls overflowed with people: "over three hundred [women] were . . . sent away. . . . It is impossible to convey any idea of the enthusiasm the doctor has excited among both ladies and gentlemen. They remain around him in crowds, for hours after his lecture is over, asking for further information, and closely examining the models."[83]

Scholars have been tempted to reduce Hollick's appeal solely to his treatment of human sexuality, reflexively assigning him to the tawdry netherworld of popular sexology.[84] This may have been his ultimate trajectory, but in the 1840s and 1850s, he had respectable supporters. Audience members were undoubtedly attracted by his bold choice of topics—which served to put an edge on the proceedings—but what they marveled at was a full discussion and exhibition of the anatomical body in toto, not just the sexual parts. In any event, the distinction between anatomy and sexology was nebulous: the body was metaphorically linked to desire. Even without venturing below the waist, the dissection of the body—even an "artificial dissection" performed on a papier maché dummy—had a sexual meaning, was regarded as a public undressing of sorts.

Hollick's popularity depended on such associations, but in a complicated way. Anticipating the regular practice of twentieth-century advertising, he cultivated and played upon the tension between his audience's longing for, and anxiety about, erotic pleasure. Audience members were simultaneously titillated and disturbed by the prospect of hearing a public discussion of sexuality, but also reassured by the prospect of the body demystified, which, Hollick promised, would attenuate troubling desire (repression was identified as the cause of sexual obsessiveness): "the culti-

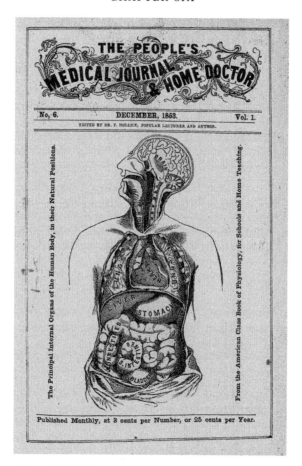

Figure 6.17. The geography of the body. *The People's Medical Journal and Home Doctor* 1.6 (1853): cover; same illustration used on the cover of F. C. Hollick, *Outlines of Anatomy and Physiology* (Philadelphia, 1847). Courtesy of the Library of the College of Physicians of Philadelphia.

vation of the mind directly decreases the animal feeling, besides providing the only agent which can properly control it."[85] Newspaper accounts lauded Hollick for approaching "his subject with . . . delicacy and reverence"; "doubts of the propriety" of his lectures "being attended by the ladies . . . were entirely dispelled."[86] In her second "Letter from New York," Lydia Maria Child rejoiced:

> it has long been a cherished wish with me that a general knowledge of the structure of our bodies, and the laws which govern it, should extend from the scientific few into the common education of the people. I know of nothing so

well calculated to diminish vice and vulgarity as universal and rational information on these subjects. . . . [T]he impure state of society has so perverted nature, and blinded common sense, that intelligent women, though eagerly studying the structure of the Earth, the attraction of the Planets, and the reproduction of Plants, seem ashamed to know anything of the structure of the human Body, and of those Physiological facts most intimately connected with their deepest and purest emotions, and the holiest experience of their lives.

Anatomical discourse provided a vocabulary in which bourgeois women could speak of their embodiedness, including the sexual body, in a refined, dignified manner, without resorting to overly delicate euphemisms, elaborately indirect allusions, or vulgarity. Child praised Hollick's lectures as "plain, familiar conversations, uttered and listened to with great modesty of language, and propriety of demeanor":

The Manikin . . . by which he illustrates his subject, is a most wonderful machine. . . . It is made of *papier maché*, and represents the human Body with admirable perfection in the shape, coloring, and arrangement, even of the minutest fibres. By the removal of wires, it can be dissected completely, so as to show the locality and functions of the various Organs, the interior of the Heart, Lungs, &c. Until I examined this curious piece of mechanism, I had very faint and imperfect ideas of the miraculous machinery of the house we live in. I found it highly suggestive.[87]

From Child's perspective, Hollick's lectures on "the house we live in" supported Alcott's medico-moral vision: physiological study providentially inspires piety, physiological law enforces morality; there can be no contradiction between physiology and Christianity. But Hollick added a twist: sexual desire is a natural property of the human species and must be allowed its correct expression, otherwise the body will sicken. If the scientific "principles of virtue and morality . . . are ever in agreement with true Religion," then the expression of sexuality is God given and moral, properly the subject for respectful public discussion and disinterested scientific administration.[88] In Alcott's *House* sexual anatomy is accessible only to the priesthood of medical knowledge. It functions as a hidden source of self. But Hollick argued that true freedom and morality can flourish only when such information is in the hands of every individual: repression breeds corrupted desire, openness delibidinizes. Anatomy, with its greco-latinate place names and cartographic conventions, constructs the body as public space, provides a "respectable" vocabulary in which to conduct a public discussion of what was customarily a "disreputable" topic. In contrast, the "vulgar" or "coarse" vocabulary of the body, especially the sexual body (cock, cunt, etc.), which anatomical discourse has negative reference to, was used by the unrefined or, if among bourgeois men, in carefully bounded homosocial settings.

If men claimed the right to speak in a sexual vocabulary denied bourgeois women, they also claimed the right to control their wives' and
daughters' sexuality. But physiological law could trump male (and also
clerical) privilege, which partly accounts for the enthusiasm of Hollick's
female audience. It was "preposterous and tyrannically unjust," Hollick
argued, that men

> sufficiently liberal to contend for their own right to know such things, . . .
> nevertheless deny the same right to women. . . . It is assuming . . . either that
> females are incapable of understanding, or unworthy of possessing such
> knowledge. . . . The present ignorance of women respecting their own struc-
> ture, and the influence of external agents upon it, produces among them a
> most lamentable amount of disease and suffering, which nothing but enlight-
> ening them can prevent. They are even more interested in such knowledge
> than men.[89]

With his eye on the market, Hollick undoubtedly knew that to go further would invite repression; he was already pushing his luck. His sexual
radicalism, therefore, was strictly limited; there was no antinomian fol-
lowthrough. He was not an advocate of free love. But critics, and a handful of more adventurous radicals, were quick to draw out the implications
of the opening made by Hollick (and other sexologists). They argued
that the self-regulating atomic individualist position covertly invited liber-
tinism or, positively, a greater scope of sexual action that was linked to
emancipatory individualism.

However, as the recurrent emphasis on the terrors of venereal disease
makes plain, in Hollick's anatomy the body was not really emancipated
for the pleasure principle. Instead, physiological regulations organized
and rationalized that which was previously thought to exceed or repel
discourse: sex. In opening sexuality and the sexual body to public scrutiny, Hollick freed it from clerical and paternal strictures. But in their
place, he instated a more thoroughgoing regulatory regime, self-adminis-
tered in one respect, but governed overall by a physiological law that
punished transgression with nightmarish venereal diseases: impotence,
sterility, syphilitic lesions, skin rashes, gonorrheic discharges, genital
warts, miscarriage, stillbirth, deformity in offspring, etc. Some of Hollick's
books featured brightly colored illustrations of faces disfigured by syphilitic caries, penises afflicted with chancres, and even an engraving showing
a surgical circumcision necessitated by a violation of physiological law.[90]
Hollick incited and catered to the public's horrified fascination with venereal disease, a fascination that, as will be discussed in chapter 9, was invested with a complicated eroticism of its own.

In focusing on the entrepreneurial logic of Hollick's relationship to his
audience, we should not obscure his work's designedly political and social

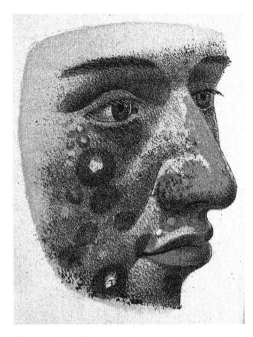

Figure 6.18. "Various forms of venereal skin diseases, secondary and tertiary." F. C. Hollick, *Popular Treatise on Venereal Diseases* (New York, 1853). Courtesy of the Library of the College of Physicians of Philadelphia.

implications. In the early 1850s, Hollick publicly supported the revolutions of 1848 and labeled himself a "medical red republican," a supporter of "Young Physic" (an echo of Mazzini's revolutionary anticlerical Young Italy movement). If the body is metaphorically associated with sexuality, it is also associated with "the people" who make up the "body politic." In 1853–1854, Hollick edited *The People's Medical Journal*, a threepenny monthly which usually featured an anatomical illustration on its cover: "Progress, Reform, Popular Instruction and NO MYSTERY!" was its motto.[91] Knowledge of the body, Hollick preached, is powerful. The people may use such information to escape the bonds of religious or state discipline: the license to discuss sex publicly is also the license to overthrow religious and political authority. Hollick's sympathies lay with the Chartists and the white American working class (in the early 1840s he aligned himself with working-class apologists for slavery).[92] He sought to expand the audience for anatomy to include "the common folk," "the mass of the people", and to expand the visual representation of the anatomical body to include the anatomy and physiology of sexual reproduction. His object, like Alcott, was to induct the nonanatomical "million" into the anatomical/bourgeois order—but, unlike Alcott, Hollick hoped to transform that order, to make it freer and more democratic, at least for white people.

Here again, this radical move had its limits. In the American context, "Young Physic" could be assimilated to anti-Catholicism and bourgeois reform. To Lydia Maria Child, an ultraist abolitionist but no social or sexual revolutionary, Hollick was expanding the domain of respectability and emancipatory rationality, not overthrowing them. Arrested in Philadelphia in March 1846 on charges of publishing a book that "corrupt[ed] the public morals" and "exhibit[ing] indecent models and pictures at his lectures," he was able to win acquittal and was awarded "a very elegant gold medal" "by the ladies who attended his lectures on Physiological Science . . . as an expression of their approbation of the knowledge therein conveyed."[93] Such women publicly denied that sexual arousal was intended, or facilitated, by Hollick's lectures. Their own "reputations" depended on it (although their public petition on his behalf also put them at risk).

In other circles, Hollick was not accepted: the trustees of the Ladies' Physiological Institute of Boston, when presented with some of his works, refused to allow them to circulate.[94] Hollick, of course, took pains to disavow any erotic effect—he did not "gratify vulgar curiosity, or minister to

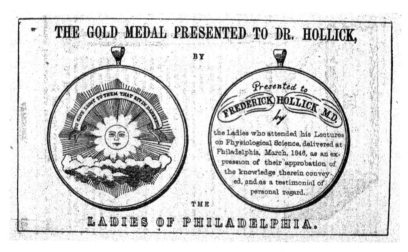

Figure 6.19. "The gold medal presented to Dr. Hollick, by the ladies of Philadelphia." F. C. Hollick, *The Male Generative Organs in Health and Disease, from Infancy to Old Age: Being a Complete Practical Treatise on the Anatomy and Physiology of the Male System . . .* (1849; New York and Boston, 1853). Courtesy of the Library of the College of Physicians of Philadelphia

a depraved taste." Rather, he insistently linked the formation of the ("human") bourgeois self to the rationalization and regulation of ("brute") sexuality:

> There are few young persons [who do not] . . . experience the sexual feeling, it arises in them from the natural laws of their development, and no mystery, or seclusion can prevent it. It is useless . . . to attempt to conceal the *main fact*. . . . We have therefore merely a choice, between giving correct information, and leaving the mind to be filled with error and vain surmise, for with one or the other it will most assuredly be occupied.

The argument was based on two parallel binary oppositions: human/animal and reason/desire.

> We are often told that the difference between man and the lower animals consists in this; that both feel the same instincts and propensities, but, in the brute they alone impel to action, while man has his reason to control or counteract them. . . . [I]t follows . . . that, whenever man acts from his propensities alone he becomes a mere brute. Now what is the fact with regard to the association of the sexes at the present time? . . . does reason have anything to do with it? Very seldom; and from the simple fact that all attempts to reason about it are condemned! Every individual is told that it is immoral to seek for, and give, any information on the subject, and that he must not even *think* about it! The consequence is, that blind passion rules alone, . . . and man becomes a mere brute, both in thought and action. Now my object is . . . to give correct information, in a simple and unobjectionable form, and so employ the reason; thus, bringing it into opposition to the mere animal propensity, which it is intended to control and regulate.[95]

Thus, even though Hollick took a risky, transgressive cultural position—an avowed willingness to openly discuss sexual topics—his logic reinforced the hegemonic bourgeois position on sexuality: the need to rationalize the body and discipline desire, an ideology shared by William A. Alcott, and, later, Anthony Comstock, leader of the New York Society for the Suppression of Vice. But logic and performance can vary widely. From the mixed responses that Hollick received, it is evident that many possibilities inhered in the anatomical body, conservative and radical, disciplinary and erotic, often within the same text: "the animal propensity" stubbornly resisted regulation and control. Public discussion of sexual desire, ostensibly a part of the medical technology of self-regulation, provided an opening through which the pleasure principle could be smuggled in, a fact that popular anatomists were well aware of, and manipulated to their benefit. The articulation of a theory of sexuality titillated audiences even as it instructed them to defer or rationalize the consummation of desire, intercourse between bodies. In this way regulation and desire fed off each other, defined each other, incited each other, as the late Michel Foucault trenchantly observed.[96] And this in turn gave rise to disputes about the regulation of the marketplace and the boundaries of professional disciplines: Who, if any one, should have the opportunity to market and buy sexual commodities (including medical advice)? Who, if any one, should have the opportunity to profit?

Hollick was a master of playing on the tension between his audience's desire to articulate sexual desire openly and their fear of doing so. On the one hand, he boldly announced that it was not only proper but necessary to speak of such topics, and condemned his critics as hypocrites who mendaciously disavowed their own sexuality. On the other hand, public speaking was justified only by the need to combat venereal disease—a category that lumped sterility, impotence, incontinence, horniness, obsession, and nervousness with syphilis, gonorrhea, warts, and sores—and that was attributed to behavioral causes: masturbation, extramarital sex, promiscuity, improper thoughts. Hollick alternated between arousing and allaying the sexual anxieties of his public, a state of suspension that his audience found compelling and even pleasurable.

Conclusion: Taking "Liberties" with "The Ghastly Looking Object"

This then brings us back to the relation between audience and anatomical performance. Hollick claimed that he did not lecture to satisfy "vulgar curiosity" or "depraved taste." Yet some of his listeners, perhaps many, must have come to gawk, be entertained, titillated, or even disgusted. In the early 1850s, Marianne Finch, an aristocratic young English tourist, reported on her visit to Boston, then the epicenter of popular anatomy. In the morning, Finch went to see an exhibition of "some anatomical figures" at Madame Sarti's:

> By paying a dollar, and joining a class, you can make four visits of an hour each. . . . Madame S— is a young and beautiful Englishwoman, whose husband dying soon after landing in America, she was left unprovided for, except by continuing his occupation of dissecting and explaining these figures. Fortunately she had acquired a sufficient knowledge of anatomy for this purpose, and is very successful.

Finch was not especially interested in the moral benefits of anatomical education, but a beautiful female dissector was a curiosity worth seeking out. Later that day, she paid a visit to the Ladies' Physiological Institute, where "about sixty ladies were present":

> Standing on the platform, beside the lecturer, was a "female manikin." It represented the human figure, *minus* the skin, arms, and ribs; thus affording

a good view of its internal structure, on which the professor was expatiating. While speaking, he frequently put his hand on the shoulder—sometimes his arm round the neck—of this ghastly-looking object. By degrees I became accustomed to it; but at first it was really startling to see him take such liberties with a lady of her appearance.[97]

Finch playfully mocked the anatomical body, "a ghastly looking object," while easily making the association between anatomy and sexuality—"it was really startling to see him take such liberties with a lady of her appearance"—an association vehemently disavowed by Hollick and every other lecturer. At the same time, she marveled at the earnest interest displayed by the female members of the Institute.

Upon his 1860 visit to the dissecting room of the College of Physicians and Surgeons, Samuel Edgerly, with whom we started this chapter, reported feeling a similar blend of curiosity, titillation, and revulsion—but also saw vivid illustrations of the lessons pressed upon him by popular and pedagogical anatomy:

> Bouncing up the stairs . . . we neared the "ROOM," . . . the Doctor asked us if we smelt the stench . . . ? Before I could answer . . . , the "Dr" flung open the door—and oh! ye gods! what a smell! "Hold us someone!" We gathered our scattered senses—disappated [*sic*] by the effluvia—and marched in—what a sight! The room was . . . about 50 ft long, and 11 ft wide and filled with tables . . . on which were placed human remains for dissecting purposes. The first thing that caught our eye in the "Charnel house," was a "*stove*" in close proximity to a table, on which reposed the different parts of a body, which however, were too decayed for recognition, and we thought immediately that the stove was heated; and then the idea of *heat!* in such a smelling room!, was too much for human endurance.

The diary entry stresses the dissecting room's impact on Edgerly's body, the overwhelming impact of the smell, heat, and sight of the disaggregated and decomposing anatomical specimens. This was what popular lectures only gestured at. They presented a safely deodorized, cleaned-up version of the human body, a representational ghost, suitable for the parlor. The manikins and charts of the popular lecture were reminders of corporeality, but only that. Compared to the dissecting room, the anatomical lecture's impact on the bodies of its audience was only a tingle, a mild arousal and/or revulsion. In the rhetoric of popular discourse, such bodily effects were said to be negligible compared to the moral benefits of anatomical study: the inculcation of piety via natural theology, the mental discipline of learning the body's place names and boundaries, the moral discipline of gaining the understanding of the need to submit to the physiological laws that govern the parts of the body. In fact, the disjunction between the corporeal body and anatomical discourse was considerable, but with some effort the two could be made to refer to each other. Anatomical representation could be made to function as an "auto-icon," an internalized representation of self.

If so, the auto-icon had an intrinsic doubleness that oscillated in parallel with the poles of self and other, text and body. Recovering his senses, Edgerly goes on to draw a series of moral lessons that could have been lifted from Alcott or Hollick. Race and the universal human subject: "The next 'Stiff' was that of a Negro of about 35 years of age, and on his limbs I saw the fact demonstrated of their having a white skin under their black one." The physiological consequences of promiscuity: "The next was apparently a *fresh* subject, a female about 22 yrs of age—On her person venerial sores were to be seen." The inexorably leveling universality of death: "And so on to the end each table having its own occupant, who but a short time ago, walked perhaps side by side with us on some public thoroughfare, little dreaming of his final residence in that aristocratic quarter of our city, [the medical college on] Fourth Avenue." Anatomy as a means of making order of the human body: "A Student was dissecting the arm and hand of a subject; working out every fibre and sinew,—muscle and nerve,—clear to the finger ends; and picking out all the fatty surrounding parts; left the other distinct and well defined." At the same time, the dominant theme here is the body's disruptive chaotic otherness. This is barely, unconvincingly, smoothed over by the final lesson. Edgerly has been improved: "I left, feeling that I had learned considerably about the human frame by my first visit to a 'Dissecting Room.' "[98]

In discussing popular anatomy, I have sought to balance supply with demand. There was a market for anatomical products and services: physicians, lecturers, writers, publishers, and museum proprietors catered to the market and attempted, with varying degrees of success, to stimulate demand for their products. The market as a whole was connected to the emergence of a reading, consuming public that was embarked on a far-ranging collective search for gestures, styles, ideology, politics, credentials, and activities that could mark a person as bourgeois (mark difference from the nonbourgeois), while universalizing bourgeois values as norms. In other words, popular anatomy was connected to the contemporary Anglo-American obsession with what William Ellery Channing deemed "Self Culture." Samuel Dickson, the eccentric British critic of mainstream anatomical medicine, went so far as to say that, although he regarded anatomy as of little use in the treatment of disease, "[c]ultivated in a proper spirit, I would . . . make it a part of the useful education of the people," to elevate "the people."[99] Anatomy became the favored vocabulary of the new self-making curriculum. With its topography and land-

marks mapped out in fine detail, personhood was defined as the anatomical body.[100]

"The modern notion of the self"—in antebellum America, a bourgeois
self—philosopher Charles W. Taylor explains, is constituted by "a sense of
inwardness":

> We think of our capacities or potentialities as "inner," awaiting the develop-
> ment which will manifest them . . . in the public world. The unconscious is
> for us within. . . . But as strong as this partitioning of the world appears to us,
> as solid as this localization may seem, and anchored in the very nature of the
> human agent, it is in large part a feature of . . . the world of modern, Western
> people. The localization is not a universal one. . . . Rather it is a function of a
> historically limited mode of self-interpretation.[101]

Taylor narrates the history of the articulation of the modern self in high
philosophy and literature. But that self was not solely or even primarily
derived from those rarefied disciplines, but rather, as he concedes, it was
forged out of "disciplinary practices . . . in the military, hospitals, and
schools as well as the related practices of methodical bureaucratic control
and organization," Foucault's domain:

> the whole . . . picture of myself as objectified nature . . . only became avail-
> able through that special kind of reflexive stance I am calling disengagement.
> We had to be trained (or bullied) into making it, not only of course through
> imbibing doctrines, but much more through all the disciplines which have
> been inseparable from our modern way of life, the disciplines of self-control,
> in the economic, moral, and sexual fields.[102]

Yet the modern self was not entirely coerced, it was desired and pursued
by people who, in search of identity and a moral order, created, agitated,
and sustained the new professions, institutions, and fields. And that desire and pursuit can be seen in the history of popular anatomy, a missing
link, an intermediate enterprise in which a kit of metaphors, practices,
and performances of self were retailed to an avid market of consumers,
assembly not included.

7

"The Foul Altar of a Dissecting Table"

ANATOMY, SEX AND SENSATIONALIST
FICTION AT MID-CENTURY

IN AN 1851 homily entitled "A Little Plain Talk for the People," published in the *American Journal of Medical Reform* ("for the people and the profession"), Dr. Frank Stewart identified the set of people who stood in need of instruction in anatomy and physiology. These were a vice-ridden "class of readers," young men "ignorant of the construction of their own bodies . . . , who generally compose the mass of sufferers." Resistant to anatomical writings, such readers were distracted by, even addicted to, an entirely different set of texts:

> [T]housands of yellow-covered emissaries of Satan . . . known as cheap novels, are . . . each month, eagerly bought up by the young; not a steamboat can be approached, or a railway station reached, but that the ever watchful news-boy appears, and tenders . . . the yellow-covered novel for only twenty-five cents or less, the latest emission of some wicked imagination on its way to debase the young men and women of this land. . . .
>
> Enter our rail-road cars—visit our steam-boats—go, if you please, into any of our large hotels—and there . . . can be seen some young man lounging on the sofa, eagerly drinking in this polluting poison until he is lost to all that is going on around him. A habit once formed for this kind of reading, appealing, as it does to the "animal man," the baser appetites, the reader eagerly craves more, until the spare time at home or behind his employer's counter is spent daily, nightly, in this to him, fascinating amusement.[1]

Stewart conjured up a sprawling and densely interconnected urban environment of boarding houses, hotels, playhouses, dime museums, saloons, and depots, where entrepreneurs incessantly hawked an ever-multiplying array of pleasures. This was a new, unpoliced sphere of consumption, a proliferating indoor network of gas-lit spaces, that continually subverted and thwarted efforts to shape and regulate the bourgeois self. For Stewart and his fellow medical reformers, new scientific methods of moral self-formation were required. The *"mass* ignorant" must be instructed in anatomy and physiology. "Animal man" must learn that violation of the "immutable laws" that govern the body has dire consequences: illness, disfig-urement, social debarment, sexual debility.

Stewart assumed that physiologically minded persons would form a class entirely apart from the devotees of yellow-covered novels. We may not be so sure: Samuel Edgerly, a young New York City merchant's clerk, read serialized fiction printed in popular newspapers, enjoyed rowdy min-strel shows and the circus, but also went to church, attended morally instructive lectures, and toured the dissecting room of the College of Phy-sicians and Surgeons.[2] The middling readers of Stewart's *American Journal of Medical Reform* may very well have succumbed, on occasion, to the plea-sures of sensationalist novels, cheap romances, and joke books—even as they sought to define themselves as anatomical and physiological beings who were "temperate," "healthy," "civilized," "cultivated," "educated," "moral," "virtuous," "intelligent," and "hygienic," the buzzwords that col-lectively signified bourgeois identity. And, if some of Stewart's readers rejected the yellow-covered novel, they were more than matched by a large reading public that respected the claims of anatomical medicine, but was bored by popular anatomy's lack of narrative impulse, its conde-scending tone, and its joyless insistence on physiological propriety.

And yet, from the sheer numbers of popular anatomical publications, exhibitions staged in respectable physiological societies and entertain-ment-oriented museums and circuses, and the enthusiastic reception ac-corded lecturers like John M. Wieting and F. C. Hollick, it is evident that the anatomical body was important to a wide swath of the American pub-lic. This importance was not quite the same thing as approval or disap-proval. Medical professionals, reformers, middle-class men and women, the indigent poor, all had different stakes in the new cultural politics of the body. Anatomy was one of many cultural goods circulating in mid-nineteenth-century America. And just as anatomy overflowed the banks of professional medical discourse, it also overflowed the banks of popular medical discourse and entered the realm of fiction, poetry, fine art, car-toons, almanacs, and political rhetoric. In such places, it often received a less than respectful reception, as in this line from a postbellum joke book: "Brown, while looking at a skeleton of the jackass, remarked, that 'we are fearfully and wonderfully made.'"[3] An 1874 cartoon in *Harper's Monthly*, a middle-class periodical that usually supported the progress of medical sci-ence, mocked the pretensions and body-snatching propensities of "Pro-fessor Jingo." And even in places where it was not mocked, anatomy could be used to serve foreign purposes. *The Gypsy Dream Book and Fortune Teller, with Napoleon's Oraculum* (ca. 1850), a slim volume devoted to "true inter-pretations of dreams and the numbers of the lottery to which they apply" and information on "how to get rich, and how to receive oracles," also promised readers instruction in methods of "prognostications and divina-

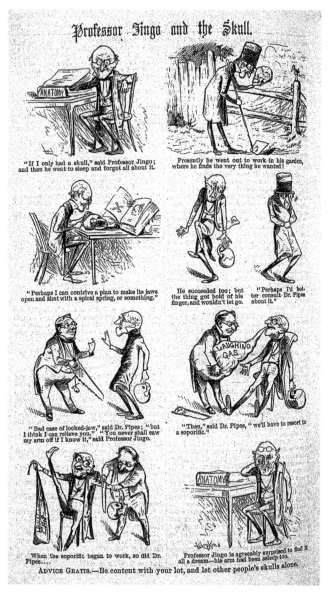

Figure 7.1. "Professor Jingo and the Skull." Anatomy did not always receive a respectful reception in popular middle-class periodicals, even in the epitome of respectability, *Harpers' Monthly*. The dissector dismembered or dissected was a common theme. *Harpers' Monthly Magazine* 49.290 (6–1874): 304. Library of Congress. (Thanks to Elizabeth Blackmar and Judy Hahn for bringing this cartoon to my attention.)

tions" through "physiology," as though that body of knowledge was equivalent to the reading of "cards, dice, dominoes, moles and marks, . . . grounds of tea and coffee cups," and other ways of producing "signs, auguries, charms, and incantations."[4]

Even yellow-backed novels were not innocent of anatomy. As the anatomical body began to become a prerequisite of bourgeois identity, it came into contact with the discourse of flesh, desire, and corruption that was articulated in Christian theology, political rhetoric, and folk narratives, but also in minstrelsy, sensationalist fiction, and melodrama. Anatomical claims to epistemological authority, established through graphic representation, greco-latinate nomenclature, dissection performances, and narratives, made anatomy an appealing product in the marketplace of cultural goods. Willy nilly, anatomy became a resource for other cultural practices—hostile, ambivalent, indifferent, or supportive.

Popular anatomy and the sensationalist novel had roughly parallel trajectories. Both took advantage of technological innovations in print and transportation to produce, distribute, and sell their products cheaply. Both found customers in the mass audience of readers and ticket buyers that clustered in cities and towns in the 1830s, 1840s and 1850s. Given their close proximity, it is not surprising then that anatomical ideas, metaphors, and narratives should crop up in the sensationalist novel. The physician was one of the regular cast of characters who inhabited the pages of sensationalist fiction. Often, he appeared as a dissector, a powerful figure (or someone desiring to be so) who wielded his scalpel on the bodies of the living and the dead, in the graveyard, the hospital, the anatomical theater, the anatomical museum, and on the dissecting table. In the sensationalist novel, as in real life, the anatomist operated at the center of a burgeoning social network that connected well-to-do patients, colleagues, striving medical students, proletarian body snatchers, and cadavers. Every identity, every act, in the anatomical enterprise had a sexual and social valence: social honor and class identity, and sexual honor and gender identity, were intertwined. Anatomy was gendered: dissectors were male; the dissected were discursively female. Anatomy was class based: the medical gentry dissected; the poor were dissected. Antebellum sensationalist novels exploited these metaphorical elements, obsessively fixing on dissection and body snatching, and on the dyad of the anatomist and the dead body, especially the dead female body.

Edgar Allan Poe famously proclaimed that "the death of a beautiful woman is . . . the most poetical topic in the world."[5] The two sensationalist fictions of the 1840s discussed in this chapter—John Hovey Robinson's *Marietta* and George Lippard's *The Quaker City*—follow this dictum and improve on it.[6] Set in the night-time world of the antebellum city, a world of unbridgeable social and gender divisions, they are necrophiliac "narratives of sexual danger."[7] Brutish body snatchers, aristocratic seducers, demonic sorcerors, and medical experimenters prey upon beautiful virgins. Mad doctors hypnotize or drug young women in order to dissect or debauch them.[8] Dark conspiracies abound: innocence is incessantly imperiled by the threat of rape or betrayal; the deflowered virgin suffers an irreparable stain, an ineradicable and contaminating moral pollution.

ANATOMICAL SENSATIONALISM: *MARIETTA*

Virtually unknown today, John Hovey Robinson (1825–1867) was a moderately successful hack novelist who churned out westerns, medieval romances, historical fiction, and mysteries. Before becoming a writer, he briefly attended Harvard Medical College.[9] His first novel, *Marietta, or the Two Students: A Tale of the Dissecting Room and "Body Snatchers,"* is set in a seedy area of Boston in 1842 and betrays some familiarity with the workings of the anatomy room.[10] The hero of the book is Levator—*levator* is an anatomical term for a muscle that raises a body part—a man of action, a man of elevated moral and social status. In the first scene, two body snatchers provide him with the body of a beautiful woman. In a long soliloquy, he agonizes over the cadaver: "How can I disfigure that angelic face—how can I cut, piecemeal, the flesh from those delicate limbs, and observe daily the ravages of the scalpel . . . converting it . . . into all that is loathesome" (3). Levator has fallen in love with his subject.

The entrance of his charismatic anatomy professor, Dr. Frene (whose name, derived from the Greek word for mind, *phrenos*, suggests that he represents pure reason unencumbered by moral restraint) and Eugene, a well-born but dissipated medical student, interrupts these cogitations. Frene asks Levator to commence the dissection. Levator refuses: he cannot, will not. Brandishing a scalpel, Eugene announces that, given his friend's indisposition, *he* will perform the dissection, beginning with the face, to prevent the body from being recognized by the friends of the deceased. Horrified, Levator interposes himself between Eugene and the cadaver. A heated argument ensues. Frene reproaches Levator for his illogic and "sensibility" (i.e., sensitivity, a noble, but feminine trait), and questions his courage and manliness:

> "[Y]ou carry your sensibility too far. What possible harm can it do that body—fair and delicate it is, I allow—to dissect it? Will it feel the keen edge of the knife? Will the tender limbs shrink from it, and give intimations of torture? Do you fear that those closed eyes there, will start open, and that clod-like hand will raise itself, and that still tongue will throw off the spell of death, at the first incision, and entreat you to desist? Fie! where is your manhood?" (6)

Mastery of the dead body—the display of clinical detachment in the dissecting room, the will to dissect—is thus equated with masculine honor. Levator, accepting the premise, rejects the charge:

> "Have you not seen me without anything like fear or hesitation, look upon death in all its awful phases—in the form of wrinkled old age—smiling infancy—and at every point between. . . .? Have I not seen it in every stage of decomposition, and in all its loathsome details? Have you not seen me sever joint from joint, and muscle from muscle a score of times, without the least symtoms [*sic*] of emotion?" (6)

Frene concedes the point, but not the argument: "I have often thought that I never knew a student so indifferent to the 'disagreeables' of a dissecting-room as yourself; but to-night you are a *woman*" (6).

Anatomical narrative here readily lends itself to the purposes of sensationalist fiction and its largely male readership. The nineteenth-century readers of sensationalist fiction expected that the reading of such texts would incite palpable bodily sensations: chills, muscular tension, relaxation, laughter. "Philosophical" fiction, history, and other high genres, in contrast, were understood to be morally and culturally superior because they principally worked on, and "elevated," the reader's mind (or spirit or soul). (Sentimental fiction did both; it moved the reader bodily to sympathetic tears, but tears that are morally redemptive.)[11] Sensationalist fiction is not quite pornography, but has affinities to porn. It works on the body of the reader through representations of bodies—more often than not, female, naked, and/or dead. Thus, much of *Marietta*'s first chapter is conducted over the body of a naked woman. There are repeated references to tender limbs, fair skin, etc., always in conjunction with a feinting movement of the scalpel: Robinson teases the reader. The scene perversely travesties the generic procedures of love poetry, the male poet's inventory of his beloved's parts.[12] Dissection, the act of penetrating the dead body with a sharp knife, is a masculine performance that gives rise to and resolves masculine anxieties: fear of death and the dead body is feminizing. The man who cannot master his fear is "unmanned"; the woman who does not fear death or the decomposing dead body is "desexed," masculinized.

Robinson portrays the dissecting room as a liminal zone where male doctors and students cross the boundary between life and death, between the exterior and interior of the body, and are initiated into an exclusive homosocial order. Among themselves they claim exemption from funerary customs and social strictures. Already marked as privileged gentlemen by their elevated diction, upright posture, and fine clothes, the shared experience of dissection binds the medical students together and marks them as a distinctive fraternity of dissectors—masters of the body through reason and force of will.

Levator's refusal to dissect undermines his place within the fraternity and disrupts the group. But behind his refusal lies a more fundamentally disruptive power, the erotic power of a sexually desirable woman (in this case a dead woman!). Typically, male homosociality defines itself in opposition to the feminine and is part of a continuum that includes or symbolically suggests homosexuality, even as it works to enforce the heterosexist order, and a shared traffic in women (and here also a shared traffic in cadavers). Scornfully dismissed as a "woman" for his refusal to dissect, Levator takes up the conceit: if he's a woman, then Frene, a ladies' man, he jokes, should cater to him in order to seduce him.

But the banter fails to restore homosocial solidarity. "[T]hat body," Levator insists, "shall not be mutilated with a dissecting knife"; Frene and Eugene are forced to sheathe their scalpels and withdraw. Left to himself, Levator resolves that the body must be returned to the tomb, "where it may crumble and mingle peacefully, and in obedience to natural laws with its kindred atoms" (9). The thought consoles him: the dematerializing dispersion into nothingness counters the horrifying prospect that his beloved's body will be rendered hideous by decay. He takes a ring off the finger of the dead woman, and exchanges it with a ring from his own hand, a symbolic betrothal.

He then travels under cover of night to another liminal zone, a filthy, decrepit waterfront tenement apartment, a dismal place that is the antithesis of the bourgeois home (there are "no chairs . . . the deficiency supplied by a rude bench and blocks. . . . You are looking for a table: there is none"). There he finds the two men who originally supplied the beautiful corpse: Gaunt, "a skeleton . . . invested with a scant covering of skin," "a wreck of a human being," and Thick, his muscle-bound, libidinous, bullying partner (10). For $30 (a hefty sum in 1846), Levator purchases another body to dissect and, with a barrage of insults and threats, directs the two scoundrels to return the cadaver to the tomb from which it was plundered.

The scene next shifts to the apartment next door, a bordello where Eugene's mistress, Cecil, lives: "several wretched beds are seen in different parts of the house. . . . One must be very tired and sleepy to rest upon such couches; and let us go farther and say that no one ever did or ever will rest upon such as these" (12). Cecil is a fallen woman, and also the object of Thick's unwelcome advances. Awakened by terrible nightmares, she discovers the body snatchers' "dead room," which is visible through a crack in the wall. There, on a slab, lies the decomposing body of her first seducer, the man who destroyed her sexual honor, now dead of advanced syphilis, a fitting medico-moral punishment for debauchery.

Meanwhile, the body snatchers scheme to sell Levator's beautiful corpse to some other buyer, so as to make triple rather than double money—and rid themselves of the work, and risk, of restoring it to its burial place. Carrying the body in a sack, they encounter Dr. Frene and Eugene; a deal is quickly consummated. Without examining the goods, the professor and student, decide to experiment on the subject with a "Galvanic battery," to study the "power of electricity on the dead body." Such experiments, sporadically conducted in the first four decades of the nineteenth century, served as a kind of medical performance art, a demonstration of the physician-anatomist's ability to manipulate the *élan vital*, even to resurrect the dead. Opening the sack, Eugene and Frene discover that they have purchased Levator's subject. Frene gloats that they will finally have their way. The erotic coding of the scene is unmistakable: "[T]hat corpse—in all its unearthly beauty is about to be offered for the advancement of science. . . . 'Make a very small incision, Eugene, just back of the ear. . . . Now place the conductor in the orifice'" (30). However, with successive jolts, the dead woman revives. She has not really been dead, or has she?

The tale continues on, but the only extant version of the serialized novel stops a few pages later, in the middle of the story. A 1945 article by F. C. Waite provides a synopsis of the full novel and tells the finish: the revived woman is restored to health and returns to her family, with no knowledge of what transpired while she was in her death trance. Later she encounters Levator who shows her the ring on his finger and explains how he came by it. They marry and live happily ever after. Waite, however, does not explain who or what caused the heroine to fall into the death trance and be prematurely buried (or where he found a copy of the novel that includes its second half).[13] In J. V. Huntington's longer and more literary *Rosemary, or Life and Death*, an 1860 novel which uses many of the same plot elements, the woman has been drugged by a mad anatomist.[14]

The body snatchers in *Marietta* represent the lowest depths of society. Socially dead, they are all body: animalistic brutes, insensitive to death's moral consequences, numb to the aesthetics of beauty and the sublimity of death. The medical students represent the upper crust of society; they constitute the social order. But within the liminal zones of the dissecting room, the derelict waterfront district, and the night-time city, their membership in the fraternity of dissectors exempts them from the moral discipline and manners required of their class. In these interstices they consort with outcastes, people who are physically and socially dead. And in such spaces, they are not always genteel. In the dissecting room the female anatomical subject is "rudely gazed upon, by the curious eye" of the dissector. Distressed at the prospect of the "rough touch of the student at work on the limbs of his beloved corpse," Levator resolves that "the coarse jest of the thoughtless and unfeeling shall never be uttered over it, or fall . . . upon these dead ears!" (9). Rationalist discourse undermines any spiritual valuation of the dead body and licenses a homosocial vulgarity.

The division between upper and lower classes corresponds to the binary self: upper-class mind versus lower-class body. (Body, in turn, is divided into two aspects: Thick represents the sexual/animal body; Gaunt represents death, the body minus soul.) But the body/mind dichotomy is disrupted by a third term, "spirit," represented by Levator and Marietta. Spirit (disembodied love) is the highest moral category; the disinterested fusing of masculine and feminine spirit is morally redemptive. Reason (Frene) and aestheticism (Eugene) are associated with the moral depravity of the body. They are coded as masculine qualities that too easily descend into tyrannizing aggrandizement, dissipation, and hubris (aristocratic vices). Their proximity to the body side of the ledger is dangerous; they are tainted with embodied desire.

Marietta also has a feminine symbolic: the woman-is-body topos. Cecil, the fallen beauty, stands for the contaminated sexual body (Eugene fornicates with her; Thick wants to rape her). Marietta, the dead beauty, represents the virginal body, frozen in its purity by death, made over into a representation. The virgin, the unpenetrated object of desire, has a transcendent value, can only be exchanged once, in a special protected ceremony (marriage), or not at all.[15] Cecil, having failed to maintain her virginal status, is implicated, tainted by desire. She is a prostitute and circulates repeatedly as an exchangeable object in the cash economy.

The gender logic, as always, has social significance. Thick's hatred for the upper-class male medical students has a sexual valence: he resents their valuation of him as "matter," which puts him into the subject position of a passive thing, a woman. Against this he asserts a manly contempt of the medical students and attempts to castrate Eugene symbolically through the rape of Cecil.

In *Marietta*, then, the sensationalist novel appropriates the constituent elements of anatomy's cultural poetics: the homosocial cult of dissectors; the contest between anatomist and the living and dead body; the body's power and its resistance to medical claims of sovereignty; dissection as rape or seduction of the cadaver; body snatching as a rape of the grave; dissection as posthumous punishment; the body reduced to the status of commodity, or demoted to inert, undifferentiated matter; the body colonized as a field for scientific investigation; and so on.

GOTHIC ANATOMY: *THE QUAKER CITY*

"It's my opinion that you'd make a bad subject for the
dissectin' table!"

DEVIL-BUG, CHOKING LUKE HARVEY,
The Quaker City (1845), 266

Marietta was a marginal work, an obscure specimen of "yellow-covered novel." But in the case of *The Quaker City, or the Monks of Monk Hall* and its author George Lippard (1822–1854), we have a literary phenomenon. Lippard was the premier antebellum narrativist of sexual danger, a leading exponent of morbid romanticism (along with his friend Edgar Allan Poe). In an 1849 article, *Godey's Ladies Book* dubbed him "the most popular writer of the day," and *The Quaker City* (published in serial form in 1844, as a book in 1845) was the best-selling American novel prior to *Uncle Tom's Cabin.*[16] Lippard, who died at the age of 32, was an aesthete, social critic, and activist (he labeled himself a "red republican").[17] Though not quite an avant-gardist (except politically), Lippard mounted a kind of revolt against bourgeois formalism. His serial novels, in the mysteries-of-the-city genre invented by Eugene Sue, are shapeless, hastily written, travel haphazardly forward and backward in time; protagonists drop out, a new hero is introduced, without rhyme or reason.[18] There are occasional poetic flights ("on the opposite side of the way, a mass of miserable frame houses seemed about to commit suicide and fling themselves madly into the gutter"), but more often hyperbole piled upon hyperbole, cliché upon cliché.[19] The relentless succession of bizarre developments quickly becomes predictable, but in the final instance the grotesque characters, bitter sarcasm, hyperemotionalism, and idiosyncratic politics (a stew of egalitarianism, fraternalism, American nationalism, and Christian sentimentalism), all combine to produce an original, oppositional, and even hallucinatory effect.

The Quaker City approximates a fever delirium. Characters sweat, spasm, ache, tremble, and hallucinate. A middle-aged merchant, for example, is seized by a rippling succession of emotions when confronted with evidence of his young wife's infidelity:

> his countenance . . . was like a mirror, in which different faces are seen, one after another, by sudden transition. At first his face grew crimson, then it was pale as death in an instant. Then his lips dropped apart, and his eyes were covered with a glassy film. Then a deep wrinkle shot upward between his brows, and then, black and ghastly, the circles of discolored flesh were visible beneath each eye. The quivering nostrils—the trembling hands—the heaving chest.[20]

Narrative developments produce effects on the bodies of his characters, providing a model of the effects of sensationalist prose on the reader (and, via the mechanism of reader identification, contributing to them). Genteel critics responded to such excesses by consigning Lippard to "the raw head and bloody bones school" of literature.[21]

Even by the elastic standards of gothic sensationalism, *The Quaker City* is extreme. Much of the novel is set in "Monk Hall," a shadowy mansion with hellish basements and sub-basements, labyrinthine corridors, trapdoors, fake walls, vaults, and concealed tunnels that reach outward to distant parts of the city. Safe from the scrutiny of the outside world, Monk Hall is a private club where the members of the male elite of Philadelphia go to gamble and drink; debauch virgins and seduce married women; play sadistic pranks; torture, humiliate, drug, and murder enemies and inconvenient partners; and laugh off their public professions of religious, political, and social piety:

> Here were the lawyers . . . , doctors . . . , and judges. . . . Here too, ruddy and round faced, sat a demure parson, whose white hands and soft words, had made him the idol of his wealthy congregation. Here was a puffy-faced Editor side by side with a Magazine proprietor; here were sleek-visaged tradesmen, with round faces and gouty hands, whose voices had re-echoed the prayer and the psalm in the aristocratic church, not longer than a Sunday ago; here were solemn-faced merchants, whose names were wont to figure largely in the records of "Bible Societies", "Tract Societies" and "Send Flannel-to-the-South-Sea-Islanders Societies." . . . Moderately drunk, or deeply drunk, or vilely drunk, all . . . kept up a running fire of oaths, disjointed remarks, . . . and snatches of bacchanalian songs, slightly improved by a peculiar chorus of hiccups. (48)

Together these "monks of Monk Hall" conspire to corrupt true Christianity and the democratic republic. In other novels Lippard connects such commercial and professional club men to a malign fraternal order that stretches back to the days of Christ (who they crucified), through the Spanish Inquisition (which they instigated and administered) and the American Revolution (which they sought to undermine and pervert), right up to the present.

Lippard has a social analysis. The Monks represent a bourgeois elite that grasps for power, that aims to set itself up as a new aristocracy. This elite victimizes the honest tradesman, the journeyman, the needlewoman. At every opportunity, the conspirators assault political, religious, and mercantile virtue—but, most insidiously, they claim a seigneurial privilege, the license to seduce and deflower "poor and innocent" young women. Such attacks on the sexual honor of virgins are not merely in addition to their felonies, but rather the most visible and depraved sign of the "colossal vices and the terrible deformities, presented in the social system of this Large City in the Nineteenth Century," the epitome of social injustice, "worse than the murder of the body, for it is the assassination of the soul" (1).

The concierge of Monk Hall, Devil-Bug, one of the most memorable characters in American fiction, is a murderer, blackmailer, thief, hangman. Sporting a working-class Irish/German/Scottish accent, he takes ghoulish delight in robbing graves:

> "The *doctor* sent for me last night; the one what wants me to steal dead bodies for him. I must go airly in the mornin'; he pays me well; and I likes the business. . . . To creep over the well o' some grave yard in the dead o' the

night, and with a spade in yer hand, to turn up the airth of a new made grave! To mash the coffin lid into small pieces with a blow o' the spade, and to drag the stiff corpse out from its restin' place, with the shroud so white and clean, spotted by the damp clay! To kiver the corpse with an old overcoat or a coffee bag, and bear it off to the doctor . . . ! Hoo, hoo! . . . sich a jolly business!" (311)

Devil-Bug is simultaneously the figure of death and a perversely transgressive "animal" vitality. His brutish callousness is morally equivalent to the scientific disinterestedness of the anatomist (who hypocritically disavows any social or moral connection to his body snatchers): "There was a great deal of the philosopher in Devil-Bug. Never a doctor of all the schools, with his dissecting knife in hand and the corpse of a subject before him, could have manifested more nerve and coolness than the savage of Monk-Hall" (311).

The Quaker City features a succession of attempted and consummated murders, mutilations, seductions, premature burials, despoiled graves, grave robberies, and dissections. Skeletons, skulls, dead bodies, and coffins prop up scenes and soliliquies—morbid romanticism runs full throttle. There are several death visions, including a premonition of an apocalypse in the America of 1950:

> phantoms of his murdered victims rose before him; the man with the broken jaw and the lolling tongue, the woman with the blood falling drop by drop from the hollow skull. . . . Then the dream became confused and wandering. Devil-Bug was surrounded by a hazy atmosphere, with coffins floating slowly past, and the stars shining through the eyes of skulls, and the sun pouring his livid light straight downward into a wilderness of new-made graves, which extended yawning and dismal over the surface of a boundless plain. (312–13)

The Gothic had always taken its requisite imagery from memento mori and the danse macabre, but never so excessively. In *The Quaker City*, these generic images are supplemented with anatomical imagery, which serves as an additional provocation (not that the reader needs any), and as a social critique. An encounter between Byrnewood Arlington, the hero of most of the book, and Lorrimer, who methodically designs to debauch Arlington's sister Mary, produces this exchange:

> [Arlington:] "Do you see this flame? Sooner than agree to leave these walls, without—my—my—without Mary, pure and stainless, mark ye, I would hold this good right hand in the blaze of this lamp, until flesh fell blackened and festering from the very bone. Are you answered?"
> [Lorrimer:] "Excuse me, sir—I was not speaking of any *anatomical experiments;* however interesting such little efforts in the surgical line, may be to you. . . . "
> (86; Lippard's emphasis)

This is a dialogue between moral sentiment and amoral objective detachment. Detachment suppresses all affect, mobilizes the body for the sole obsessive purpose of a genital satisfaction that destroys its object: virginity and the virgin, the goal of the sport of male conquest. Moral sentiment circulates throughout the body, can even burn the flesh off a hand. The two stances cannot coexist in the same person. Byrnewood is inundated by a tidal wave of emotion. His detachment has been shattered by the news that Lorrimer has deceived and is about to debauch his sister Mary. Lorrimer replies with undentable cool, tells Byrnewood that the invocation of self-mutilation, Byrnewood's strongest figure of speech, amounts to a trifling "anatomical experiment."

In a later scene, Mary's distraught parents beg Lorrimer to marry her, to "Save her from public shame." But, for the high-born Lorrimer, such a request only provides an easy opportunity to inflict another humiliation. He replies "with withering politeness," that is, without bodily affect: "Why the fact is my friends, I'm not a marrying man. . . . This affair is quite unpleasant and—your family and mine, are quite different in their style. You are not of our 'set'" (468). The command of intellect over emotion, and accomplished sexual predation, are emblems of masculine aristocratic social practice. Female peers and superiors receive protection; everyone else is fair game, even those only a notch lower on the social scale.

Lippard links this predatory sexuality to science. Without the constraint of emotional ties and moral sentiment, the operation of mind is economical and precise, but monstrous, annihilating. Reason is a genital force of will, directed toward the penetration, the hostile takeover, of female or feminized bodies. Knowledge reduces its objects to the status of playthings, and invariably destroys them in play. Dissection (via the scalpel), mesmerism or seduction (via the gaze), and rape (via the phallus) are its representative and morally equivalent operations. Recurrent allusions to dissection reinforce the point:

> Lorrimer looked at him . . . and then, taking a small pen-knife from his pocket, began to pare his nails. . . . He wore the careless and easy look of a gentleman, who having just dined, is wondering where in the deuce he shall spend the afternoon.
>
> "I say, Byrnie my boy —" he cried suddenly, with his eyes fixed on the operations of the knife—"Devilish odd, ain't it? That little affair of yours, with *Annie?* Wonder if she has any *brother?* Keen cut that —"
>
> . . . Byrnewood shivered at the name of Annie, as though an ague-fit had passed suddenly over him. The "cut" was rather keen, and somewhat deep. This careless kind of intellectual surgery, sometimes makes ghastly wounds in the soul, which it so pleasantly dissects. (86–87)

Byrnewood's emotional outpourings undo the homosocial bond between him and Lorrimer, a bond constructed around their shared interest in

sexual conquest. Byrnewood had been a debaucher himself, and frater-
nally cheered Lorrimer on in his debauchery, until learning that the
woman to be seduced was his sister. Then emotion, a feminine trait that
disorders the commanding masculine ego, overtakes it. As in *Marietta*,
emotion demasculinizes, but here it is infantilizing rather than feminizing. Lorrimer condescendingly begins to address Byrnewood as "Byrnie
my boy," a speech act that castrates him.

Lorrimer, for his part, mockingly celebrates deception, seduction, rape,
defloration, as a disciplinary practice: "Woman—the means of securing
her affection, of compassing her ruin, of enjoying her beauty, has been
my book, my study, my science, nay my *profession*" (88). Science and professionalism, unencumbered by moral sentiment, are linked to male desire. Lorrimer has made a science of debauchery, takes his virgins in the
same way that the anatomist cuts up his subject. A page later, the anatomical metaphor recurs: "the consciousness that he [Byrnewood] was in the
power of this libertine . . . came stealing round his heart, like the prob-
ings of a surgeon's knife" (89). Byrnewood, too, has become Lorrimer's
anatomical subject; the loss of sexual honor destroys not only the virgin
but also her family members.

Lorrimer's science has its most profound effect on its chosen object,
Mary Arlington. It operates via an appropriating, penetrating "read" or
"gaze": "[Lorrimer] knew every leaf of woman's many-leaved heart, and
knew how to apply the revealings, which the fair book opened to his gaze.
His gaze, in some cases, in itself was fascination . . . " (77). According to
Foucault, anatomical dissection is the key performance of an epistemological revolution, a transformation of the relationship between medicine
and its object (the body). The characteristic methodology of the new
medicine is a disciplined, systematic form of looking, a surveying, penetrating "clinical gaze" that is trained to regard the living and dead body as
the same class of objects. This purposeful but avowedly disinterested view
taxonomizes the field, constitutes objects of discourse, and, like dissection, penetrates the opaque material object, makes it transparent, legible.[22]
In the nineteenth century, the performance of the gaze becomes a characteristic feature of masculinist bourgeois subjectivity and, as it diffuses to
a wider public, comes to be identified with modernity—and science.

Lippard plays on the disjunction between the discourse of the new
medical epistemology and its performance. In *The Quaker City*, the gaze is
not disinterested, but murderously possessive, erotically charged, a contradiction that implicitly discredits medical authority on the very grounds
on which it is constituted. At the same time, Lippard's critique performs
an important job for the author: the narrative of the subjugating gaze—
and its subjugated object—arouses and pleasures the reader. To both its
exponents and its critics, the gaze, the emblematic procedure of rationalist science, is a sexual procedure.

Lippard expounds at length on the phenomenology of the erotic gaze. Prior to her capture by Lorrimer's gaze, Mary's "soul" is "stainless." Her love for Lorrimer is disembodied, pure, immaterial:

> [W]as there aught of *earth* in this love? Did the fever of sensual passion throb in the pulse of her virgin blood? Did she love Lorimer [*sic*] because his eye was bright, his form magnificent, his countenance full of healthy manliness? No, no, no! . . . She loved Lorimer for a something which he did not possess, which vile worldlings of his class never will possess. For the magic with which her fancy had enshrouded his face and form, she loved him, for the wierd [*sic*] fascination which *her own soul* had flung around his very existence, for a dream in which he was the idol, for a waking trance . . . , for imagination, for fancy, for any thing but *sense*, she loved him. . . . (72–73)

She is innocent of "sense," meaning embodied sensation and sexual desire, but the coolly deceptive Lorrimer plays like a surgeon on the flesh of his female victims. "[L]ooking her steadily in the eye, with a deep gaze, which every instant grew more vivid and burning" (109), Lorrimer seizes Mary, scopically enters her. His technical command of the gaze enables him to embody the disembodied virgin, to raise her "animal nature," the carnal body of "pulsing" and "feverish throbbings," to warm her heart with "convulsive beatings"—the code words that stand for the rhythm of genital excitation.

These are unrepresentable in her consciousness (and only barely representable in the text). In *The Quaker City*, the female capacity for sexual sensation, for sexual pleasure, is a dangerous potential:

> She knew not that . . . the blood in her veins only waited an opportunity to betray her, that in the very atmosphere of the holiest love of woman, crouched a sleeping fiend, who at the first whisperings of her Wronger, would arise with hot breath and blood shot eyes to wreak eternal ruin on her, woman's-honor."
>
> For this is the doctrine we deem it right to hold in regard to woman. . . . Unlike man her animal nature is a *passive* thing, that must be roused ere it will develope [*sic*] itself in action. Let the intellectual nature of woman, be the only object of man's influence, and woman will love him most holily. But let him play with her animal nature as you would toy with the machinery of a watch, let him rouse the treacherous blood, let him fan the pulse into quick, feverish throbbings, let him warm the heart with convulsive beatings, and the woman becomes, like himself, but a mere animal. *Sense* rises like a vapor, and utter darkens *Soul.* (73)

The disinterested heart or spirit protects the female body from bodily desires. Female desire lies dormant as long as the pure "intellectual nature" is kept ignorant of the knowledge of its underflowing "animal na-

ture." With knowledge comes desire and the fall. At the moment of seduction and defloration, the polluted innocent either dies or becomes a
prostitute or virago, socially dead beings who take vampiric pleasure in
passing the taint on to undefiled virgins:

> How many of the graves in an hundred churchyards, graves of the fair and
> beautiful, had been dug by the gouty hands of the vile old hag, who sate
> chuckling in her quiet arm-chair? How many of the betrayed maidens, found
> rotting on the rivers waves, dangling from the garret rafter, starving in the
> streets, or resting, vile and loathsome, in the Green-house ["the house for the
> unknown dead"]; how many of these will, at the last day when the accounts of
> this lovely earth will be closed forever, rise up and curse the old hag with
> their ruin, with their shame, with their unwept death? (66)

The liquidation of virginity results in both orgasm and death, the ultimate extinction of the feminine body. Seduction transforms the "fair and
beautiful" into "hag" and corpse.

THE CABINET OF DR. McTOURNIQUET

The Quaker City narrates social and gender relations within a literary vocabulary that draws on the characteristic moves of anatomical performance and discourse: the unearthing and exhibition of dead bodies, dissection, clinical detachment and the gaze, science, professionalism. It also
takes issue with anatomy itself. In the 1840s, Philadelphia was famously
the capital of American medicine, the nation's premier center for the
study of anatomy. Lippard detested the city's large medical establishment
and mocked the anatomical basis of medical authority through a series of
vignettes featuring a character named Dr. McTourniquet, a buffoonish
medical professor. In one scene, the doctor gives Livingstone, the cuck-
olded merchant, a tour of his anatomical museum. McTourniquet prattles
on about his prize specimens, all of them pathological curiosities:

> "A little of every thing from all parts of the world. In that jar a negro child
> with two heads. Preserved in spirits. Capital specimen of a double-headed
> negro. Ought to have been at [Surgeon's] Hall this morning; cut off a poor
> fellow's arm. Took it quite lively. . . . Singular specimen of an arm that. In
> that long jar. Took it off the body of a man who was hung for robbing the
> mail. Hand had seven fingers." (177)

Livingstone, who intends to murder his unfaithful wife, leads McTourniquet into a discussion of deadly and untraceable poisons. The thick-
headed surgeon informs him of a poison that makes the "victim lay as
though he (or she) had but fallen asleep" (179). He has a treatise in his
collection on the subject and shows it off, "surrounded by shelves piled

with surgical curiosities, preserved in jars, or hanging by parti-colored strings, or, yet again, huddled carelessly together . . . ":

> Dead men in fragments, in great pieces and little, in all shapes and every form, were scattered around. In the full light of the window, fashioned in the ceiling of the room, stood a grisly skeleton, one hand placed on his thigh-bone, while the other, with the fingers stuck in the cavity of the nose, seemed performing the stale jest, common with the boys along the street. "You can't come it Mister, by no manner of means!" that gesture said, as plainly as a skeleton's gesture can say. (179–80)

Just as the street kids delight in offending bourgeois propriety, the dead anatomical exhibits taunt the living, mock Livingstone's cuckoldry and McTourniquet's banalities. Compared to Lorrimer and Devil-Bug, Mc-Tourniquet is a lightweight, obtuse but not terribly evil.

In a later chapter, "The Dissecting Room," McTourniquet blithely invites Byrnewood to "witness a dissection of the human subject": "It's quite a treat to the uninitiated" (370). Byrnewood accepts—he is obsessed with the image of his sister's dead body "laid on the foul altar of a dissecting table" (368)—and they enter "Dissecting Hall." The "treat" turns out to be a spectacle of decomposing bodies and body parts, attended by a jeering chorus of students. The passage, one of the most extraordinary in nineteenth-century fiction, is worth quoting at length:

> Around the room . . . were placed some twenty oblong tables. . . . Bending over each table was a young man, whose long hair and characteristic look of frankness and recklessness combined, betrayed the Medical Student of the Quaker City. At some of the tables were groups of two and three, talking earnestly together, knife in hand all the while, and the whole body of students wore the same dark apron reaching to the shoulders, and each arm was defended by a false sleeve of coarse muslin. And on each table, sweltering and festering in the sunlight, lay the remains of woman and child and a man. . . .
>
> Here a ghastly head, placed upright, with the livid lips parted in a hideous grin, received the gay light of the sun, full on its glassy eyeballs, there a mass of flesh and sinews and bones, shone in the beams of the morning, as corruption only can shine. A Soul once shone from those eyes, a voice once spoke from those lips!
>
> Here lay an arm, whose soft and beautiful outlines, were terminated by a small and graceful hand, and over the alabaster arm and the snowy hand, the blue taint of decay spread like a foul curse, turning loveliness in loathing. There in the full glare of the sunlight was spread a reeking trunk, lopped short below the waist, with loathsomeness and beauty combined in one horrible embrace. The head had been severed and below the purple neck two white globes, the bosom of what had once been woman, were perceptible in

the light. And the Rainbow of corruption crept like a foul serpent around that bosom. For Corruption has its Rainbow; and blue and red and purple and grey and pink and orange were mingled together on that trunk in one repulsive mass of decay. And on this fair bosom hands of affection had been pressed, or sweet young children had nestled; or maybe the white skin had crimsoned to a lover's kiss!

The multiple references to a corrupting or ghastly light should be read against the conventional tropes of "enlightenment" illuminism: spirit, light, reason, and progress are a grotesquely contaminated riot of carnage and carnality, materiality run rampant.

"I say Bob, this must have been a jolly old chap!" cried a young gentleman whose snub nose harmonized with his wide mouth and cross eyes. "No doubt these lips have opened with several thousand jolly grins in their time—now look at them! Pah! How blue and livid."

And he tossed the head of the old man down upon the table, twining his fingers in the white hairs, while his knife severed the flesh from the brow.

"Sweet girl, this was once upon a time! Many a poor devil has been dying for love of her eyes and lips. Just now she dont look altogether loveable. The eyes staring from their sockets and the lips falling to pieces! And then the bosom, ha, ha! The Scalpel makes love to it now!" And the sunbeams glistened upon the blade of the knife as it plyed briskly over the livid flesh.

"Wonder how many people have shaken hands with this old fellow?" muttered another student, with dark eyes and stiff lank black hair. "Just look at this hand—old and withered and hardened by toil. How these cramped fingers have clutched at the dollars and the pennies—ha, ha!" . . .

"He, he, he!" laughed a young Student in tow-colored hair and a pear nose. "Jist look at that—good, capital!"

He had placed the mangled body of a dead man, against the wall in a sitting posture, with the knees drawn up to the chin, and the right hand fixed between one knee and the face, with the fingers outspread and the thumb pressed upon the nose, in a gesture very much the vogue among dirty little boys, rowdies, and cabmen.

"Is'nt that the touch?" laughed the tow-haired Student. "Does'nt he say 'Cant come it!' plain as chalk? And then that eye half shut—is'nt the wink perfect!"

"Ha, ha! Ho! Ho! Good—capital!" chorused some dozen students, as grotesque mockery streamed the yellow sunshine coloring the leaden eyeballs and the hanging lips with hues of vivid gold. (370–72)

The students are the pupils of the mysterious Signor Ravoni, an anatomist-sorcerer-alienist-theologian-messiah, who becomes the central figure of the last section of the book. McTourniquet detests him:

"[T]his Italian or Frenchman or Turk or Jew, no sooner puts his foot on the soil of the Quaker City, than he astonishes the Faculty; strikes Science dumb; plucks Theology by the beard, and in fact walks over everybody's notions on everything—"

"How does he do all this?"

"That's the mystery. He walked into our Medical Halls unbidden, and proved himself a great Anatomist, a splendid Surgeon. No one has had the bravery or impudence to question him concerning his former life, because there's a cold impenetrable gleam in his eye, that few men would like to brave. . . .

"An unknown Pretender appears in the Quaker city, and lo! Everybody hastens to entrust him with their own lives, and the lives of those they love. You ask how? He gives out that he will cure the Insane, and before a day is past he has an hundred patients under his care."

"Does he cure them?"

"Ha, ha! The ugly ones he cures, and returns to their relatives with all possible despatch. But the women, and the *handsome* women, ho, ho! 'It will require *time*,' is his invariable answer. And then he has established a Lecture Room, where he gives lectures on Anatomy. Egad! Our students are crazy with the fellow. . . . " (369)

Ravoni stands as a reproach to professional medicine, to scientific reason itself. Other anatomists just map the body, flatten it out. Ravoni extracts its essence, plumbs its depths. Against the superficial neoclassicism of au courant anatomical medicine, he practices a superior, dark, ancient science. His gaze is of the highest intensity, "alive with the rays of magnetic power" (375). Women are irresistibly drawn and held in its field. It even subjugates Devil-Bug, up to this point the novel's incarnation of evil. The hitherto indomitable monster becomes the wizard's cringing lackey. Ravoni's powers are so great that he can even arrest death: he himself is hundreds of years old.

In another extraordinary scene, the medical establishment of Philadelphia, five hundred students and professors, assemble at an anatomical theater, to see Ravoni demonstrate "some important discoveries in Anatomy. . . . some new Theory of the origin of life," illustrated "by the dissection of a subject" (369). The body snatchers (one of them Devil-Bug) produce a body, stolen from the almshouse graveyard.[23] Ravoni unveils the cadaver, which he himself has not yet seen:

There was an awful silence. Every eye beheld the corpse, and every heart grew cold with dread. Ravoni himself at the sight of that hideous spectacle started backward with a pale cheek and a trembling lip. Then . . . a murmured cry of horror shook the room. . . . From head to foot, along the trunk and over each limb, that corpse was all one cankering sore, one loathsome blotch. Features on the face there were none; brow and lip and cheek were all one hideous ulcer. The eye-balls were spotted with clotted blood; the mouth a cavern of corruption; the very hair was thick with festering pollution. I[t] was the corpse of a man who had died from . . . the most infectious of all epidemics, a curse at whose name beauty shudders and grave science grows pale—the small-pox. Better to look into the plague-pit where man and woman and babe lay mingled together, one reeking mass of quick lime and gory flesh, than to have gazed upon that corpse extended on the Dissecting table before the eyes of five hundred living men! . . .

Ravoni stood silent and pale. . . . There he stood with eternal youth in his veins but in his twelve brief hours, he might lay a foul thing of ulcers and blotches, like the corse before his eyes. For the common phases of this disease, there were remedies; but let a single infectious atom breathed from the lips of a corse like this, enter the lips of living man, and no arm under God's sky could bring relief.

. . . A wild cry of horror shook the room, and . . . in one mass the audience rushed toward the door. It was a living picture of a panic. . . . [T]he dense throng rushed against the door, crushing all who stood near its panels until they howled in very agony. . . . There was a wild crashing sound; the door gave way; splintered into fragments it fell before the living mass, and through the opened passage, the panic-stricken crowd rushed from the place of death. (373–75)

The cowardice and hypocrisy of scientific medicine stand revealed. The anatomical effort to enclose the body is a puny thing beside the profundity of bodily corruption, the corporeal sublime. Devil-Bug laughs: "Ho, ho, ho! . . . The doctor and the students all skeered to death by a bundle o' small pox!" (375). Against the bantering mockery of the dissecting room, against the anatomical pose of detachment, death and the body prevail. Science is exposed as vain and ineffectual. The disenchantment of the flesh is futile.

This critique of reason is conducted in the vocabulary of body and bodily affects that genteel discourse excludes. The diseased and desirous body far exceeds the inert anatomical cadaver of texts and the dissecting table. The carnal body bursts with moral and immoral significance, articulates longing, fear, hatred. The members of the medical profession claim to stand above and outside corporeality. But for all their contempt of the dissected body and the working people who stand in a "mass" against the "intelligent" individual, "a mass of gory flesh" reduces the physicians themselves to a "living mass," a body of humanity. The entire audience (including McTourniquet) stampedes out of the anatomical theater. Ravoni remains standing beside the corpse. Byrnewood Arlington, "with long black hair and a flashing eye," stands by his side: "'Thou hast a firm soul,' spoke the Sorcerer, . . . his eyes shone and his brow warmed with a sudden enthusiasm, 'By the Soul of Ravoni thou shall be one of the Chosen; thou shalt be a Priest of the Faith!'" (375).

Ravoni has cast himself as a messiah who will overthrow Christianity with a new cult of knowledge that is both religion and science. This "new Faith" will recuperate the forgotten, dormant power of ancient magic, even the power to resurrect the dead:

> "That Faith, buried for long, long centuries which man in the olden time, in the world's youth of promise, loved and cherished, which raised him to godhead, and made the Universe itself his own, that Faith will we raise from the grim ruins of fable and superstition! And the old Faith, revised and recreated shall be our New Religion of hope to Man!" . . . The words of the Sorcerer were wild and strange. . . . *"This hour shalt thou behold the dead arise!"* (375)

This proto-Nietzchean creed does what the anatomical narrative of reason versus superstition only trifles with: resurrects the dead, destroys "superstition" (redefined to include Christianity), brings on a new millennium. Unchecked by moral encumbrance, the new order promises a boundless expansion of human agency, fusing reason, desire, and revelation—a triumph of anatomical Will far beyond the reach of contemporary anatomy.

"The Most Poetical Topic in the World"

> "And sich a purty corse!" cried Mrs. Wilson, "Jist look there! Did ever ye see sich hair? So curly and long, and so like gold. Did you ever see sich a mouth?"
>
> Mrs. Wilson, to Ravoni, *The Quaker City* (348)

In the end, however, the new anatomical cult is also thwarted. Devil-Bug's improbable love for an innocent young virgin (it is revealed that he is her father) leads to Ravoni's undoing. Christian spirit wins out over embodied, desirous reason. Yet the text's performance does something very different from what the text says. *The Quaker City* ostensibly narrates the war between flesh, mind, and spirit, a perilous struggle in which moral sentiment enjoys a victory over voracious reason and the embodied self. Lippard's motives in writing the book, he claimed, were "pure," "destitute of any idea of sensualism" (2).

But such claims are hardly credible. The sensationalist novel has many affinities to pornography, and *The Quaker City* has many suggestive passages involving a beautiful young woman who is dead or seems so:

[O]n the altar, lay a stiffened corpse, whose outlines were dimly seen through the folds of a white cloth, flung lightly over each icy limb. There was a beauty in that corpse, and grace, for the cloth was moulded into soft folds, as though it veiled a woman's form. The feet were thrust upward, the arms folded over the chest, and the globes of the bosom rose gently in the light, even beneath their thick disguise. (377–78)

Antebellum readers well understood the erotic coding of the "soft folds," "globes of the bosom," and emergent "worms":

Yet she was dead, ah, cold and dead! And the light streamed warmly over the marble whiteness of that uncovered form, revealing beauties which the worms were soon to riot. Over the round limbs, over the white bosom, over the beaming face the worms would crawl, marking their progress with the blue taint of decay. And Ravoni could raise this corse to life again? (382–83)

The particulars of this have much to do with nineteenth-century cultural taboos on the representation of the sexual body. In *The Quaker City*, the only bodies permitted erotic representation are dead, asleep, or inanimate (quasi-dead) women. Public display of unclothed female flesh was taboo in the antebellum era. Only in anatomy and fine art could the naked body find legitimate representation, and in those domains, whose erotic potential was evident, this was circumscribed, a matter of tricky negotiation.

Death provided anatomy and fine art with their subject and legitimized the representation of flesh:

It was the corse of a young beautiful woman. There was a smile on the lips, a calm glory beaming from the face, around whose swelling outlines, a warm mass of golden hair curled and twined and glistened. The round arms folded on the breast, the white fingers gently clasped, and the snowy bosom with the blue threaded veins, that bosom whose fulness bespoke the mother—ah! Death was there in holy beauty. Fairer form than that, did painter never shape, sweeter limbs than those did sculptor never carve. (383)

In death, the body becomes a naked or lightly veiled statue, identical to the classical representations that, by long-standing convention, carry both an erotic and moral valence. Death aestheticizes the body. The body is frozen (for a moment) into a representation that draws on a stock of classical imagery: the clothing of everyday life is replaced by a shroud, which is reminiscent of classical drapery. Death whitens the skin: in the antebellum era, aesthetic convention dictated the paler the better. Death quiets the body, makes it fall into an exquisite, unshakeable repose that approximates the feminine ideal of beautiful passivity.

In death, the virginal female body, unclothed or dressed in a veil-like translucent shroud, undergoes a transformation that fixes its status,

places it for eternity outside the "traffic of women." The dead body becomes the object of moral contemplation. But paradoxically, its very un-
availability is easily converted into desirability: in death, the female body
becomes a scarce commodity.

But, again, only for a moment. The commodity is perishable. In narratives of the productive bourgeois self, the dead female body is initially
deployed in opposition to the chaos and destructiveness of death. The
eroticized cadaver simultaneously articulates and represses the knowledge
of the disordering, destroying pleasure of sexual desire. But as the dead
body undergoes decomposition, it undergoes a moral metamorphosis, becomes a source of pollution. Neither subject nor object, the decaying
corpse is an "abject," an ontological category that stands outside discourse as the opposite of value, the antithesis of productivity and repro-
ductivity. The decaying body disrupts labor and reproductive discipline.

Death, in both stages, is a boundary breached, just like sexual intercourse, where the boundary between bodies is breached (the special case
that intensifies this erotic effect is the defloration of the virgin, a double
boundary breached). Death, stereotypically represented as a masculine
figure, invades the body and strips it of its will, its independent subjectivity. Like the mesmeric trance or even rape, death extinguishes the
agency that opposes male appropriation and penetration of the female
body. The antebellum fascination with the dead body, like the mesmerized body, stands as the expression of a desire to surrender the boundaries that define bourgeois personhood, a willful annihilation of the prop-
ertied self.

The regulation of female sexuality almost requires that Eros and
Thanatos become equivalents. For women, the loss of virginity outside of
marriage, or the violation of the marital bed by infidelity, is a social death.
The debauched virgin and the adulterous wife, like the dissected dead
body, are sources of contamination and sites of desire. Defloration, like
death, strips the female body of any defense against male sexual predation, but also gives rise to a pathological fecundity.

Death then, like sex, epitomizes self and other. Death purifies and reveals, but also corrupts and contaminates. Death is the telos of the narrated life, a life navigated by a purposeful, moral self. A beautiful life
requires a beautiful death; its representative figure in sentimental fiction
is the beautiful child (who is innocent of sexuality); in sensationalist fiction, the beautiful woman. But death also liquidates the self/other binary
in a dialectical big bang. In the erotics of death, the early stages are
iconically feminine and beautiful and pure; the latter stages masculine
and ugly and contaminating. As decomposition proceeds, worms consume the dead body—a metaphor that encodes the destructive phallus
and the consummation of desire. The body generates foul odors, loses

symmetry and uniformity of coloring, etc. Death, like sexual desire, is
what bourgeois morality and aesthetics cannot contain. Those without
honor, those who lack moral sentiment, revel in ugly death (e.g., Devil-
Bug). And this phenomenology recapitulates the negative Christian afterlife: the decomposed body is a hell where negations are articulated, with
no hope of redemption.

The Body Turned Inside Out, and Back Again

As we have seen, the procedures of gothic sensationalism stand as a reproach to the hegemony of mind over matter. In operating on the reader's
body, sensationalism evades bourgeois self-discipline, the regulatory action of reason, and produces its own bodily effects. For Lippard, anatomy
is a refusal of deeper knowledge, a vain and illegitimate attempt to coerce
the body. The language of carnality, corruption, and desire acts as a sol-
vent on the pretensions of anatomy. In hackwork like *Marietta*, visceralism
serves as the technical vocabulary of sensationalism. In *The Quaker City*,
and other works of Lippard, it is elevated to the status of aesthetic principle and political program. His own disavowals notwithstanding, Lippard
turns the body inside out. Instead of reason penetrating, organizing, and
purifying the body, corruption, feeling, and desire pour out of the body.
This is the revenge of matter over mind.

   Even so, gothic sensationalism and anatomy had some affinities. Within
medical texts as well as sensationalist fiction, the mesmeric or seductive
gaze was barely distinguishable (or not at all) from the clinical gaze: both
appropriated their objects, constituted them, mastered them. Anatomy
overlapped the gothic—both operated in a liminal zone between death
and life, both deployed memento mori. Both worked the same tropes: the
problems of material power, immaterial will, and the boundaries of self.
(Recall that mesmerism was a staple of the gothic novel and a specialty of
antebellum medical performance.) In early-nineteenth-century anatomy
museums, doctors' offices, hospitals, anatomical theaters, and dissecting
rooms, physicians exhibited skeletons, crania, anatomical objects, and
death figures and assumed facial and bodily poses that signified willful
vital mastery of the material world. Such icons and poses were also designed to engineer physical and emotional effects on the bodies of patients, colleagues, and the public, to elicit fear, awe, respect, acquies-
cence, and perhaps desire. In practice, the affectless clinical gaze was not
highly developed in the medicine of the 1840s, only a potential. The
mockery of the medical students in "The Dissecting Room" was not yet
that detachment which ruthlessly suppresses expressive gesture, orna-
ment, metaphor, rhetorical flourish, and romantic narrative in favor of

methodological rigor, reductionist narrative, schematic illustration, and tabular columns.

Lippard sought to discredit anatomical (and all professional and class) authority, and to credit his own, via the romantic narrative of literary genius, the republican narrative of conspiracy against the people, the masculinist narrative of honor defended. But both Lippard and the anatomists operated on their subjects through parallel discursive practices: Lippard on the bodies of his readers, anatomists on their patients and cadavers. In order for the physician to authorize himself, he must dissect. His subject must be rendered speechless and helpless, inert (just as the characters in *The Quaker City* are rendered inert through hypnosis, drugging, burking). Lippard opposed anatomy as a rape of the body and the grave, but his very critique exerted a sexual power that titillated and shocked the passive reader through erotic narratives of sexual danger and descriptions of dead female bodies. He may have seen through the anatomist who cloaks desire in the rhetoric of disinterested science, but Lippard's own avowals of disinterestedness have even less credibility.

However, it would be too easy to dismiss Lippard as a crank and hypocrite. His writings are eccentric, but were powerfully evocative by virtue of their reference to real social experiences. Lippard's tales of dark conspiracies of physicians, body snatchers, secret orders, assaults on funerary and sexual honor, and a rapacious elite resonated with antebellum readers. They *were* subject to powerful, invisible, and inexplicable forces—the market economy, backroom party politics, the cloistered social and professional activities of new elites, and the speculative machinations of finance capital. These received representation in a fantasy discourse that dreamed of powerful secret cults, most famously the Masons and the Roman Catholic church, which controlled and violated their victims at a distance through hypnotism, druggings, false preachment, and desecration of bodies. But dissection rituals and resurrection conspiracies (unlike Masonic and Catholic conspiracies) *did* actually exist, were even common occurrences. In a variety of ways, then, Lippard's fantastic creations gestured toward "the real." Even Devil-Bug, his most bizarre creation, corresponded to figures who could be found in the social reality of his readers: ghoulish characters like George T. Alberti, a body snatcher, fugitive-slave catcher, kidnapper, and sometime hangman, who ended his career as an extortionate petty politician in the Southwark district of Philadelphia, and William Cunningham ("Old Cunny"), the ghoulishly notorious leader of a Cincinnati body-snatching gang.[25]

Not surprisingly, sensationalist rhetoric traveled from literature back to political discourse. Thus, in the New York legislative debate on the 1854 "Bone Bill" (which granted medical schools the right to dissect the bodies of people who died in poorhouses and prisons), assemblyman Joseph

Cook charged that the law was "a nefarious plot against the repose of the dead" that would license "the immolation of this sacred image [the human body] upon the altar of science." Imagine, he asked his fellow assemblymen, that your own "wife or daughter" wanders from home "in the moment of delirium": "Would you wish her body—in the event of death—conveyed from the hospital to the dissecting block?" In recognizably Lippardian rhetoric, Cook denounced the medical profession as "a class of men who . . . have neither hope of heaven nor the fear of hell before their eyes—who laugh at the jest and top off the bowl, while before them quivers the flesh of inanimate humanity."[26] Sensationalist discourse therefore had a resonant interpretive function. It provided a descriptive vocabulary and narrative which helped its audience make sense of its experience.

8

The Education of Sammy Tubbs

ANATOMICAL DISSECTION, MINSTRELSY,

AND THE TECHNOLOGY OF SELF-MAKING IN

POSTBELLUM AMERICA

• • • • • •

We have thus far focused on antebellum anatomical performances, contests, and negotiations—the anatomization of American medicine, debates over anatomy law, the incorporation of the anatomical body into the curriculum of bourgeois self-making, and the general cultural fascination with dissection and grave robbery. The remainder of this book continues the study into the postbellum era, but first we must pause to consider the "bellum." How did the War Between the States affect the cultural politics of anatomy?

During the Civil War, the cultural politics of anatomy fell dormant; the war took priority over, disrupted, or restructured other cultural concerns. Between 1861 and 1865, there were few medical grave robberies, no body-snatching scandals, no debates over anatomy law. There was no need. Bodies were mass produced: over 150,000 men died of wounds; over 350,000 from illness. Given the carnage, poor sanitary conditions, and rampant disease, the need for physicians was pressing. Thousands of medical students and doctors enlisted as medical officers in the Union and Confederate armies, where they had plenty of bodies to work on. Lacking staff and students, medical schools found it difficult or impossible to operate during the war.

For novice and even experienced doctors, the war represented an opportunity for advanced practical training, especially in surgery (and a risk; they were in harm's way). The sudden demand for able surgeons starkly revealed the short-comings of American medical training. Many diplomaed practitioners were exposed as incompetent, unable to perform amputations, set fractures, remove bullets, and do other basic surgeries. But, over the five years of war, many medical officers developed surgical expertise. In general, the experience of wartime served to strengthen advocates of higher standards, state licensure laws, anatomy acts, and increases in the length, rigor, and rationalization of medical training. The Civil War visibly demonstrated the need for anatomical training in surgery, and so intensified the anatomization of American medicine.[1]

We should not, however, make too much of the war's impact. The anatomization of medicine was a project that was centuries in the making. In the 1850s, its progress further accelerated as the locus of advanced medical research and education began to shift from France to Germany, and the dominant paradigm began to shift from clinical to laboratory medicine. Postbellum medicine continued these trends. As anatomical medicine became increasingly complex and specialized, the prestige of gross anatomy and pathological anatomy began to wane and professional enthusiasm shifted to the more sophisticated specialties of physiology and microbiology (typically referred to as "microscopic anatomy").

Ultimately, the war's greatest impact on the cultural politics of anatomy was political. Vindicated by Emancipation and the Northern victory, in the postbellum era, a coalition of radicals and professionalizing reformers buoyantly tried to implement and expand their vision of an improved society. In many domains the professionalizing reformers triumphed; the war experience bolstered the authority of anatomical medicine. But, as the following chapter shows, after a crescendo in the mid-1870s the momentum of radical reform slowed. Powerful reactionary forces, nurtured by the failure of Reconstruction and a general atmosphere of disillusionment, ultimately checked the advance of cultural radicalism and disrupted alliances between professionalizers and radical reformers based on anatomy and identity.

• • • • • •

THE NINETEENTH CENTURY, proverbially the era of the "self-made man," can be more accurately characterized as the era of the man-made self. Beginning in the 1830s, and gathering force in the 1840s and 1850s, discourses and technologies of self-making proliferated, touching in some fashion nearly every segment of the American population. As we have seen, this occurred very visibly in a movement of popular anatomists— lecturers, teachers, physicians, and writers—who argued that a "true and rational course of human conduct, in all respects" required "a universal diffusion of a knowledge of human anatomy and physiology."[2] While they differed considerably about what constituted a "true and rational course of human conduct," all agreed that the dispersion of natural knowledge about the body was the necessary foundation for social, political, cultural, and moral reform, for an improved or even perfected humanity.

During the Civil War, not much was heard about the need to teach anatomy and physiology to schoolchildren, workers, women, and savages. Popular anatomists and their constituency were distracted by wartime duties and issues. Afterward, the cultural politics of anatomy resumed, with some modification: in the 1870s and 1880s, popular discourse began to absorb the motifs and narratives of evolutionary theory, cellular physiology, microbiology, and scientific experimentalism; the term *physiology* replaced *popular anatomy*.[3] This chapter is about one postbellum physiologist, Dr. Edward Bliss Foote, and his now obscure but extraordinary "novelty in literature," *Sammy Tubbs, the Boy Doctor, and "Sponsie," the Troublesome Monkey*.[4]

In the 1870s, the boundaries and content of the bourgeois self were

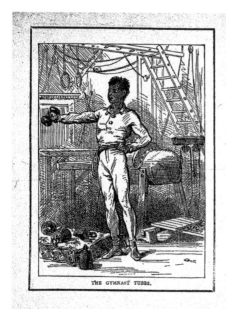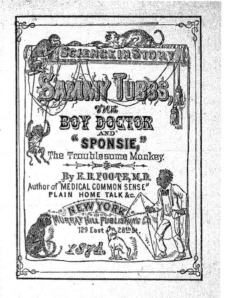

Figure 8.1. *Sammy Tubbs, the Boy Doctor and "Sponsie," the Troublesome Monkey* (New York: Murray Hill Publishing Co., 1874–75; rpt. 1887) All illustrations from *Sammy Tubbs* are by Henry L. Stephens, except for anatomical diagrams. Courtesy of the Department of Rare Books and Special Collections, University of Rochester Libraries.

sharply contested in an exuberant and often transgressive cultural politics of anatomy.[5] The anatomical body, seemingly "scientific," value-free, and outside the domain of social contention, was from its inception full of complexity and contradiction, and available for appropriation by a variety of contending parties. The cultural politics that attempted to draw its logic and legitimacy from physiological discourse was problematic. In some ways it was socially subversive, even emancipatory. But in other ways it ratified and enforced the regnant social hierarchy and moral economy of capital. And in still other ways it produced and enlarged new domains of professional, state and entrepreneurial social power.

The stakes were high. The acquisition and performance of bourgeois social identity continued to be a pressing problem for many Americans. People urgently demanded materials that might help them—and their children—to become "cultivated," "civilized," "intelligent." Such qualities could be signified outwardly through conversational and literary use of anatomical and physiological terminology and logic, attendance at physiological lectures, and purchase and reading of anatomico-physiological texts, but, more importantly, through an "inner," ideological performance. Anatomy and physiology provided the terminology, linkages, and figurations out of which a narrative of social and physical identity could be constructed and represented to one's self as well as others, the substance of an internal dialogue. The acquisition of bourgeois identity then was not epiphenomenal, not just a putting on of anatomical clothes. Individuals experienced the anatomical body—as taught in schools, public lectures, and popular scientific books, and given powerful reinforcement in medicine, naturalist fiction, art, and journalism—at a phenomenological, cognitive level. The anatomical self was learned, experienced, and performed—and there was a growing market for books, lectures, and exhibitions that could impart and rehearse that learning.

The *Sammy Tubbs* books bulge with physiological ideas, arguments, and obsessions. Some 1,200-odd pages long and profusely illustrated, the series is a complicated read, brimming over with figurations of nation, society, cosmos, and self, and commentaries on race, gender, eugenics, corporal punishment, diet, child labor, medical licensure, philanthropy, and physical fitness: the anatomical body fairly bursts with meaning. Given this textual richness, much could be said; in this chapter I want to concentrate on Foote's idiosyncratic blend of minstrelsy, anatomical instruction, and juvenile fiction. *Sammy Tubbs* offered itself as a program for producing a universalized bourgeois self that explicitly included black people and women—even as it served to reinforce prevailing hierarchies of race and gender. I will end the chapter with a consideration of Foote's career as entrepreneur/activist and the strategic difficulties involved in a radical cultural politics based on the anatomical body.

DR. EDWARD BLISS FOOTE

Edward Bliss Foote (1829–1906) of New York City, an irregular "medical and electrical therapeutist" of the eclectic persuasion, was among the most popular physiologists of the postbellum era. Historians know him mainly as the self-proclaimed inventor of the "womb veil," a rimless contraceptive diaphragm or cervical cap made out of "india rubber,"[6] and as a victim of Anthony Comstock's moral crusades: in 1876 Foote was found guilty of having sent "obscene matter" (a birth control tract entitled *Words in Pearl, For Married People Only*) through the mails.[7] But Foote's career, as unorthodox healer, medical entrepreneur, and social activist, surely deserves greater scrutiny. Taking advantage of federal measures that reduced postal rates and extended mail delivery to new regions, Foote built up a highly successful mail-order medical practice and publishing company.[8] An article in the *New York Independent* described the operation. Foote and his assistants received walk-in patients at "elegantly furnished" offices, located at 120 Lexington Avenue and East 28th Street in Manhat-

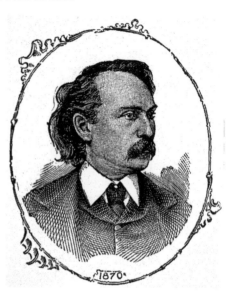

Figure 8.2. Portrait of Edward Bliss Foote, 1870, from Theodore Burr Wakeman, *In Memory of Edward Bliss Foote, M.D.: A "Beloved Physician," of the New, Scientific, Human, Social, "Agnostic" Faith. . . . The Funeral Address Delivered . . .* (New York, 1907), 60. Courtesy of the Library of the College of Physicians of Philadelphia.

tan, but most of the building was devoted to the manufacture of patent medicines and processing of medical correspondence. One floor was "occupied by stenographers" who, "under the direct dictation of the Doctor," attended to "the immense correspondence, which often exceeds one hundred letters per day." The mail-order operation was systematic and lucrative: "The Doctor has originated and perfected a series of questions related to invalids. These questions are so thorough . . . that when they are answered by patients at a distance, the Doctor is able to make a complete diagnosis and prescribe for his patients with about the same facility as if they were present."[9] Such advice was free (except for letters in German which cost a dollar). The remedies, generally unorthodox and of Foote's own manufacture, were not. Offered for sale were "magnetic anti-bilious pills," "botanical medicines," "electro-magnetic machines," the "womb veil," and a variety of other devices to prevent conception, cure ailments, and improve functioning (sexual and otherwise).

Foote's medical practice operated in conjunction with his publications. An unceasing self-promoter, he was one of the most popular medical journalists of his day. His books, pamphlets, and long-running monthly journal amounted to thousands of pages, and were avidly read. He frequently boasted that *Medical Common Sense* (1857–1858) and *Plain Home Talk* (1869–1870) combined to sell more than 750,000 copies, while *Dr. Foote's Health Monthly* had tens of thousands of subscribers.[10] Foote advised his readers on health, hygiene, sex, and politics, and promoted his medical practice, publications, and products. He championed a cranky jumble of

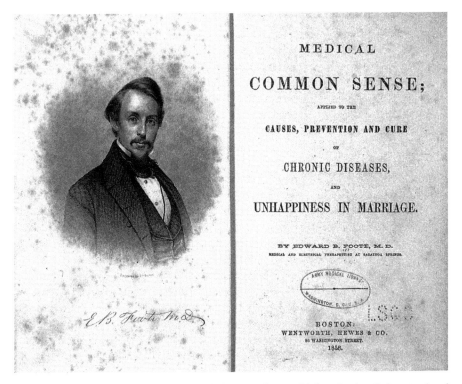

Figure 8.3. In various editions, *Medical Common Sense* sold hundreds of thousands of copies over several decades. Courtesy of the National Library of Medicine.

causes and ideas: dietary reform, feminism, tobacco temperance, dress reform, paper money, physical fitness, phrenology, racial egalitarianism and "amalgamation," cremation, divorce reform, eugenics, evolution, agnosticism, sex education, positivist medical science, and unorthodox medicine. He saw himself as an evangel of progress and keeper of the faith: the secular perfectionism and scientific faddishness of the antebellum era, the cultural revolution of the 1830s and 1840s.

It is worth considering Foote's social origins, class identity, and filiations. Linda Gordon says he was "born into a poor family" and stresses his working-class origins as "a printer's devil and then a journalist."[11] But a contemporary biographical sketch reports that Foote's father Herschel, an early migrant from Connecticut to the Western Reserve, was "the village merchant, the postmaster, and the squire," his home "literally a free hotel for ministers, school teachers, and singing masters," where "on one Sunday three of the Beechers were entertained." An entry on E. B. Foote in D. M. Bennett's 1876 biographical encyclopedia of *The World's Sages,*

Thinkers and Reformers describes Herschel Foote as "a strict Presbyterian" who introduced "book-binding and the teaching of sacred music in Cleveland," while *The Biographical History of Westchester County* stresses Foote's descent from two lines of Revolutionary War officers, and his father's status as "a prosperous and esteemed merchant" and long-time Justice of the Peace.[12] Raised among the provincial gentry, Foote's teenage apprenticeship as a printer was an instance of a restless and rebellious young man settling in trade over the objections of his parents. In the printshop he came into contact with the freethinking tradition of Paine (hence *Medical Common Sense*) and renounced his parents' Calvinism. After finishing his apprenticeship, at age 20 he became editor of the *New Britain Journal*. For the next few years he worked as a journalist and editor, ending up in the 1850s at the *Brooklyn Morning Journal*.

By his own account, Foote then had a medical revelation, which called him to a lucrative career in unorthodox medicine as both practitioner and author.[13] His Murray Hill Publishing Company began in the 1870s with an authorized capital of $20,000. By 1877 an R. G. Dun & Co. credit investigation rated him as "well off," with a house on Lexington Avenue worth $30,000.[14] He also invested in an oil company and was its president.[15] Hal D. Sears calls him "the principal bank-roller" of the postbellum freethought/free-love movement: Foote posted bail and paid fines for activists arrested under the Comstock laws and helped finance their publications and organizations.[16]

He became eminent enough to merit an entry in the *National Cyclopædia of American Biography*; yet he must have been socially unwelcome in many homes. His avant-garde cultural politics and entrepreneurial medical practice gave him a more than comfortable income, but depended on the manufacture and sale of devices for use in "sexual hygiene," and cheap literature treating sexual topics. He had the pedigree, income, and cachet as a member of a learned profession to be solidly bourgeois, but his hands were soiled with disreputable trade—and his 1876 arrest and conviction at the hands of Comstock surely did not help his reputation.

His medical filiations and political enthusiasms were suspect as well. In the 1870s and 1880s, eclectics were an insecure minority in the medical profession. Foote's exuberant proselytizing for phrenology, physiognomy, electrotherapy, and animal magnetism marked him as a bit vulgar if not a crackpot, by the standards of the 1870s (such ideas, although marginal in medical discourse, remained current among reformers, writers, and artists).[17] His politics also placed him near the edge, if not over it. Foote was an early supporter of the Republican party when it was the party of antislavery, but in later years sympathized with the Greenback, Populist, and Democratic parties; in 1894 he ran a quixotic race for Congress as a Populist.[18] The range of articles published in his *Health Monthly* (written mostly by Foote and his son) reflect the unwieldy coalition of cultural reformers he attempted to hold together: feminists, physiologists, spiritualists, positivists, antivaccinationists, teetotallers, antivivisectionists, eugenicists, greenbackers, free-lovers, and freethinkers.[19] In the words of George E. Macdonald, Foote belonged to "every party that never carried an election. . . . But his favorite reforms were not such as any political party would put in its platform—the divorce of the Church from the State without alimony, the freedom of thought and the unrestricted distribution of knowledge on all subjects, religious, social, industrial, and especially medical."[20] He was, however, not terribly sympathetic to the working class and the poor, arguing that "tramps" and "molly maguires" were "evils" that should be dealt with eugenically by "preventing the increase of these pauper classes by propagation" through contraception, in the same way that "farms and stock-raising pastures" only retained the best animals "for breeding purposes."[21]

Apart from these sources, we also have Foote's depiction of himself as Dr. Hubbs in *Sammy Tubbs*. Drawn to resemble Foote by the able comic illustrator Henry L. Stephens, Hubbs is the masculine center of a bourgeois household, with neurasthenic wife, Irish servants, and colored office-boy. His home (located, like Foote's, at Lexington Avenue and East 28th Street) is furnished in high Victorian style, with all the requisite trappings and amenities, plus a doctor's office equipped with suitably scientific chemical apparatus and anatomical cabinet. The Doctor himself wears a dignified gentleman's suit and is a model of comportment. Immaculate, wise, unflappable, he tends with fatherly authority to the disruptive children, servants, lower-class supplicants and women who deferentially orbit around him.[22]

Sammy Tubbs the Boy Doctor

In 1874, at the height of his popularity, Foote wrote *Sammy Tubbs, the Boy Doctor, and "Sponsie," the Troublesome Monkey*, a five-volume series on anatomy and physiology aimed at "children from 10 to 15 years of age who are entirely ignorant of the wonderful mechanism of their bodies," and also "such busy adults as are too hardly worked in the never-ending treadmill of business-life to spend the leisure they need for mental and physical relaxation in the pursuit of abstruse science."[23] Designed to "especially meet a popular want," the books were printed on cheap paper and priced low: in a variety of editions.[24] Unlike other postbellum works of popular anatomy, *Sammy Tubbs* was not a textbook or lecture in pamphlet form, rather a generic hybrid that Foote called "Science in Story" (what would now be termed an "edutainment"). The basic plot is Pygmalion without any reversal or irony: Sammy Tubbs, a young emancipated slave possessed of great native intelligence and resourcefulness, comes north with his mother (a washerwoman) and father (a whitewasher) and enters the service of the kindly Dr. Samuel Hubbs as a "door-tender." The doctor tutors Sammy in anatomy, physiology, and hygiene, and the boy turns out to be a prodigy. Sammy becomes a lecturer, a lay medical missionary, and a hero to a black community that has long been denied medical treatment and physiological instruction because of prejudice and poverty.

Each chapter features an anatomy or physiology lesson interspersed with the antics of Sponsie "the troublesome monkey" (actually two monkeys, Sponsie 1 and Sponsie 2) and other characters. In the fourth book, Sammy, now about 15 years old, lectures on anatomy to a racially mixed audience at "Lincoln Hall" and dissects Sponsie 1 (who has been acciden-

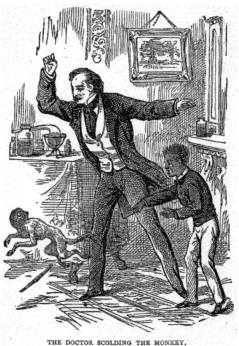

THE DOCTOR SCOLDING THE MONKEY.

Figure 8.4. "The Doctor scolding the monkey," *Sammy Tubbs*, 2 (1887): 100. Note Dr. Hubbs's strong resemblance to Foote. The room is decorated with items connoting the doctor's class and professional status. Courtesy of the Department of Rare Books and Special Collections, University of Rochester Libraries.

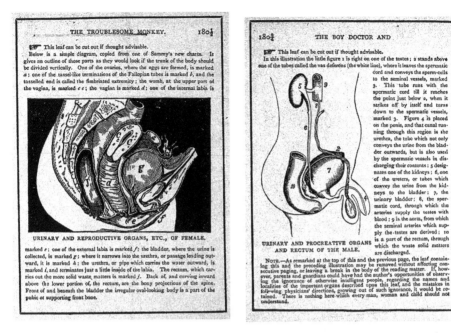

Figure 8.5. Anatomical diagrams of male and female genitals, *Sammy Tubbs*, 5 (1876): 180½–180¾. The unconventional page numbering is designed so that parents can remove the pages and not destroy the consecutive pagination. In the small print, Foote urges them to refrain from doing so. Courtesy of Florida State University Library.

tally shot dead by Sponsie 2), using the monkey's brain to demonstrate cerebral anatomy. A fifth volume, published in early 1875, covers the topic of "Reproduction and Elimination" ("for private reading")—and is probably the first anatomically explicit sex education book for preadolescent children. In that book, a gymnasium for black people is constructed according to a utilitarian plan devised by Sammy: the exercisers in the gym provide power, via belts and pulleys, to a textile factory that gives employment to widows and unemployed men. Sammy undertakes a strenuous program of gymnastics and muscle building (a self-making corollary to the study of anatomical texts and objects), and speaks on the physiology of reproduction and sexuality to racially integrated audiences of young men and women at "Gymnasium Hall." As Sammy lectures, Sponsie 2 accidentally becomes enmeshed in the gears of the factory and dies; his elimination leads to an autopsy that illustrates the physiology of "elimination" (urination and defecation). The series ends with Sammy preparing to go to medical college and the suggestion of a budding romance between Sammy and a young white girl, the daughter of a cotton manufacturer (ever the controversialist, Foote favored interracial breeding

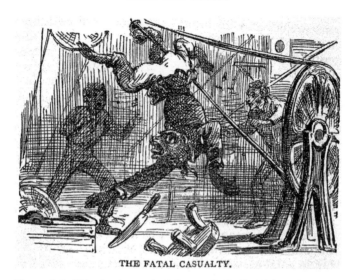

THE FATAL CASUALTY.

Figure 8.6. "The fatal casualty," *Sammy Tubbs*, 5 (1887): 189; Sponsie 2 dies in the conveyor belts that connect the gymnasium to the
factory. Courtesy of the Department of Rare Books and Special
Collections, University of Rochester Libraries.

on eugenical grounds). Sammy comes of age sexually and racially, having attained intellectual and physical maturity through his mastery of
anatomy.

"Formatory Processes": Anatomical Embodiment and the Bourgeois Self

A year after the publication of the final *Sammy Tubbs* volume, in the
spring of 1876, Foote was prosecuted by Anthony Comstock. In a letter to
the *New York Times*, he defended himself: "Brother Comstock and [I] are
engaged in what each regards as humanitarian reforms. He is trying to
make people better by reformatory measures, and I by formatory processes; he playing the role of the moralist, and I the part of both moralist
and physiologist."[25] Foote's avowed mission was to mold his readers into
disciplined anatomically conscious individuals. Thus the first volume of
Sammy Tubbs is taken up with an extended exploration of "the curious
construction of the parts which, joined together, made the material body
of the boy Sammy Tubbs" (1:36). Foote wanted to "captivate the youthful
mind" with "anatomical and physiological knowledge" (1:iii). The unregulated body must be subjected to a higher, disembodied physiologico-
moral law—the mind must subordinate the body through a knowledge of
anatomy. And insofar as mind is a material part of the body, and unac-

quainted with anatomical knowledge or moral ideals, it too must be stamped with the anatomical template. Like his predecessors Alcott and Hollick, Foote adapted anatomical discourse to the broadest sociocultural domain—the making of the bourgeois self.

The critical period in the formation of social identity was childhood. Though not "an admirer of popular tales or novels"—he claimed to have only ever read one work of fiction,[26] "and that one in childhood" (1:ii–iii)—Foote ventured into the burgeoning market for morally instructive juvenile fiction because his "formatory processes" required it. A modicum of entertainment was needed, he argued, to overcome "the average" child's "instinctive . . . criticism . . . of civilized life" (1:ii), a necessary accommodation to the pleasure principle. "Books of anatomy and physiology . . . have been justly considered dry reading" but given children's "passion for works of fiction," "the dry studies . . . might be woven into a story"; the entertainment would function in the same way that "pill-vendors" use an "envelope of sugar" to coat foul-tasting remedies (1:ii). Foote's inspiration here was likely the 1865 appearance of Lewis Carroll's *Alice in Wonderland,* the first bestseller expressly written for the entertainment of child readers, with John Tenniel's brilliant drawings complementing the text. (Foote secured the services of comic illustrator H. L. Stephens for the *Sammy Tubbs* series.)

Like other nineteenth-century health reformers, Foote insisted on the importance of instruction in anatomy for children and called for the adoption of anatomy in the school curriculum alongside geography. It was a physiological commonplace that, as T. S. Lambert put it, anatomy is "the geography of the body."[27] Anatomy uses the same representational vocabulary as geography: names, borders, regions, islands, topography. Like geography, it locates the body in space and represents space in the body. It inscribes a social and moral order, a set of boundaries on the body. To be "human," "civilized," or "intelligent" (interchangeable terms in *Sammy Tubbs*), one must know this internal geography. Anatomy maps the body's internal borders, its regions and terrains, its diverse inhabitants, characteristics, and laws. The body figures and naturalizes the social; the social figures and disciplines the body. Foote variously depicts the body as a business, economy, nation, empire, or (citing Buffon) "a world in little" (4:231). The constitutional structure is federal: the body is ruled and regulated by a metropolis ("the Capitol of the Nervous System—the Brain," Foote announces in several places).[28] A network of "nerve-telegraphs" connects the regions and informs the brain, which balances and restrains competing bodily interests. Pathways of blood and lymph transport materials from the provinces to the center and back; various organs construct the bodily structures, process food, and eliminate waste (there are even "contractors" and "sub-contractors" [4:202]).

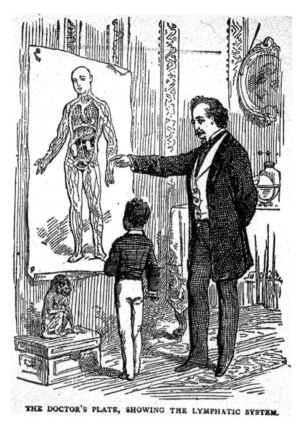

THE DOCTOR'S PLATE, SHOWING THE LYMPHATIC SYSTEM.

Figure 8.7. "The Doctor's plate, showing the lymphatic system," *Sammy Tubbs*, 2 (1887): 118. The sequential placement of the figures emphasizes the developmental/evolutionary/racial sequence from monkey to child to adult, and from animal to black to white. Courtesy of the Department of Rare Books and Special Collections, University of Rochester Libraries.

"Without your bones you would fall together in a shapeless mass," Dr. Hubbs tells Sammy (1:28). Anatomical knowledge makes the body over into a "well-ordered" person, an internal organizing principle that renders external regulation (state and religious policing) of the body unnecessary. The anatomical self must conform to natural law, in harmony with moral law, or it sickens, a disciplinary arrangement that makes possible and desirable a "liberal" economic and political culture. Foote strongly identified with freethinking "liberalism"—Wakeman remarks that "In everything the Doctor is liberal"—which he associated with progressive reform, sanitarianism, and secular radicalism.[29]

Without anatomical self-knowledge, the body becomes "badly-organized," an unregulated chaos, prey to sickness, violence, and accident: "the majority of people never get the nerves of their brains and bodies into such well-ordered action" (4:219). Foote makes the point by trotting out a parade of characters who lack anatomical consciousness: superstitious (but good-hearted) Irish maids; an Italian immigrant couple who exploit and abuse their children and organ-grinding monkey (exemplifying also those who need instruction in eugenical contraception); the lazy and dimwitted Louis Napoleon Bonaparte ("bone-apart"), a liveried "boy," who serves as Sammy's negative mirror image; and the two Sponsies, whose "troublesome" antics continually disrupt Dr. Hubbs's bourgeois household while endangering their own health and well-being. Unlike Curious George, there is nothing lovable about the monkeys: they function as entertaining foils and object lessons for the heroic Sammy—and ultimately become his dissecting material.

In contrast to the popular anatomies of the antebellum era, the anatomical self in *Sammy Tubbs* is set within an explicitly evolutionary frame-

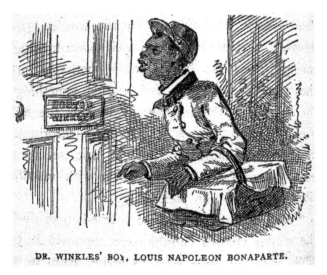

DR. WINKLES' BOY, LOUIS NAPOLEON BONAPARTE.

Figure 8.8. "Dr. Winkles' boy, Louis Napoleon Bonaparte," *Sammy Tubbs*, 1 (1887): 134. Sammy's mirror opposite has big lips and cringing posture, and is dressed as a liveried servant. Unlike Sammy, he is fearful, conniving, and utterly incapable of learning anatomy. His employer, the mirror opposite of Dr. Hubbs, is a conservative regular physician who regularly tries (and fails) to put Sammy in his place. Courtesy of the Department of Rare Books and Special Collections, University of Rochester Libraries.

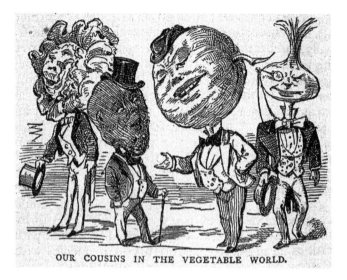

Figure 8.9. "Our cousins in the vegetable world." The human
body recapitulates vegetable and animal biology, *Sammy Tubbs*,
5 (1887): 8. Courtesy of the Department of Rare Books and
Special Collections, University of Rochester Libraries.

work that refigures the mind/body binary as the civilized/primitive dichotomy and the human/animal/vegetable triangle. Extending Haeckel's
principle of "ontogeny recapitulates phylogeny" (Foote acknowledged
Haeckel as a great influence), the evolutionary continuum from vegetable to lower animal to higher animal to primitive to civilized human is
recapitulated within the human body and within the nervous system.[30]
(And within the narrative, in the progression from Sponsie to the boy
Sammy Tubbs to Dr. Samuel Hubbs.) The cerebrum corresponds to "intellectual man"; the cerebellum is "animal man"; the medulla oblongata,
"vegetable man."[31] It is anatomical self-knowledge, and our psychological
capacity for such knowledge, then, that makes us distinctively human.
Animals, with their inferior mental development, can not know or control
their bodies or the world. Humans who never learn anatomy or other
sciences "die as animals do, unconscious of . . . all enjoyments excepting
those which proceed from sensuous pleasures" (2:50), while "trained
monkeys appear to nearly as good advantage as uncultivated men" (4:65).
Atop the natural hierarchy is not just the human but the anatomically
embodied human and, above all, the dissector. And this hierarchy is recapitulated within the anatomical individual as well as in the natural and
social world.

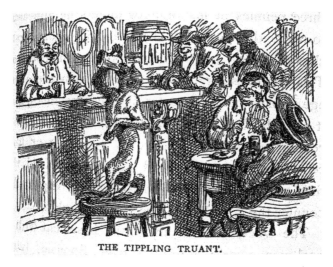

THE TIPPLING TRUANT.

Figure 8.10. "The tippling truant," *Sammy Tubbs*, 3 (1887): 25. Intemperance is animalistic; the two Sponsies represent undisciplined desire. Courtesy of the Department of Rare Books and Special Collections, University of Rochester Libraries.

"Them Is Only Dead Bones": Minstrelsy and Anatomy

The anatomical demarcation of the internal boundaries of the body and its properties is a metaphor of the self-containment and self-discipline that shapes the impulsive child/self into the rational bounded individual of Victorian parlor liberalism.[32] Foote registers his radicalism by allowing his young black hero to attain and exercise anatomical mastery over the body, by arguing that black people are capable of such mastery. But that position is subverted by the blackface minstrelsy that the story evokes (Sammy = Sambo). The implausibility of the black boy as anatomist is the comic effect that draws a mass (white) readership (or so Foote hoped).[33] At the same time, Sammy's parity with or superiority to whites undercuts the racial logic of the minstrel show. Sammy's maturation, from child to young man, contradicts one of the central tenets of minstrelsy (and the evolutionary discourse of the 1870s): the Negro race is in a state of arrested development, a race of children.

Sammy Tubbs, then, is both minstrel show and anti–minstrel show. An introductory illustration has Sammy and Sponsie on stage, commencing the performance, and references to minstrelsy are scattered throughout the text.[34] According to Eric Lott, the minstrel show originated as a working-class entertainment that "staged class" through "stale patter and bad

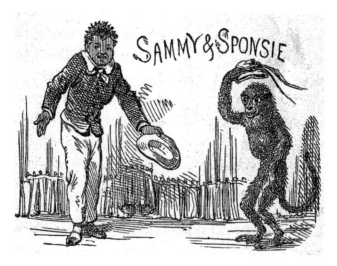

Figure 8.11. "The firm of S. & S.", *Sammy Tubbs*, 1 (1887): 23. Sammy and Sponsie are introduced on the minstrel show stage. Courtesy of the Department of Rare Books and Special Collections, University of Rochester Libraries.

puns and achieved grotesquerie . . . [,] sliding from racial burlesque into class affiliation or affirmation."[35] Minstrelsy was a technology of anti-self-making. The performance of "African"-ness licensed white performers to display ostentatious vulgarity—sexual innuendo, tumult, insult, dirtiness, lack of manners, grand and uncontrolled gestures—all in defiance of bourgeois gentility. Minstrel show players enacted the opposite of drawing-room refinement. Chaotic and undomesticated, the black body in such shows spoke a body language of slouching, stuttering, shuffling, and jerky motions and gait. Exaggerated lethargy alternated with undue speed—the perverse contrary of the predictable, disciplined middle-class body and the charted fixity of the anatomical body.

Blackface performances, Eric Lott tells us, "constantly deflated the pretensions of an emerging middle-class culture of science, reform, education, and professionalism."[36] Minstrel show "stump speeches" mocked bourgeois professors and reformers (and the obscurantist language of science), even as they ridiculed black people for their supposed inability to comprehend and correctly use scientific concepts: "psychological irrefragibility . . . is deribed from a profound contemplation ob de irregability ob dose incessimable divisions ob de more minute portions . . . dat become ana-tom-catically tattable in de circumambulatin commotion."[37] The minstrel show thus depicted science as legitimate—a sophisticated, technical body of knowledge that blacks were constitutionally de-

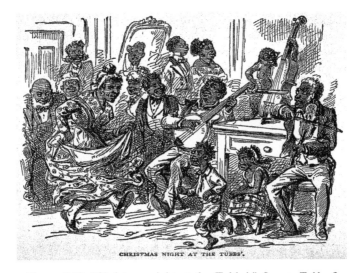

Figure 8.12. "Christmas night at the Tubbs'," *Sammy Tubbs*, 3 (1887): 224. The Tubbs family, dressed in their Sunday best, dance and assume the antic postures of minstrelsy; Sammy is not pictured but Sponsie avidly participates. Courtesy of the Department of Rare Books and Special Collections, University of Rochester Libraries.

barred from acquiring—and illegitimate—pretentious bourgeois double-talk.

Foote, who wanted to democratize medical science and use medical science to democratize society, found the minstrel show a congenial vehicle. No form had more appeal to children or working- and lower-middle-class audiences. But its deployment for moral and educational purposes, within the pages of a book of pedagogical juvenile fiction, contained and domesticated its wilder impulses:[38] anatomy, with its methodical, sober description of the penetration of the body, is the antithesis of minstrelsy's carnivalesque preoccupation with skin color and surface.[39] At the same time, readers were asked to identify with Sammy as the child protagonist and secondarily with the Negro, the child race: a chain of figuration that undercut the racial comedy. The moral was that if blacks can learn anatomy and become civilized by it, then so can white children: "Do not let a little black boy do better than you. Be sure, when you have finished reading these pages, that you know as much as he does of the human system." [2:15] However, the reverse also holds. If children can be taught anatomy, so can the "masses of the people" [2:75] and those members of society who discursively correspond to children: blacks, manual laborers, and, more ambiguously, women.

In this way Foote challenged the minstrel form. By series end, Sammy,

about to go to medical college, is the doctor's equal, morally equipped to
kiss Julia Barkenstir, a respectable white girl (is there another such scene
in nineteenth-century American fiction?); Dr. Winkles, a racist colleague
of Dr. Hubbs, has been publicly assaulted and humiliated for his efforts to
embarrass Sammy by appearing in blackface at Sammy's lecture.[40] The
characteristic disruptions of minstrelsy are displaced from Sammy to troublesome monkeys, other black characters, Irish and Italian immigrants,
native-born poor whites, even Dr. Winkles. Minstrelsy itself is disrupted by
Sammy, who confounds the stereotypical expectations of the genre at
every turn.

   The figure of the negro in minstrelsy, and nineteenth-century American culture generally, stands for the unregulated body, the unclean body,
and is also associated with fear of the body, particularly the dead body
and the spirits that inhabit it. In minstrel shows and popular entertainments, black people were typically portrayed as filthy, impulsive, intem-
perant, oversexed, overly sentimental, superstitious, and morbidly afraid
of cemeteries and medical schools with their dissecting rooms. Narratives
of black and Irish terror of the dead body circulated widely on the stage,
in popular fiction, and the press, as in this anecdote from an 1874 issue
of the *New York World*:

> Dr. Trenchard, of Greensburg, Pa., keeps a skeleton in a closet in his office
> . . . , a real bony preparation boiled and cleansed and hung on wires. A
> nigger on burglarious thoughts intent made his way into the office, and in
> the dim religious light thought he heard a noise, pulled open the closet-door
> and plunged in. Groping about with extended arms he disturbed some of the
> wires and the jaws of "the thing" closing upon his hand, he made out that he
> was in the grasp of death itself, shrieked for help, and fainted, in which
> condition he was found by Dr. Trenchard, who, with a constable's assistance,
> kindly released him.[41]

In such stories, the physician and the apparatus of anatomy invariably
personify the superiority of commanding reason over black and Irish
emotionalism, superstition, and fecklessness. Sammy's journey from racial
stereotype to universal human is predicated on his overcoming his fear of
the dead body and his emotions generally, including sentimental attachments. In a crucial scene in book 1, Sammy is confronted with two skeletons belonging to Dr. Hubbs and receives a lesson from the doctor on
dissection's importance in the epistemology and progress of medical science. The doctor's plan to dissect Sponsie (who they wrongly believe to
be dead) precipitates a moral crisis for Sammy:

> With all [Sammy's] attachment for the mischievous monkey he one moment
> felt that he could see him . . . dissected, . . . in order that he might know
> better how the machine . . . or the animal organism . . . was constructed. But,

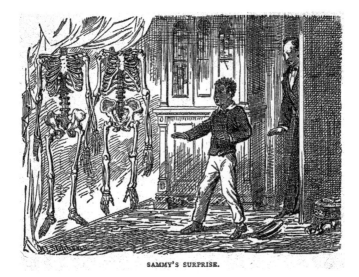

SAMMY'S SURPRISE.

Figure 8.13. "Sammy's surprise," *Sammy Tubbs*, 1 (1887): 64. The skeleton on the right is an ape's. Courtesy of the Department of Rare Books and Special Collections, University of Rochester Libraries.

quickly taking back this cruel thought, and putting in the place of it one which suggested that there might be monkeys already dead, whose bodies might be taken apart for his instruction, he mentally begged Sponsie's pardon for even thinking of making a subject of him. . . . [T]he remark of the Doctor as to what constitutes an anatomist popped into Sammy's mind: "Studying the formation of the human body in all its parts while dissecting it!" Is it quite so . . . that the doctors ever cut folks up? This thought made him involuntarily shiver. . . . He tried the best he could to go to sleep. (1:36–37)

Sammy is an emancipatory figure precisely because he works against stereotype. After an uneasy night, the "little anatomist" overcomes his attachment to Sponsie and his aversion to the dead body: "them is only dead bones and can't hurt nobody" (the last time he talks in anything approaching dialect) (1:66). After this decisive moment, Sammy begins to develop clinical detachment and appropriates the dead body's power and mystique for himself: he learns to perform a disinterested inventory of his own skeleton—"two hundred and sixty bones" (1:125)—and determines that he has "the heart to cut up Sponsie's body" (1:71). His pet monkey (Sponsie 1), in contrast, is terrified of the doctor's two skeletons (1:70–71) and ultimately ends up on the dissecting table.

In nineteenth-century racial discourse, blackness was a powerful contaminant, like the decomposing dead body, a form of "social death" (a phrase William Wells Brown coined to describe slavery).[42] Novels, minstrel show skits, and newspapers stereotypically represented black people as the dissected rather than dissectors (and, in fact, blacks involuntarily supplied a disproportionate number of subjects for medical school dissecting tables), as outcaste bodysnatchers rather than anatomists, and (paradoxically) as superstitiously afraid of the dead rather than scientific.[43] In turning this pattern on its head for laughs, Foote makes a serious moral argument, geared to the highly charged racial politics of Reconstruction-era America: black people can be taught to be dissectors.[44] Anatomical dissection is a democratic technology for the making of self. In overcoming his fear of the dead body and attaining anatomical knowledge, Sammy overcomes the stigma attached to the black body.

This black body, according to Eric Lott, is powerful, an Other, but "contained by representation, by imitation" (in the same way as the human body in *Sammy Tubbs* is powerful and contained by anatomical outlining).[45] But unlike the minstrel show, with its critique of bourgeois pretension and absolute "othering" of blacks, Foote aims to bourgeoisify the non-bourgeois, in the most extreme instance, black people. His universalist method of self-making centers around anatomical dissection as a civilizing epistemology. To be human is to dissect the body, the "animal organism": Sammy signifies his humanity by dissecting a frog, a dog, and (standing in for humanity) the two monkeys. (It should be noted that, Foote's universalism notwithstanding, bourgeois identity (like racial identity) still requires Others: the Irish, Italians, black people (other than Sammy), "monstrosities." Above all, animals and the body figure the anti-bourgeois Other negatively, even as children do positively.)

Dissection, a kind of critical deconstruction of the body, becomes then the constitutive operation of spirit, a triumph of mind over obdurate matter, a means of empowerment. Dissection breaks the skin and penetrates to the body's essential core. The dissector surveys the body's topography, mines the body for meaning, inscribes boundaries, and names various regions and formations. Anatomical terminology takes on an almost magical significance. Children in particular, Foote continually preached, must learn the technical nomenclature, the Greek and Latin terms for the parts, including the sexual parts, the vagina, clitoris, penis, etc.[46] The anatomical procedure of penetrating, dividing, and naming is a mental discipline, an inner performance. More than a metaphor, dissection is both a model of analysis and an embodiment: one knows and controls one's body, as national, colonial, and imperial powers know and control the world, by cutting it apart into clearly named, bounded, and regulated regions, and by enforcing local, regional, and super-regional laws conducive to social and hygienic utility. As Sammy learns and lectures on human anatomy, the reader is encouraged to perform an imaginary self-vivisection. Anatomy/analysis empowers human subjects to act on the world and themselves—as animals cannot—in order to become fully human.

Dissection is also one of the foundational performances through which medical authority is established. Early on in the proceedings, Dr. Hubbs teaches Sammy the history of anatomy as the triumphant struggle of medical progress against superstition and prejudice.[47] In this millennial narrative, dissection takes on the character of a sacrament, a civic ritual. Everyone should dissect, especially school children. Everyone should offer themselves up for dissection—a medical imitation of Christ. To be taken apart on the dissecting table is not an ignominious death but a noble sacrifice for the progress of humanity. Democracy and morality require that the dissector willingly offers himself up for dissection. Foote cited approvingly the case of William Byrd Powell, a Kentucky phrenologist whose request that his brain be dissected after his death was honored only after his survivors took the case to court.[48]

"SIDE BY SIDE IN THE LOWER PORTIONS OF THE TRUNK": DEATH, SPIRIT, AND THE ANATOMICAL BODY

The discussion of dissection, like everything else in *Sammy Tubbs*, figures as a coded meditation on relations between mind and body, and their social and moral corollaries, but in a few spots Foote explicitly theorizes the spirit/matter dichotomy. In those passages, he is inconsistent, or maybe undecided, as to how he should theorize the cohabitation of spirit and matter in the human body. In the first book, Dr. Hubbs tells Sammy that the body without spirit is dead, "no more to us than the shell is to the tortoise" (1:172). In some passages he equates electricity or "animal magnetism" with spirit itself, but mostly describes it as a medium: mind/spirit animates the body through "galvanism": "the mind sets in motion a wave of animal magnetism upon those muscles it desires to contract" (1:164).

In the fourth book, Foote stages a full-blown rehearsal of the mid-1870s debate over materialism in the form of a dialogue between Sammy and Dr. Hubbs. Foote evidently was struggling with the issue, but felt constrained to respect the boundaries set by his liberal evangelical allies: materialism was much more heretical than racial radicalism. Citing Fernand Papillon's "Physiology of the Passions," Hubbs argues that "the brain is the centre of passional as well as of intellectual phenomena," but that "nothing can be found in the nervous ganglia or brain to fully account for them," and so there must exist "a psychic faculty or soul" (4:78–79). (This in reply to the "too materialistic" Ludwig Buchner who argued that "the peculiar function of the brain is to secrete thought, just as it is the function of the liver to secrete bile" [4:79].) Hubbs concludes: "Thus does science ever lead us back to that eternal and mysterious thing we call force, and, beyond force, to that which we call spirit" (4:81–82).

But a page later, Sammy has the last word and argues for the materiality of thought: "the brain is an organ . . . [that] seems to have a way of working up into ideas the food it extracts from the blood which in turn has had its supper from the food received by the stomach." Thoughts, Sammy says, are a material part of the bodily economy; according to T. H. Huxley "every word uttered by a speaker cost him so much bodily loss." The set piece on materialism ends, unconvincingly, with Hubbs's assertion that Huxley and Papillon "can be easily reconciled" (4:82–83), but Foote never tells how.

Here, as elsewhere in the text, the untheorized entity is medical authority itself. Medical authority floats above the text as a disembodied voice that is both spirit and privileged mediator *between* spirit and matter. By mastering the body, by dissecting, naming, narrating, and regulating the parts and translating them into text, the anatomist sets himself up above and outside bodily existence. The body can then be assessed according to utilitarian principles, for the convenience of the mind/anatomist, without superstitious awe or obfuscating sentiment; reason is the moral principle. The body is nothing more than a "complicated mechanism" regulated by the brain (here characterized as "the most wonderful telegraphic station on earth" [4:199]) via the nervous system: "the pneumogastric nerve reaches down from the skull . . . , much as the arm of the engineer reaches out to the levers, valves, etc., of an engine, and exercises more or less of a guiding power" (4:202–03).[49] Mind and the physician are discursively identified with each other: both survey, operate and regulate the body.

But in the fifth book, Foote describes another, more dynamic, relationship between matter and spirit, between death and life, that derives from contemporary physiology and cellular pathology: "death and life lie side by side in the lower portions of the trunk" (5:192–93). Death is no longer an absolute condition—and certainly not the moral conclusion of the life narrative—but rather an ongoing process, intrinsic to life. Dr. Hubbs tells Sammy that:

"Particles of matter are all the time dying in your body, and fresh ones are as constantly taking their places, when you are in a condition of health. Some physiologists say that we change our bodies completely as often as once in seven years. I think that some active ones change theirs much oftener, while more sluggish people do not change theirs so often."

"Then," said Sammy, with a look of surprise, "the body I was born with has been buried, and in smaller pieces and more places than if it had been cut up by the physicians!"

"[Y]ou are right. . . . The body with which you were born has . . . died in instalments. . . . The old body, while undergoing the process of dissolution, produced the blood of which your new body has been rebuilt. If you live, your present body must undergo a similar change until every particle of bone, muscle and flesh which is in you to-day, will pass away, giving place to new matter altogether." (2:25–27)

This notion of "the daily dying body" (5:40) is congenial to the project of self formation. Enterprising, anatomically educated people can quickly remake themselves in their entirety by adherence to physiological laws of improvement. And if the body is a delicate economy of continuous construction and destruction, full of "microscopic beings" and forces (5:62), then the need for anatomical and physiological knowledge—and professional guidance and intervention—becomes paramount.

Such notions attenuate the distinction between the contaminating dead body and living body, between pathology and physiology, between matter and spirit. "Waste matters" (urine and feces) and cadavers, Foote argues, should be a problem of sanitary management and aesthetics, requiring efficient action, not dread, grief, and avoidance: "There is nothing herein of an uncleanly nature. But because [bodily wastes] are dead matters they must be put out of sight with as much care as the beautiful corpse of a deceased friend, for they will undergo changes which are not agreeable to our senses" (5:200).[50] Anatomical embodiment decontaminates the dead body (as it does the black body). Thus a potentially universalizing component emerges for the reader: We (the bourgeois "we") are all in part black (animal, uncivilized); we are all in part dead (or continuously dying), with contaminants constantly circulating within our bodies. This is no longer popular anatomy, a boundary-making practice, but a popular physiology that at least potentially leads toward the overcoming of ontological and social boundaries.

"Morbid Mandates": The Problem of Desire

There is then a recuperation of animism. The body is not an inanimate robot operated by outside forces, but rather the site of multiple agencies and complex interactions, "like a huge ant-hill, full of insect life" (3:109): "each distant part makes known its wants to the brain; and though the latter like a good ventriloquist makes the call for food appear to come from the stomach, there is no question but that complaints from the parts suffering from starvation are first reported to the Capitol of the Nervous System" (3:78). All parts (animal and vegetable) should defer to the brain, but in book 5 (on sexuality and "elimination") the problem of chaos arises. The multiplicity and speed of bodily transactions evoke the accelerating technologies and increasing complexity and productivity of postbellum society, modernity itself. By sheer accumulation of anatomical detail, the body is revved up, productive but careening out of control.

According to Foote, positive sexual desire—"awakened by a worthy and attractive object"—originates in the brain, not the groin. But there is a repression hypothesis: denial of this "natural excitement" leads to "sexual starvation," a blockage that causes a reversal of flow. Sexual impulses travel "from the feverishly active secretory tissues upward through the nerve-tracts, to inflame and brutalize the mind" (5:113), a state of animalistic "unnatural excitement" (5:185). The human organism is then plunged into anarchy or insurrection, leading to venereal diseases or the disease of masturbation (which undoes the internal economy of the nervous system). The moral reconstruction of the body depends on the restoration of the mind's authority over the body. For an individual to be truly human, the internal chain of command must flow from top to bottom, from mind to groin:

> [T]o render man's sexual characteristics distinct from those of lower animals, . . . men and women must be drawn together in the performance of the reproductive function by an impulse proceeding from the psychic faculty telegraphing its message of love downward, rather than by an impulse originating in starving, congested, and overloaded ovaries and testes telegraphing their morbid mandates upward. Till a new and regenerate humanity is born, it were well if all relations between the sexes could be made fruitless . . . by carefully intercepting the union of the germ-cell and sperm-cell by judicious means of prevention. (5:113–14)

Thus, though the larger narrative ends triumphantly with Sammy's coming of age, a contrapuntal uneasiness enters in: the body, like the nation-state, capitalist economy, and social hierarchy, is precarious, easily disordered and sickened. This bodily disorder, moreover, has external social consequences. Through a Lamarckian evolutionary transformation, moral turpitude, intemperance, and undisciplined sexual desire shape future generations biologically, producing "monstrosities, physical and moral" (5:211). Such "human weeds" (5:230) are resistant to anatomical embodiment and physiological morality, contemptuous of bourgeois niceties.[51] Sexual desire therefore requires not suppression, which only further destabilizes the body, but constant self-scrutiny and regulation (and contraception!), until the physiological millennium, which by Foote's reckoning will take awhile, "two or three centuries" (5:112–13).

The discussion of sexuality centers on the problem of desire as a matter of self-regulation—but at the same time picks up a powerful, though unacknowledged, erotic charge through its violation of the taboo on public discussion and representation of explicitly sexual topics. This erotic effect exceeds the design of the narrative, which confines undisciplined desire

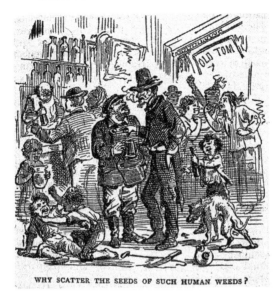

WHY SCATTER THE SEEDS OF SUCH HUMAN WEEDS?

Figure 8.14. "Why scatter the seeds of such human weeds?" *Sammy Tubbs*, 5 (1887): 230. Courtesy of the Department of Rare Books and Special Collections, University of Rochester Libraries.

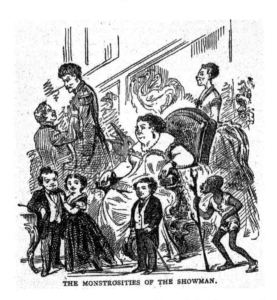

THE MONSTROSITIES OF THE SHOWMAN.

Figure 8.15. "The monstrosities of the showman," *Sammy Tubbs*, 5 (1887): 213. The dysgenic consequences of undisciplined desire. Courtesy of the Department of Rare Books and Special Collections, University of Rochester Libraries.

to Sponsie and other supporting characters. Sammy is always polite and judicious, ever ready to defer and subordinate the gratification of his desires. His libido is channeled into a passion for anatomy, physiology, and especially dissection. But this takes on a sexually inflected urgency—"I can't bear the idea of seeing Sponsie brought home dead . . . but if he really is dead, I want his body to dissect" (1:170)—and has sexual, and racial, consequences: Sammy's mastery of the body arouses the admiration of young women of both races. The ostensible moral of the interracial love affair at the end of book 5 is that physiologically regulated, rationalized sexuality can overcome an irrational and unjust social taboo, but here again desire overflows its banks: Sammy and Julia Barkenstir's kiss packed a wallop for nineteenth-century readers. H. L. Stephens's uncaptioned illustration (a love that dare not speak its name) alludes to this reception by including a set of eyes peering at the two lovers through Venetian blinds.

THE ANATOMICAL STATUS OF WOMEN

This raises a final textual problem: the ambiguous status of women in *Sammy Tubbs*. Foote, a self-identified feminist, called for "able women to adorn all the professions," including medicine.[52] Yet middle-class females are excluded from the male fraternity of dissectors in *Sammy Tubbs*, figuring as passive spectators, comic relief, and love interests. (Nonbourgeois females are active but disruptive and prey to the disfiguring vices of men; their "intemperance" and "indelicacy" fix their lower-class status and make them eligible for eugenical management.) Notwithstanding Sammy's efforts to instruct the ladies and Hubbs's support of women's right to dissect, dissection has in *Sammy Tubbs* a masculinist coloring that cuts against the feminist grain. Anatomy is something that men do together. The book's strongest relationship is between men, Sammy and Dr. Hubbs, and even the creatures that Sammy dissects are male. More generally, the positive value attached to dissection draws on anatomy's larger cultural identification with phallic, "sharp-edged," analytical wit and manly "masterful" intellect.

Foote identifies women, like black people, with the body, but the bourgeois female body is not a contaminant but sacralized—a potential object of desire rather than a corrupt and desiring subject. Like the child races of evolutionary discourse, women are categorically infantile, characteristically associated with innocently undisciplined desire and impulse. And like the child races, women stand in need of anatomical embodiment, but for very different reasons: the analogy between women, children, and child races no longer holds. Women suffer from diseases of overcivilization—Mrs. Hubbs, the doctor's wife, has a "nervous condition." Their

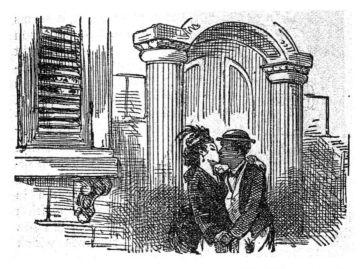

Figure 8.16. Uncaptioned, *Sammy Tubbs*, 5 (1876): 203; perhaps the first positive representation of an interracial kiss in nineteenth-century American illustrated fiction. Foote believed that robust hybrids would result from interracial mixture; the progeny would have the best qualities of both races. Other eugenicists accepted this logic but their idea of an acceptable interracial hybrid was a Scottish-English mix; most eugenicists strongly condemned black-white couplings as leading to degeneration. Courtesy of Florida State University Library.

bodies are overdisciplined but underdeveloped, and their sensibility is correspondingly overdeveloped. They are forced (or choose) to wear restrictive clothes; they are denied (or choose to forgo) physical exercise; they are coerced into sexual acts or denied sexual pleasure (or deny themselves). Unlike other discursive categories identified with child and body (black, Irish, working class, animal), women suffer from repression of the body, a repression enforced by institutions like the church and marriage, but also through women's own self-inflicted conformity to social convention and fashion.

Sammy's anatomy and physiology lectures (and a corollary program of gymnastic exercise), then, are calculated to have a reverse effect on his female audience, endowing them with a rigorous anatomical consciousness of the body to counterbalance the oversensitive, but undisciplined feminine mind. Foote believed such instruction especially necessary as a step toward rationalizing (though not desacralizing) the female body and sexuality. Anatomical self-making in *Sammy Tubbs* functions as a critique of the female culture of consumption, a highly problematic domain for the bourgeois self, the realm of pleasure for pleasure's sake, pleasure

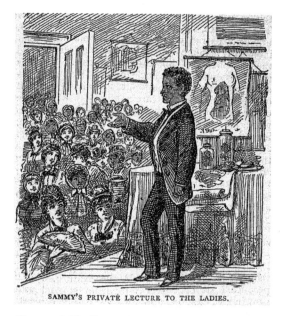

SAMMY'S PRIVATE LECTURE TO THE LADIES.

Figure 8.17. "Sammy's private lecture to the ladies," *Sammy Tubbs*, 5 (1887): 199. Courtesy of the Department of Rare Books and Special Collections, University of Rochester Libraries.

without reason. Anatomical knowledge also functions as a kind of empowerment, enabling women to resist or regulate their own frivolous desires and more importantly intemperate male sexual desire—and to prevent the dire eugenic consequences of such intemperance. At stake is nothing less than the biological production of humanity and the progress of "civilization," "the moral and physical redemption of the human race" (5:211). Such notions won Foote a large female readership, if the testimonial letters published in *Foote's Health Monthly* are any indication.[53] They also worked to expand the field of female sexuality as a medical domain, establishing the physician as an authority, in competition with husbands and fathers, the church, the state, and nonphysiological cultural critics, foremost among them "Brother Comstock."

"HIGHLY COMMENDED":
THE RECEPTION OF *SAMMY TUBBS*

From the foregoing discussion it should be clear that *Sammy Tubbs* is an extraordinary work. How did it do? The answer is: at first, fairly well. A promotional advertisement that ran regularly in the *Health Monthly* touted books 1 through 4 as "Highly Commended by The N.Y. Independent, Beecher's Christian Union, Mother's Magazine, Moore's Rural New Yorker, N.Y. Graphic, Medical Eclectic, Domestic Monthly, N.Y. Daily Times, World, Evening Express, Commercial Advertiser, Church Union, Talmage's Christian at Work, N.Y. Methodist, Chicago Inter-Ocean, Cleveland Leader, Pomeroy's Democrat and more than 200 other first-class papers"—mainly the liberal, greenback, and evangelical press.[54]

This approbation did not, however, extend to book 5. The *New York Independent*, the popular religious newspaper that fellow-traveled with the physiological movement, endorsed the first four volumes, but "question[ed] the advisability" of providing instruction on the topic of sex to children in the yet-to-be published fifth volume, "since information" on the subject could "be better given by judicious parent than by any printed words."[55] The *Independent* and Henry Ward Beecher's *Christian Union* declined to review volume five. And this seems to have been the general pattern: the *New York Times* warmly praised the first four books of *Sammy Tubbs*, but never reviewed the fifth. After his 1876 arrest by Comstock, the *Times* dismissed Foote as a "quack doctor" and ally of "abortionists" (even though Foote vehemently opposed abortion).[56] Comstock's campaign against the free-love wing of the physiological movement—and the movement's own accelerating radicalism, of which the last book of *Sammy Tubbs* is only one example—worked to fracture the physiological-evangelical alliance.[57] In the December 1876 issue of *Health Monthly*, Foote boasted that a "Western clergyman" had placed *Sammy Tubbs* in his "Sabbath School Library," but also noted that an offer of the books as a premium to subscribers by the publisher of "a popular religious paper . . . gave offence in some prudish quarters."[58] Given such difficulties, Foote could take solace in the fact that, by his own reckoning, the series sold more than 25,000 volumes the first year (book 5 came out early the next year) and in succeeding years "held its own." The series stayed in print for more than 25 years. Ultimately, however, sales disappointed, never matching his big sellers, *Medical Common Sense* and *Plain Home Talk*.[59]

Sammy Tubbs was a money-making venture and probably turned a profit. But Foote rarely let the bottom line stand in the way of cultural politicking. Even if the profits from the sale of sex education materials outweighed the dangers of public censure and prosecution—an arguable proposition in this period—a more commercially calculating author would not have larded the series with sermons on the politics of medical licensure, interracial breeding, and so on, and certainly would have avoided explicit anatomical diagrams in a book ostensibly aimed at ten- to fifteen-year-olds. The transgressive fifth volume, then, should be seen as part of Foote's public performance as a social critic, a shot across the bow that bolstered his radical credentials. He could not have been surprised, and may even have been pleased, that it inflamed the opposition. But he must have been disappointed with the press's determination to overlook it. Upstaged by Comstock's 1876 arrest of Foote for selling a pamphlet on birth control through the U.S. Mail, book 5 hardly made a stir.[60]

As we have seen, sexual radicalism was always a potential theme of popular anatomical discourse. The natural laws of the body could model and enforce social hierarchies, but they also could render external disciplinary forces unnecessary, thereby empowering the individual and destabilizing the existing social order. And if anatomy and physiology, like geography, were to become part of the curriculum that produced bourgeois social identity, there were troublesome questions absent from geography: how much of the body should be taught, how should it be taught, to whom, and for what purpose? Should children, women, the lower classes and races be taught anatomy? Who should be allowed to dissect, to have "unmediated" knowledge of the body? Who should be allowed to view anatomically detailed representations of the body?

Unlike geography, the body had forbidden zones. "Respectable" anatomy and physiology texts for women, children, or "the public" omitted mention of sexuality, or heavily coded them through euphemisms and discussion of flower reproduction. Foote sent up this genre in the original edition by presenting an illustration of the "reproductive organs of the morning-glory" next to illustrations of an anthropomorphized singing vagina (a musical note hovers over it) and an erect penis. In nineteenth-century pedagogical anatomy, the space between the legs was left blank, a *terra incognita*, or placed entirely outside the pictorial frame; sexual anatomy was denied representation.[61] Like the pornography of the *ancien regime*, the breaching of taboos on the public discussion and representation of sexual organs—especially in the domain of formal education for children—signified an attack on the authority of the state, religion, and fathers and husbands (and more ambiguously professional authority). On this terrain most physiologists stepped carefully, fearful of repercussions.[62]

Foote's position (delivered by Dr. Hubbs), however, was unequivocal: "The text-books for the common school I would so revise as to have them take in and explain all the organs and functions of the body, not omitting those through which humanity enters the world" (5:224). Foote even made a timid gesture toward the pleasure principle (an even more dangerous topic; hence he assigned the words to Sammy):

> "All our functions . . . seem to have been so devised that when our bodily health is perfect their performance is attended with a sense of pleasure. . . .

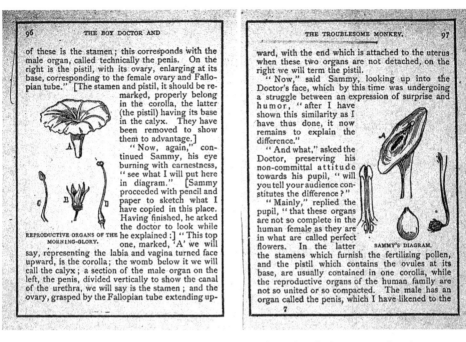

96   THE BOY DOCTOR AND

of these is the stamen; this corresponds with the male organ, called technically the penis. On the right is the pistil, with its ovary, enlarging at its base, corresponding to the female ovary and Fallopian tube." [The stamen and pistil, it should be remarked, properly belong in the corolla, the latter (the pistil) having its base in the calyx. They have been removed to show them to advantage.]

"Now, again," continued Sammy, his eye burning with earnestness, "see what I will put here in diagram." [Sammy proceeded with pencil and paper to sketch what I have copied in this place. Having finished, he asked the doctor to look while he explained:] "This top one, marked, 'A' we will say, representing the labia and vagina turned face upward, is the corolla; the womb below it we will call the calyx; a section of the male organ on the left, divided vertically to show the canal of the urethra, we will say is the stamen; and the ovary, grasped by the Fallopian tube extending up-

REPRODUCTIVE ORGANS OF THE MORNING-GLORY.

97   THE TROUBLESOME MONKEY.

ward, with the end which is attached to the uterus when these two organs are not detached, on the right we will term the pistil.

"Now," said Sammy, looking up into the Doctor's face, which by this time was undergoing a struggle between an expression of surprise and humor, "after I have shown this similarity as I have thus done, it now remains to explain the difference."

"And what," asked the Doctor, preserving his non-committal attitude towards his pupil, "will you tell your audience constitutes the difference?"

"Mainly," replied the pupil, "that these organs are not so complete in the human female as they are in what are called perfect flowers. In the latter the stamens which furnish the fertilizing pollen, and the pistil which contains the ovules at its base, are usually contained in one corolla, while the reproductive organs of the human family are not so united or so compacted. The male has an organ called the penis, which I have likened to the

SAMMY'S DIAGRAM.

7

Figure 8.18. "Reproductive organs of the morning glory," the conventional way to graphically represent human sexuality through flower anatomy, and "Sammy's diagram," Foote's send-up of the genre; 5 (1876): 96–97 in some 1874 imprint editions. Courtesy of Florida State University Library.

> So, too, the function of reproduction is one attended with highly pleasurable emotions, provided the organs used in its performance have not been injured by self-induced excitation . . . , or by excesses, or by neglect." (5:183–84)

However, in deference to the legal and social difficulties that such a commitment entailed, in some editions Foote omitted the anatomically explicit diagrams of penis and vagina, and in others omitted the erect penis and singing vagina, or omitted both.[63] Foote self-referentially anticipated the problem in the written text, using a dialogue between Dr. Hubbs and Sammy to present the issue, as he does elsewhere when discussing the almost-as-transgressive topic of materialism. And in this case, as in other parts where he playfully argues with himself, Foote has Sammy act as the spokesman for the radical position. The boy-anatomist makes the traditional flower sexuality analogy explicit by drawing human genitalia (the illustration captioned "Sammy's Diagram"), while Dr. Hubbs frets over the political consequences: "'Why, Sammy, you surprise me! I fear you are going to undertake more than you will clearly be able to perform,' replied the Doctor, with an anxious countenance. '*I think I would hardly feel bold enough to lay out such a programme for myself if I were to stand in your place. . . . Be careful, my boy, that you do not impair your growing popularity by some injudicious or inconsiderate step*' " [my emphasis].[64]

From our perspective, the irony is that, though critics branded Foote an advocate of free love (in fact he was more of a fellow-traveler of the free-love movement), he espoused an obsessively regulated sexuality that in many ways reinforced conventional morality. *Sammy Tubbs*—for all its radicalism—can be considered a representative text, part of a collective project to anatomically embody, and discipline, "the masses of people." Notwithstanding the book's prolific idiosyncrasies, stock popular anatomical arguments and stock anatomical illustrations crop up in every section—directly lifted from predecessor popular anatomies or common sources.[65]

In the postbellum era medical professors and reformers continued to campaign for the wide dispersion of a moral anatomy and physiology that would educate and uplift the northern working class, women, emancipated slaves, and young people, and that would forestall the emergence of sexual desire and social unrest.[66] Sarah Hackett Stevenson, a professor of obstetrics at the Women's Medical College of Chicago, argued that "In human development there are two essentials, matter and method—anatomy and training. . . . This is the way in which man conquers the world."[67] Instruction in the internal boundaries and functions of the body was seen as a form of self-discipline, a scientific legitimation of, and adjunct to, temperance and other reforms. Anatomical dissection, far from being butchery as its opponents insisted, was the quintessential epistemology of scientific, "civilized" man, a systematic and careful division and reduction of the material world, a triumph of mind over matter, reason over emotion, an exemplary method of analysis.

Although the millennial, perfectionist hopes of the physiological movement went unrealized, at Foote's funeral in 1907, T. B. Wakeman made this assessment of Foote's contribution:

Text books on Physiology, Hygiene, Alcohol, etc., are now considered necessary in all schools of public and general education. Lectures and publications and private instruction have followed to such an extent that a person who does not now know more on these subjects than most doctors did fifty years ago is not intelligent or no longer considered so. How far this wonderful change from popular ignorance to intelligence has been due to Dr. Foote, the circulation of nearly a million of his works, large and small, goes far to show. In the Americas, Europe, Asia, and even Africa and the Isles, wherever civilization has gained a footing, it has seemed that . . . Dr. Foote's health books were sure to follow.[68]

Wakeman's appraisal of Foote's influence is undoubtedly exaggerated, but the cultural transition it marks is not. Whatever the reception of *Sammy Tubbs*, during the span of Foote's career a vast swath of humanity adopted some version of anatomical personhood.

CONCLUSION: EVERY MAN HIS OWN ANATOMIST

I have argued that the anatomical body was a "civilized," domesticated body: disciplined by physiological regulations, as bounded as the nineteenth-century bourgeois home, front porch, and picket-fenced yard. Purified of the stigma of carnality, of proliferating flesh and corruption, the innards were figured within a medicalized aesthetics and subjected to utilitarian principles. It was this social identity that Foote sought to market, a low-cost technology of self-fashioning—even as he attacked exclusionary, hierarchical, and coercive tendencies within bourgeois ideology. His emphasis on self-regulation against state and religious compulsion led opponents, both within and without the cultural reform movement, to accuse him of physiological antinomianism.[69] In this, they had some, but only some, justification. Foote urged only a relaxation or revision of social discipline (dress, diet, sexual activity and discussion of sexuality, etc.)—the internalization and rationalization of disciplinary morality—but opened the door for more thoroughgoing critiques.

More confusingly, opponents lumped radical physiology with elements of mass commercial culture—pornography and sensationalism—that resisted or ignored bourgeois social discipline and appropriated anatomical discourse for their own purposes. The connection is not fanciful: Foote's medical entrepreneurialism was only a rung up the ladder from the suspect physicians who ran anatomy museums to advertise practices in the treatment of venereal disease and "spermatorrhea" (also Foote's specialties). A rung below these were the purely sensational, entertainment museums with their displays of naked bodies, horrific diseases, freaks, and medieval torture that reinstated the connection between butchery and dissection and reversed the privilege of mind over body. (Popular anatomical museums are discussed at length in the next chapter.)

Like other middle-class reformers, Foote called for a bounded capitalism that philanthropized the worthy poor and sequestered privileged spheres of home, body, and professions from the market. He too attacked the frivolity, indiscipline, and moral corruption of unbridled commerce and consumerism; he shared and extended the antebellum reformers' opposition to prostitution and slavery, their advocacy of dress reform versus fashion, and diet reform versus gluttony. But Foote was also a creature of the market economy, a subversive capitalist who commercialized sexual advice, fertility regulation, and medicine. He capitalized on the demand created by taboos and social barriers, even as he called for their overthrow or rationalization.

His critique of regular therapeutics, the monopolization of medical knowledge, and exclusionary licensure legislation, his openness to knowledge claims coming from outside the medical establishment—above all, his willingness to challenge social and cultural conventions of race and gender—were genuinely oppositional. However, his physiological radicalism was always more ambivalent than his enemies would allow. *Sammy Tubbs* is studded with citations from Agassiz, Cuvier, Harvey, Oliver Wendell Holmes, Sr., etc.—hardly icons of subversion. Foote legitimated himself in large part by his display of familiarity with authoritative medical texts. Such texts, highly technical and often written in foreign languages, were unintelligible to the lay public. Foote presented himself to his mass readership as an indispensable intermediary, even as he argued that such knowledge should be accessible to all.[70] As one might expect, in citing such canonical works, Foote just as often buttressed the social (and medical) order as undermined it (and even in opposition, Foote was often more argumentative than revolutionary). If the battle cry of critics of the medical profession had long been "every man his own physician," Foote and his physiological colleagues added two twists: "every man his own anatomist" and "every man his own anatomical subject."[71] But his egalitarian anatomy actually instated medical authority at a much more fundamental level than his opponents ever imagined—the embodied self. Foote imagined a social universe of self-disciplined anatomical subjects, ordered within a rationalized hierarchy based on the distinction between "the animal plane of development" and "the human" (5:112), dissected and dissector. This anatomical self naturalized (but also revised) the social order, authorizing the physiologist as cultural critic and technocratic arbiter of self, racial, sexual, class, and professional boundaries.

The nineteenth-century bourgeoisie, of course, expended much energy in constructing and patrolling such boundaries, as evidenced by calling cards, guest lists, private social clubs, and professional accreditation, as well as by racial anatomy. Bourgeois culture was obsessed by the idea of social and natural taxonomies and zones (remember Sammy's original employment by Dr. Hubbs as a door-tender). In claiming authority in matters anatomical and physiological, Foote set himself up as a privileged surveyor and crosser of boundaries—the boundaries between sickness and health, white and black, the living and the dead, male and female, animal and human, pleasure and obligation, savagery and civilization, private and public discourse, doctor and patient, learned profession and trade. Such claims licensed Foote to carry on a lucrative business in advice literature, remedies, contraceptive devices—and earned him a small fortune.

Foote then was a paradoxical figure, a critic of bourgeois social pretension and privilege who made a successful career as a retailer of authoritative physiological advice on the acquisition and maintenance of bourgeois identity. His politics and methodology of self-making, his solution to the problem of social identity and difference in a democratic society, was an egalitarian expression of a consolidating anatomical consensus. In the last quarter of the nineteenth century, anatomical embodiment decisively prevailed: the anatomical body became the modern body. But the building of a radical, universalizing political project based on anatomical embodiment was fraught with difficulties. Opposition came from within the bourgeoisie, from Anthony Comstock and his allies, but also from the American Humane Association and its 1895 campaign against dissection and vivisection in the schools.[72] If Foote defined humanity as mastery over the animal body, most powerfully signified through the metaphor of the dissected animal, antivivisection defined humanity by an empathic fellowship with animals, and a refusal to dissect. Antivivisectionism, and to a lesser degree antivaccinationism, posed immense difficulties for Foote's project—both movements had largely female and liberal middle-class followings that overlapped Foote's own. Despite his medical scientism, he was forced to adopt a fellow-traveling, conciliatory tone toward antivaccination and called for limits on vivisection.[73]

At the same time, Foote's egalitarian anatomy was contradicted by the undemocratic practice of late-nineteenth-century medicine. Many poor people, especially blacks and the Irish, continued to fear dissection and resist anatomical embodiment, with good reason: In the 1870s and 1880s the medical establishment exploited a succession of body-snatching scandals to secure the passage of state anatomy laws consigning the bodies of the indigent poor to medical schools—laws which Foote also advocated. In a society that placed great emphasis on the importance of a "decent burial," such measures were seen as a posthumous punishment for poverty and lower-class (social and racial) status.[74] Equally problematic for non-whites, immigrants, and the poor was the emerging science of eugenics—vigorously promoted by Foote in *Sammy Tubbs* and elsewhere—which naturalized difference and inequality through its proliferating taxonomies, and which served to expand state and professional power over "deviant" or "unevolved" races and social categories. And, finally, within the medical profession itself, a reform movement was gathering force that would have profoundly undemocratic consequences: the exclusion of unorthodox practitioners, women, and blacks from medical school and the dissecting room, in the name of improved educational standards.

9

"Anatomy Out of Gear"

POPULAR ANATOMY AT THE MARGINS IN
LATE-NINETEENTH-CENTURY AMERICA

> [T]he side shows . . . depend upon some morbid relish
> of the public. Abominations, congenital or artificial, are
> their specialties: five-legged *quadrumans*, double-headed
> hybrids, human abortions, diseased men and women,
> are here held up to view on the supposition that it must
> pay, because everywhere else in the world these things
> are hidden by pity and decency. The things themselves,
> . . . when finally overtaken by death, are by no means
> released from the fate of exhibition. They are then pre-
> pared for a permanent display in the Anatomical Mu-
> seum, and will continue to smile, ghastly and horribly, in
> alcohol or glass case, to the new crowds who feed the
> same appetite with a pathological excuse.
>
> "CHEAP AMUSEMENTS," *The (New York) World,*
> 4–5–1868: 3

A SHORT ACCOUNT of the campaign against anatomy museums appears in the *New York Tribune* of 10 January 1888. In the early days of the new year, a police inspector walked around the Bowery "and casually dropped into all the places that had . . . gaudy signs . . . that told the wayfarer . . . there were human monsters of all kinds within, that could be inspected for the small sum of ten cents." In most places, the "ordinary museums," Inspector Williams found nothing objectionable, but when he entered an "anatomical museum," the Egyptian Musée, "he was startled to see on every hand wax figures of both men and women without any clothes on . . . grouped so as to show the anatomy of the human body." Continuing down the Bowery, Williams came upon another anatomical establishment, the European Museum, "where he saw a figure in the window about to be cut up with hundreds of knives, representing a method of old time torture" and where inside "the things on exhibition brought the blush of modesty to his cheek."[1] The Inspector then cut short his investigation in order to consult with Anthony Comstock, leader of the New York Society for the Suppression of Vice. On 9 January 1888, warrants were issued against the aforementioned Egyptian Musée and European Museum, plus the Parisian Museum and Kahn's Museum of Anatomy—"all the so-called anatomical museums" not connected to the city's "recognized medical colleges."[2] Between 4:00 and 8:00 p.m., the police, assisted by the Society for the Suppression of Vice, mounted raids against the museums. The proprietors and employees were arrested, fourteen men in all, and charged with "exhibiting obscene figures and images." The "hideous specimens," including some "five or six van loads of female figures in wax and clay," were confiscated, and most of them later destroyed.[3]

The popular anatomical museum, a once familiar part of American urban life, is now little known outside a small circle of curators and collectors. Inspired by the success of commercial medical museums in Britain and France, popular anatomical museums sprouted in New York in the 1840s and later in Boston, Philadelphia, Chicago, San Francisco, Baltimore, and elsewhere. Until recently, historians of medicine have considered them as part of the history of quackery, or not at all.[4] A few historians of popular culture have paid them glancing attention, putting them (dismissively or nostalgically) within the dime museum or medicine show tradition, at the rock bottom of the cultural hierarchy of entertainments, with no consideration of their links to the high medical museum tradition.[5] And historians of the museum have never included them in the narrative that goes from Charles Willson Peale to the American Museum of Natural History and the Smithsonian.[6]

The urban netherworld was certainly where the popular anatomical museum ended up, but in its early career in America it aspired to a higher status. That aspiration will figure prominently in this chapter. I will argue that the popular anatomical museum needs to be placed in the context of medical museum practice, as a commercial appropriation of professional (closed to the public) medical exhibitions; and also in the context of bourgeois self-making and social reform discourse. Such an understanding is a prerequisite for a richer appreciation of the popular anatomical museum's changing audience, and changing relation to other institutions and entertainments: its race to the bottom.

BUILDING THE CABINET:
THE EARLY HISTORY OF THE ANATOMY MUSEUM

Late-nineteenth-century popular anatomical museums may have been tawdry, marginal enterprises, but they were the issue of an ancient and illustrious lineage: the "cabinets of curiosities" of Renaissance princes, scientific gentlemen, and medical faculties. These haphazard assemblages of objects, manmade or natural, featured rarities and "sports of nature," things with unusual qualities or histories which, by their very irregularity, were thought to shed light on the workings of the natural world.[7] Collection was part of the performance of early modern science: cabinets of curiosities were repositories of esoteric "facts," and often connected to scientific societies, both formal and informal. As the word "cabinet" implies, they were enclosed rooms or closets, open only to gentlemen and their collaborators. In their private space, virtuosi and their patrons displayed and expounded upon their scientific treasures to a select audience of social peers.[8] At the same time, the cabinet of curiosity and its eighteenth- and nineteenth-century successor, the anatomical museum, responded to and fostered a pleasure principle. Collection was a quasi-erotic quest to obtain the most precious and hard-to-obtain specimens. The collector prided himself on his erudition and acumen, cultivated a love of the grotesque, beautiful, and obscure, and took sensuous delight in the fine craftsmanship, creative presentation, and quality of anatomical objects, whether taken from real bodies or molded in wax or other media. Anatomical wax figures gave off a particularly voluptuous, fleshy glow; the anatomical waxes of eighteenth- and nineteenth-century Florence were especially prized for their high artistry.[9] It is also worth noting that, even in the most elite and scientific eighteenth- and nineteenth-century museums, a portion of what was collected was purely curious, not scientific at all. The tibia of a soldier killed at Waterloo, displayed in Valentine Mott's Surgical and Pathological Museum in New York, was valued not for its unusual conformation or indications of pathology, but for its connection to a world historical event.[10]

As we have seen, in the nineteenth century public interest in the anatomical body was stoked by the development and expansion of the medical profession and the extraordinary proliferation of medical schools. The anatomy museum was a standard feature of these schools, even a selling point, invariably mentioned in circular advertisements that were designed to attract medical students. A well-equipped museum, it was argued, was an indispensable supplement to the dissection of cadavers; the museum was a place of study. It was especially important that rural schools have such a museum, since they typically had the most trouble obtaining live patients and dead bodies for their students to practice on. But more than that, the museum itself played a vital role in the production and progress of medical knowledge, as a repository of facts and cases. The museum collection was an institutional locus in the fields of general and pathological anatomy, experimental physiology, phrenology, and craniology, the disciplines that have been called the "new analytical sciences" of the early nineteenth century.[11] Aside from the anatomical museum's usefulness in the education of medical students, museum displays and collecting activities served to legitimate antebellum medical colleges and professors and students—to themselves and to the public—by asserting the scientific identity of the medical enterprise. The possession of a museum was a claim of filiation with science.

The medical anatomy museum depended on the practice of anatomical dissection, and the careers of dissectors depended on the production of objects for collection. The advanced student who mastered the art of dissection, and then the techniques of producing anatomical objects, could begin to amass his own "anatomical" or "pathological cabinet," or supply anatomical objects to other members of his network, with a view toward becoming a preceptor or professor of anatomy. The prerequisite for all this was access to a sufficient number of cadavers and "interesting" cases. Here again it was mainly the urban poor, criminals, and colonized or conquered peoples who supplied the raw "anatomical material"— procured almost entirely via illegal and/or coercive methods, usually without the consent or knowledge of the deceased and kin. So that, in producing and exhibiting such objects in a cloistered, professional space, the anatomy museum articulated a powerful cultural trope: the learned professional or bourgeois collector as pure Mind; the working class, indigent poor, savage, or miscreant exhibited as the material, and often pathological, Body. Not surprisingly, the mobs that invaded medical schools, seeking to reclaim and rebury their dead, often vented their fury by destroying anatomical collections.

Anatomical museums attached to medical colleges, and the private collections of professors, attracted public notice and were sporadically opened for viewing by a trickle of respectable lay visitors.[12] From the 1720s on, anatomical exhibitions, mainly waxworks, were mounted in London and Paris, for a spectatorship of gentry and aristocrats (judging from the steep admission prices).[13] In the decades that followed, exhibitions of varying quality, and for broader audiences, traveled around Europe. In the 1760s, and for three decades thereafter, Rackstrow's Museum in London displayed anatomical objects to a plebeian and middling audience, anticipating the formula that later museums would follow. Among its treasures were a number of sculptures in wax and also actual specimens, including the penis of a sperm whale and several human penises preserved in spirits or "injected to a state of erection" with wax—"preparations" no different from those in the cabinets of medical colleges and proprietarial anatomy schools, but with a disproportionate emphasis on the reproductive organs. (The penises were arranged to provide a racial comparison between "white men," "black men," and the "mulatto.")[14]

Anatomical models and specimens were also exhibited in North America. In the 1770s in Philadelphia, Abraham Chovet exhibited wax anatomical models, to both medical students and the genteel public (Chovet was said to be "severe on vulgar people").[15] In 1781, in British-occupied New York, a Dr. Anthony Yeldall gave a lecture at City Hall, to "the curious," on "the Nervous System" and "the five senses," illustrated by "a figure . . . prepared in wax shewing where every nerve originates" and "a large eye."[16] Decades later, in 1817, the Reverend William Bentley, a Unitarian clergyman and scientific gentleman who corresponded with Thomas Jefferson, recorded in his diary a description of a traveling exhibition of "anatomical preparations in wax" at Stetson's Essex Coffee House in Salem, Massachusetts:

> They are in the best style from H. Williams of Boston, the first in America who has made such attempts to represent parts of the human body in wax. . . . He has twelve articles in separate glass cases, representing sections of the heart, of the brain, of the feet and hands, a small complete anatomy of the form and view of the intestines, and several partial preparations.[17]

Such waxes, Bentley noted, were unlike the "ordinary catch penny playthings" that typically toured Britain and America. And this was important: The artistic quality of an exhibited object was linked to the social quality of its spectatorship.

In the late 1820s and 1830s, a number of wax displays, often featuring "Anatomical" or "Florentine Venuses," were mounted in London. Across the Atlantic, similar traveling exhibitions were mounted in New York and other cities. In 1830 the *New York Medical Inquirer* reported that "a handsome collection of anatomical figures, beautifully prepared and well imitated in wax, are [*sic*] exhibited for inspection at the Masonic Hall," and recommended that physicians and "every scientific man" should examine the figures (which came with "a small explanatory manual").[18]

In the 1830s and 1840s public interest in anatomical exhibitions was fueled by a confluence of trends: the contemporary medical enthusiasm for anatomy in London, Paris, Philadelphia, and New York; the growing consumer demand for anatomical instruction as part of the curriculum of bourgeois social identity; and the growing audience for titillating and sensationalist entertainments and displays. An 1846 editorial in the *Boston Medical and Surgical Journal* complained that "Numerous lecturers have been itinerating through the country, with casts, models, drawings, and preparations, which they dignify by the name of anatomical museums, their most attractive specimens appertaining to the delicate subjects of conception, gestation, manual and instrumental labor, deformed genitals, &c."[19] In 1846, after several permanent anatomical museums had been established in London,[20] Dr. Wooster Beach imported a collection from England and founded the New York Anatomical Gallery. In the decades that followed, popular anatomical museums and exhibitions popped up in cities all over America.

The period from 1820 to 1860 was critical in the formation of the American middle class: growing numbers of people were anxious to distinguish themselves from the laboring classes, anxious to identify themselves through all sorts of cultural performances with disembodied moral and aesthetic principles, with Mind, not Body. But we are embodied be-

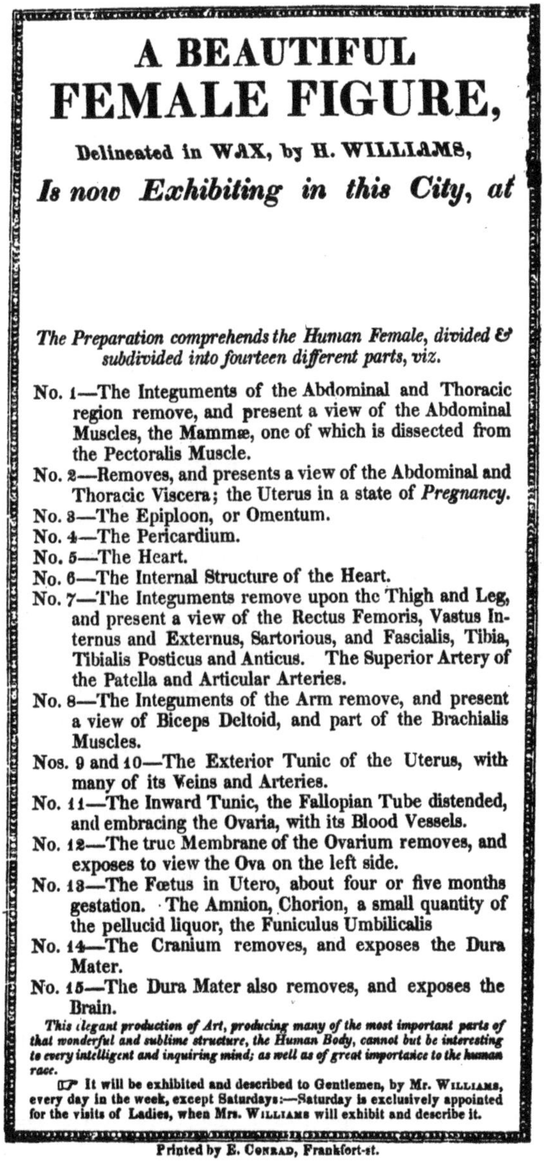

A BEAUTIFUL
FEMALE FIGURE,

Delineated in WAX, by H. WILLIAMS,

Is now Exhibiting in this City, at

The Preparation comprehends the Human Female, divided &
subdivided into fourteen different parts, viz.

No. 1—The Integuments of the Abdominal and Thoracic region remove, and present a view of the Abdominal Muscles, the Mammæ, one of which is dissected from the Pectoralis Muscle.

No. 2—Removes, and presents a view of the Abdominal and Thoracic Viscera; the Uterus in a state of *Pregnancy*.

No. 3—The Epiploon, or Omentum.

No. 4—The Pericardium.

No. 5—The Heart.

No. 6—The Internal Structure of the Heart.

No. 7—The Integuments remove upon the Thigh and Leg, and present a view of the Rectus Femoris, Vastus Internus and Externus, Sartorious, and Fascialis, Tibia, Tibialis Posticus and Anticus. The Superior Artery of the Patella and Articular Arteries.

No. 8—The Integuments of the Arm remove, and present a view of Biceps Deltoid, and part of the Brachialis Muscles.

Nos. 9 and 10—The Exterior Tunic of the Uterus, with many of its Veins and Arteries.

No. 11—The Inward Tunic, the Fallopian Tube distended, and embracing the Ovaria, with its Blood Vessels.

No. 12—The true Membrane of the Ovarium removes, and exposes to view the Ova on the left side.

No. 13—The Fœtus in Utero, about four or five months gestation. The Amnion, Chorion, a small quantity of the pellucid liquor, the Funiculus Umbilicalis

No. 14—The Cranium removes, and exposes the Dura Mater.

No. 15—The Dura Mater also removes, and exposes the Brain.

This elegant production of Art, producing many of the most important parts of that wonderful and sublime structure, the Human Body, cannot but be interesting to every intelligent and inquiring mind; as well as of great importance to the human race.

☞ It will be exhibited and described to Gentlemen, by Mr. WILLIAMS, every day in the week, except Saturdays:—Saturday is exclusively appointed for the visits of Ladies, when Mrs. WILLIAMS will exhibit and describe it.

Printed by E. CONRAD, Frankfort-st.

Figure 9.1. Broadsheet for a traveling anatomical exhibition (New York, 1818). Courtesy of Francis Countway Library, Harvard University Medical School.

ings and our identifications inevitably refer back to the body. The display of manikins and preparations in the anatomical museum provided an opportunity for spectators to imaginatively identify with a scientific body that was fixed and controlled, mapped with place names and boundaries, subjected to a disembodied natural law and medical supervision, a body that was cleaned up and demystified and fixed in authoritative texts and objects.

This conception of self had powerful appeal for the emerging middle class, but also an unsettling undertow. Both fearfully and seductively, it suggested that beneath the orderly cognitive surface, the body might be a savage, superficially colonized region of desire, impulse, messy affect, and disease—a nightmarish domain in which the regime of reason and morality was constantly under siege. Moreover, the anatomical self also contained, from the very inception of its popular discourse, the possibility of appropriation for purposes irrelevant or counter to the project of bourgeois class formation. The anatomical body could be a foreign land, full of disease and grotesquery. Anatomy's crowd might come merely to gawk at or wallow in the body's otherness. Such spectators might be ambivalent or even hostile to middle-class self-making. Given the anatomical body's inevitable association with the body of flesh and desire, the public might seek out anatomy in order to experience shock and arousal. Thus from the outset, in a good part of popular discourse—and almost always in the anatomical museum—anatomy was staged for the profitable purpose of meeting public demand for visual representations of the sexual and pathological body. Operators of anatomical museums claimed that such representations had morally instructive and even emancipatory effects on their patrons. But to critics, and many museumgoers, the popular anatomical museum was nothing more than cheap sensationalism and pornography.

"The Moral Purpose of an Anatomical Museum"

The *New York Times* report of the 9 January 1888 raid on the Egyptian Musée tells us that

> while the confiscation was in progress a man came in who said he was the proprietor and that his name was Frederick I. Tilton. . . . Mr. Comstock asked him if he thought the figures and casts that lay about served any moral purpose. Tilton had no answer ready . . . , except that he had run the place unmolested for two years.[21]

Implicitly, the newspaper account depicts Tilton's failure to rise to Comstock's challenge as a sign of the popular anatomical museum's depravity, its utter lack of moral purpose, but historical evidence shows that anatomical museums did in fact participate in the project of bourgeois self-making and did make moral claims, and that such claims were not just window dressing. From 1847 to the 1920s, museum proprietors commonly sold or handed out catalogues that offered statements of moral purpose. In fact, the 1876 catalogue of Philadelphia's European Anatomical, Pathological, and Ethnological Museum begins with the precise formula demanded by Comstock: "The moral purpose of an anatomical museum. . . ."[22] Such catalogues, which frequently plagiarized or para-

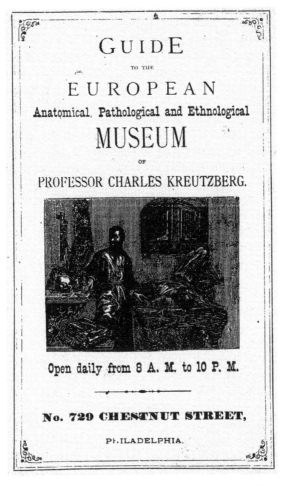

Figure 9.2. Title page, Charles Kreutzberg, *Guide to the European Anatomical, Pathological and Ethnological Museum of Professor Charles Kreutzberg* (Philadelphia, 1876). Courtesy of the Atwater Kent Museum.

phrased each other, testify to the social origin, audience, and ideology of the popular anatomy museum. Some are quite extensive: the 1854 catalogue of New York's Grand Anatomical Museum runs to sixty-four pages, of which six pages are devoted to an introductory essay full of moral purpose.[23]

How was the "moral purpose of an anatomical museum" characterized in these publications? Surveying catalogues and pamphlets published between 1847 and 1876, one finds language that is of a piece with the popular anatomical writings of the period: "to improve the intellect and elevate the morals of the people by the dissemination of a minute and intimate acquaintance with Human Physiology and the laws of life."[24] The "civilized" and "intelligent" person should know the body's boundaries, place names, and topographical features, a geographical vocabulary corresponding to those marks by which Europeans came to know, claim, and colonize the "external" non-European world. Self-knowledge is defined as domination of the body by reason; it leads outward to imperium: "[M]an stands, by his genius and his self-consciousness upon the highest platform of earthly perfection, and it is his task to bring, by his abilities, all other beings under his command, and to rule over them." Knowledge of the body is necessary for the extension of human moral and scientific agency, a prerequisite to "progress" and "improvement." And this knowledge requires an increased consciousness of the body, a monitoring self-surveillance: "Every intelligent man will consider the perception of his own body, the basis of his mental life and through self-knowledge only will he attain the height of human perfection."[25]

"No book of wisdom can compare to the strict scrutiny man can take of his own construction."[26] The body generates a secular, material, scientific theology, a body of physiological law that accords with the revelation of Scripture, and provides evidence of the hand of "the Divine Architect." Anatomy inscribes the social order and the authority of law on the body, rationalizes the body. It also domesticates it, even beautifies it. The catalogues tell us that the body is "the house we live in" (without attributing the phrase to Alcott). The body is a virtual built environment, reshaped by reference to the same aesthetic principles that many antebellum Americans were applying to their homes and yards and cities. We are wonderfully, beautifully, made.[27]

But also fearfully made, and fearfully unmade. The body is prey to "numerous lesions, contagions, and disorders which infest all the parts of this beautiful mechanism; maladies [of] . . . the skin, the muscles, the joints[,] the glands, and all the internal viscera; every disease which deranges the functions, which corrupts the blood, which decomposes the tissues, deforms the structure, and defaces the beauty of the human form divine."[28] The museum, then, can serve as a "great school of prudential and moral instruction . . . in which parents may teach their children, in the most impressive manner . . . truths which will live in their memories and hearts forever, and which will prove an effectual shield in the hour of sore temptation."[29] Disease naturally enforces moral law.

AN ANATOMICAL WALKING TOUR

Such was argued in the catalogues. What was staged in the displays? Like its medical counterpart, the popular anatomical museum exhibited skeletons; wax and papier-maché models; paintings; engravings; plaster casts; "wet" preservations (body parts sealed up in glass jars filled with preservative solution); "dry" preservations (body parts dehydrated and injected with colored wax); statuary of anatomical, moral, or historical interest; displays of human and animal body parts and products (kidney stones, gall stones, etc.); stuffed animals; etc. The displays were usually in glass cases, sometimes freestanding on pedestals or table tops. There was surprising little variation between museums: objects in one museum might be similar or even identical to objects in another. Many items were produced in multiples—we know that in the 1880s a loft on the Bowery churned out "mummies and monsters of all descriptions" for dime museums—and there was much copying from museum to museum.[30] Other workshops must have specialized in "artificial" objects for dime museum presentation. The names of Kahn and Jordan frequently recur among museum proprietors, so similarities between museum collections may reflect the itineraries of proprietors and collections, as Louis Kahn went from London to New York to San Francisco and back to New York, and Henry Jordan from London to New York to Philadelphia.[31]

The 1850 catalogue of Wooster Beach's New York Anatomical Gallery and Academy of Natural, Medical, and Moral Science is arranged in something like the form of a walking tour. It begins with displays illustrating female reproductive, urinary, and excretory anatomy; the stages of pregnancy and fetal development and their pathologies; comparative female reproductive anatomy (featuring birds and monkeys); mammary glands and placenta; and includes an "exquisitely wrought . . . Anatomical Venus, under glass, and reclining on a couch, representing the Foetus in Utero, with all the surrounding organs" (10). A smaller group of exhibits represent male urogenital anatomy. There then follow exhibits illustrating human anatomy, both male and female (including, again, the sexual organs and reproductive system). In this section, displays of female sexual anatomy outnumber male by twenty to three, an imbalance which is typical of popular anatomy museums, and which almost certainly reflects a commercial calculus. Male patrons (who formed the bulk of the

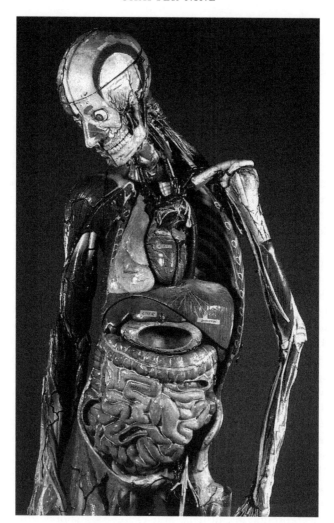

Figure 9.3. Anatomical model, male, papier-maché, ca. 1890, purchased by the Smithsonian Institution for display at the 1892 Columbian Exposition, Chicago. Like many mannequins exhibited in popular anatomical museums, it was made in the Parisian workshop of Louis Auzoux, the celebrated anatomical model maker. Models were produced with or without genitalia, depending on the customer's preference (this one is without). Courtesy of the National Museum of American History, the Smithsonian Institution.

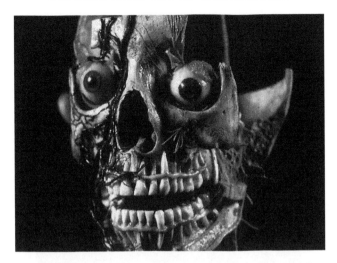

Figure 9.4. Lymphatics of the head and neck, wax model,
Vasseur & Tramond, Paris, ca. 1885. Courtesy of the Mütter
Museum, College of Physicians of Philadelphia.

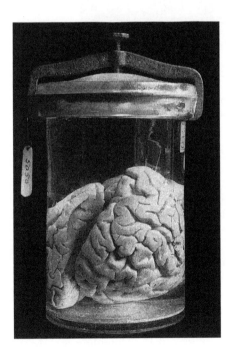

Figure 9.5. "The Murderer's Brain."
Wet preparation in jar, the brain
of John Wilson, hanged for murder at Norristown, Pennsylvania,
1887. Photo: Olivia Parker. Courtesy of the Mütter Museum, College of Physicians of Philadelphia
and Olivia Parker.

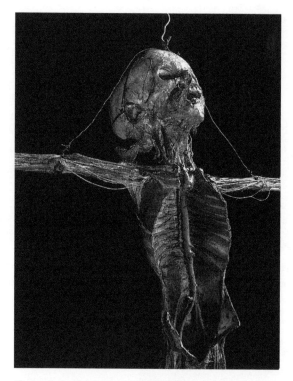

Figure 9.6. "McLellan Child." Dried preparation, ca.
1880s. Photo: Olivia Parker. Courtesy of the Mütter
Museum, College of Physicians of Philadelphia and
Olivia Parker.

anatomy museum's audience) likely preferred the overrepresentation of
female body parts.

Great emphasis is laid on inventorying the body: the exhibit attempts
as thorough an account as possible: "Sixty-four bones of the upper extremities. In the shoulders: two clavicula,—collar bones," and so forth.
"National" differences are also inventoried: we go on to "twenty-six skulls
of different tribes of Indians in the South-West": "Some of them are skulls
of chiefs, and indicate very marked traits of character. . . ." Each Indian
group receives an analysis, confirmed by (or derived from) phrenological
examination of the skulls: "Uchee Indian. . . . These people are shrewd
and cunning; have small heads, and are much less impulsive than most
Indians"; "Shawnee. The head of this people is more intellectual than is
common to Indians"; etc. Indian practices of skull molding are shown
and discussed, along with a warning that "Artificial deformities of the
brain may become congenital, may be transmitted" (30–32). Another
twenty-five skulls, also *national* in their phrenological characteristics"

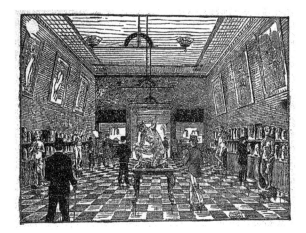

Figure 9.7. Anatomical Preparations and Dissections Department. *Catalogue, Dr. Baskette's Gallery of Anatomy* (Chicago, n.d. [ca. 1875]). Courtesy of William H. Helfand, New York.

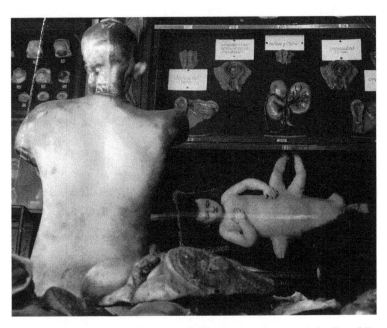

Figure 9.8. Anatomical objects, probably wax or plaster, originally exhibited in the European Anatomical, Pathological and Ethnological Museum, Philadelphia. The pieces are listed in museum catalogues that date back to at least 1876. The photograph was shot in an antique store in the late 1930s or early 1940s. Photo: Sol Mednick. Courtesy of the Atwater Kent Museum, Philadelphia, and Mrs. Miriam F. Rothman.

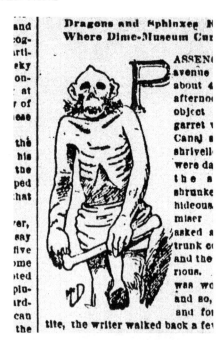

Figure 9.9. Manufactured monster. "The Sea-Serpent Factory." *New York World*, 11-6-1887: 1.

(32), come from South America, Java, South Africa, India, the Caribbean, Arabia, the South Pacific, Mongolia, and China. And, finally, there are the skulls of "a Caucasian, or White Man," "a Hottentot Venus," and two "Druids . . . found at Meudon," near Paris, in 1845.

Next comes "the Department of Morbid Anatomy," featuring hermaphroditic anomalies, venereal diseases, and diseases of the sexual, excretory, and reproductive organs:

> observe those Models on the West end of the Long Counter and under Glass Globes, some of them representing various stages and appearances of Venereal disease or Syphilis in the female, and other inflamed states of the sexual organs of the female which may arise . . . either from weakness, or irregularity of the menses. These Models, though loathsome and disgusting enough to any mind not entirely lost to every moral and virtuous sense, are far from exhibiting the most aggravated forms of this horrid disease. (36)

Other sections follow, somewhat repetitively and in no systematic order: viscera; anatomy of the brain; female and male sexual and reproductive organs and anatomy ("Virgin Breasts . . . those rare beauties so peculiar to the female form, without which she would be despoiled of one half her elegance and loveliness" (50); "external organs of Generation of the Hottentot Female showing remarkable enlargement of the Clitoris—generally called the *Natural Apron*" (51). There are also special sections on

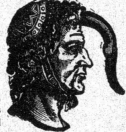
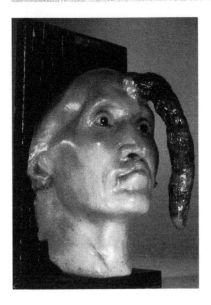

Figure 9.10. (above) Advertisement for Dr. Baskette's Gallery of Anatomy, Science, Art, and Nature, featuring "Madame Dimanche," the horned woman (back matter, *Catalogue, Dr. Baskette's Gallery of Anatomy* (Chicago, n.d., *ca.* 1875). Courtesy of William H. Helfand, New York. Wax busts of Mme. Dimanche are featured in the extant catalogues of several popular anatomical museums.

Figure 9.11. (left) Wax bust. Mme. Dimanche, possibly of French manufacture, 1859 or earlier. Courtesy of the Mütter Museum, College of Physicians of Philadelphia.

diseases and deformations of the face, skin diseases, and unusual diseases, conditions, and "monstrosities"—"horns growing on the forehead of a woman 80 years old, and having grown in 4 years 23 centimetres in length"— plus a display showing the "Consequence of Masturbation on a young female" (59).

Sprinkled throughout are displays dealing with historical and contemporary themes and figures, temperance, religion, comparative anatomy, and paleontological relics. A few miscellaneous items finish up the tour:

"Inflammation of the stomach, produced by *Rum*. . . . The Drunkard's Stomach"; "Fac simile [*sic*] of the Penis of the celebrated Gibbs the Pirate, in perfect health" (64); etc.[32] The criminological reliquary was a regular feature within the anatomical museum. The 1867 New York Museum of Anatomy boasted possession of "THE HEAD AND RIGHT ARM OF ANTON PROBST, who was recently executed in Philadelphia, for the murder of the Deering Family." "This is no plaster cast taken after death," the catalogue claimed, "but the *bona fide* head and right arm, prepared by the Professors of the Philadelphia College of Surgeons, to whom the body was delivered after execution, and purchased from the College by Dr. Jordan, certificates of which are appended to the glass case under which they stand" (6). Also on display were the skeletons of Henri Jacques, a Parisian who was executed for having murdered his wife and three children ("an inspection of his phrenological development will show the great preponderance of the animal passions"), and the Aspinall children, whose father, a London railroad clerk, "starved them to death, and was executed in July, 1856." Such objects could serve multiple purposes: "Child No. 95 shows the effects of starvation on the intestines, and also the anatomy of the arm" (6).

"THE UTILITY, . . . EVEN *NECESSITY*" OF REPRESENTING FLESH

Clearly the popular anatomy museum, even in its most respectable versions, contained contradictory impulses and appealed to a variety of tastes. The museums' excesses amply demonstrated anatomy's antinomian potential, its materialism, sensationalism, eroticism. Catalogues therefore tended to take on a defensive, self-justifying tone, addressing customers, but also critics, who attacked the museums for capitalizing on the public's taste for entertainments relating to the most debased aspect of human existence, the life of the body—and especially sex. Thus, an 1850 New York City police crackdown on shows that featured nudity also resulted in an indictment against Horace B. Tolles and Dr. Wooster Beach of the New York Anatomical Gallery for "exhibiting divers figures of men and women naked in lewd, lascivious, wicked indecent, disgusting and obscene groups attitudes and positions to the manifest corruption of morals in open violation of decency and good order to the great damage and common nuisance of the good and worthy citizens of the State of New York."[33]

To what degree, then, was the disciplinary moralism of the anatomy museum a cover for pandering? Certainly, moral and pornographic elements commingled in every anatomy museum. Proprietors could capitalize on the moral agenda of the anatomical museum only to a limited degree; survival depended on attracting male patrons who wanted to see sexual and sensational material. In the nineteenth century, the anatomy museum was one of only two public arenas where naked bodies were permitted representation. Fine art was the other, but anatomy museums went much further, displaying sexual organs.[34] Such public representations of flesh were licensed by the assignation of scientific names and categories for body parts and functions, by the claim of filiation with science. Under the governance of a physiological jurisprudence, the sexual body could be shown for purposes of moral formation, reformation and improvement. The popular anatomical museum then was a hybrid. Its dual nature is evident in the differing responses of Tolles and Beach to prosecution: Tolles, the commercial proprietor, pleaded guilty; Beach, the physician and former owner of the museum who continued to lecture there, pleaded not guilty and swore out a deposition attesting that the models in question were "of the most scientific, useful and instructive character," intended "to elevate the morals of the Public." According to F. C. Hollick, "public sentiment . . . was [in 1850] somewhat enlightened" and the attempt to suppress the museum failed, in part due to "a celebrated Professor of Anatomy and Surgery in the College of Physicians and Surgeons," who "volunteered evidence in favor of such establishments, and argued for their utility, . . . even *necessity*." The prosecution against Beach was dropped and the museum continued in operation.[35]

The popular anatomy museum's moral agenda, then, despite its detractors, had some credibility. But it tended to operate along different lines from Alcott's *The House I Live In* and Catherine Beecher's *Treatise on Domestic Economy*, which mainly featured illustrations of the universalist, ideal anatomical body. While a portion of the museum displays were devoted to specimens illustrating "normal," "general," or ideal anatomy, the bulk of the museum's collection was oppositional and pathological, illustrating the antiprinciples of asymmetry, deformity, indiscipline, disease, ignorance, promiscuity, and criminality. Mind/body was the dominant binary from which could be derived parallel, congruent pairs: health/pathology, learning/ignorance, respectability/vulgarity, civilization/savagery, etc.

Problematic in this was the male/female binary. Anatomy museums marked the difference between the sexes and displayed female bodies and body parts for the male gaze. For the male patrons of the museum, the representations of females, female body parts, and anomalies like hermaphrodites served to define masculine identity in opposition. The feminine was Other, the Body. But at the same time, in the cultural logic of antebellum bourgeois culture, the feminine principle was linked to civilization: Science (reason) and Woman (spirit) together domesticated the recalcitrant male body. Thus the Anatomical Gallery's catalogue asserted its moral and intellectual respectability by reference to the qualities of its visitors: "the most learned and distinguished scientific men in this country, and of other lands; . . . men and women of the highest standing; . . . male and female students of Medicine; . . . distinguished lecturers in popular assemblies and colleges" (6).

The suitability of viewing by women asserted the bourgeois character of the museum. It also publicly asserted the museum's allegiance to, and participation in, the movement for medical and social reform, as evidenced by the reference to female medical students, a controversial topic in the 1840s and 1850s, and for many decades to follow. Wooster Beach was a well-known medical reformer, one of the founders of the eclectic sect of alternative medicine (see chapter 5 above). His museum also had a "phrenological office"; in the late 1840s and 1850s, phrenology still had a large following among men and women who identified with medical, social, and moral reform. William Byrd Powell, a phrenological physician who was associated with eclecticism and medical reform, loaned his skull collection to the museum.[36]

But such partisan cultural political affiliations were subsumed by the museum's larger commitment to "science." Science in mid-nineteenth-century America was bankable. The popular appetite for scientific marvels, often backed by some form of scientific authentication (no matter how dubious it might seem to us), elicited no shortage of entrepreneurs, in a vast range of social niches, ranging from snake-oil salesmen to elite professors. Thus, early in his career, in October 1836, P. T. Barnum packaged a touring troupe of minstrel acts, magicians, and curiosities, under the title "Barnum's Grand Scientific and Musical Theatre." Over the course of his career, Barnum, like other exhibitors of freaks and anomalies, often obtained testimonials from scientific authorities, including Oliver Wendell Holmes, the eminent professor of anatomy at Harvard and one of the most well-known essayists of his time, who in the 1870s certified the authenticity of the tattoos of Djordji Costentius, the "noble Greek."[37] Such testimonials are telling indications of the authority and credibility of the medical professoriate—and of the boundaries and uses of that authority.

Beach's museum and Barnum's American Museum were contemporaries of the minstrel show, where rowdy audiences hooted and cheered performers and many female audience members were prostitutes. Barnum attempted to reconfigure theatrical presentations and spaces as morally beneficial and safe for "respectable" women, in part by encouraging male patrons to observe decorum and discouraging prostitutes from attending his museum.[38] Beach's museum aimed to be even more respectable than that: its emphasis on science, education, and reform was in-

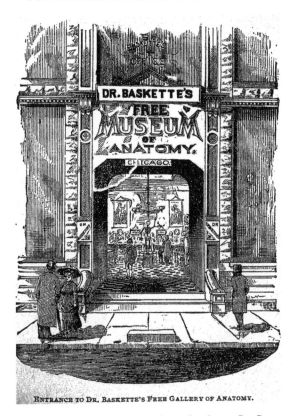

ENTRANCE TO DR. BASKETTE'S FREE GALLERY OF ANATOMY.

Figure 9.12. Cover illustration. *Catalogue, Dr. Baskette's Gallery of Anatomy* (Chicago, n.d. [ca. 1875]). Courtesy of William H. Helfand, New York.. The museum's respectability is asserted by a representation depicting women and children entering and viewing the exhibition. But the crudity of the catalogue's illustrations, and the cheapness of the paper it is printed on, undermine the assertion.

tended to appeal to a low to middling audience's desire for improvement, respectability, and morality. Public commercial spectacle was by its very nature suspect, but the Gallery's catalogue insisted on its scientific and moral vocation. So did other anatomical museums. Their cultural mission was embedded in the grandiose names they assumed: the European Anatomical, Pathological, and Ethnological Museum; the Grand Anatomical Museum, or National Academy of Natural, Anatomical and Pathological Science; etc.

"For Gentlemen Only": The Devolution
of the Anatomical Museum

Thus the first popular anatomical museums could plausibly claim a place in the larger project of bourgeois self-making. Their special role was to instruct men and women in the natural and moral science of their own bodies:

> it is not so easy to get a knowledge of the inner construction of our body, because we have to first become acquainted with and learn to designate the different organs under guidance of a competent person, and only a few have the opportunity to study the construction of the human body in a dissecting-room, where man is often disgusted with his own image. The necessity of exhibiting a museum, which is satisfactory and in which everybody can view [the parts of the body] and distinguish them in an æsthetic form, is therefore obvious.[39]

However, by the late 1880s most anatomical museums could no longer credibly claim to be educational or disciplinary institutions. They now appealed to an audience of "adolescent youth and green countrymen," as the *New York Star* had it, mainly of the working class.[40] They also, perhaps, retained a small audience of young middle- and upper-class men, ambiva-

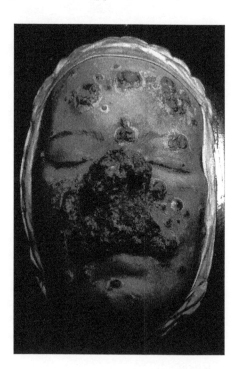

Figure 9.13. Face with tertiary syphilis, wax moulage. Possibly of German manufacture, late nineteenth or early twentieth century. Courtesy of the Mütter Museum, College of Physicians of Philadelphia.

lent about the bourgeois identity they were assuming, who sought out the anatomical museum as a momentary refuge from the feminized culture of overdecorated parlors, sentimentality, religion, and manners, a place where men could (safely) test their courage by confronting the horrors of the pathological body. Most tellingly, *not* everybody was permitted to view the displays: unlike Beach's museum, later anatomy museums were typically "For Gentlemen Only."[41] The anatomy of the anatomical museum had come to signify not the domination of mind over body, but the body itself, and this was not fit viewing for women and children.

Felix Riesenberg's *East Side West Side*, a 1927 novel set in turn-of-the-century New York, depicts the Bowery anatomical museum as a nightmarish enclave devoted to sexual grotesquery and disease. In one scene, the working-class heroine discusses the museum's exclusion of women:

> "I couldn't go in. . . . It says, 'For Men Only.'" They stood in front of Fandyke's Museum. . . .
>
> "Come away from here." He . . . led her south along the west side of the Bowery, but she continued . . . to harp on the museum and its mysterious signs. "Say," she snuggled close . . . , "what's inside? . . . Sadie Marks, my friend, went into one of them places once. She put on her brother's clothes, that's how she got in. Now Sadie says she won't never get married."[42]

How did popular anatomical museums arrive at such a debased cultural position? How did they lose their audience of earnest middle-class men and women? One of Wooster Beach's contemporaries is reported to have remarked that, although Beach "collected great museums," he "never realized any pecuniary advantage therefrom"; after a few years in operation, Beach sold his collection to Ralph Pomeroy, a sarsaparilla importer.[43] As Charles Willson Peale and sons discovered earlier in the century, museums might start with a lofty cultural mission, but could survive only by appealing to a larger audience and cruder tastes.[44] The museums of Beach and a few other proprietors tried to define themselves as places where the spectacular displays had a moral self-making purpose, but after the Civil War there were new definitions of what counted as respectable, and what counted as spectacular: the bar was getting higher. From one direction, Barnum seized the broad middle ground, presenting elaborate spectacles with vastly superior showmanship—responding rapidly to the public's escalating appetite for novelty.[45] From another direction, a new museum establishment of not-for-profit art and natural history museums, financed by wealthy elites, set a new standard for scientificity, aesthetics, and moral probity of display, and operated on a spectacularly larger scale. The American Museum of Natural History, for example, founded in 1869 by A. S. Bickmore, a student of the celebrated naturalist Louis Agassiz, was backed by Theodore Roosevelt, Sr., Benjamin A. Field, Robert Colgate, Morris K. Jesup, William E. Dodge, and J. P. Morgan—the leading magnates of the city (and the same crowd who originally sponsored and funded Comstock). Such museums had no need to earn their keep; they were above the sordid world of mass entertainment and commerce. Their appeal to upper- and middle-class men and women was as a cultural refuge: the popular anatomical museum was no competition.[46]

On its own turf, anatomy, the popular anatomical museum was also losing legitimacy. As medical science advanced, and reforms in medical education slowly took hold in the postbellum era, distinctions between high and low medicine sharpened. Public schools and sanitary fairs were sanctioned by the state and elite-sponsored voluntary associations to take up the mission of anatomical and physiological instruction to the public—albeit in a more distant and disembodied way: the anatomy and physiology of plants, animals, and cells. They too occupied a moral position above the marketplace, and by virtue of that location—and their refusal to treat sexual anatomy—such institutions undermined claims that the anatomy museum provided a unique public service.

Given these conditions, it is not surprising that anatomy museum proprietors raced to the bottom. Increasingly, their displays were taken up

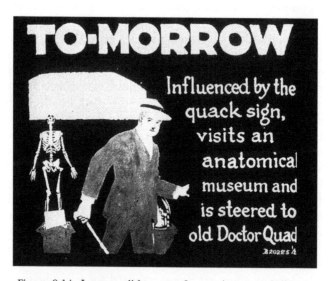

Figure 9.14. Lantern slide, part of an anti–venereal disease campaign, produced by the Army Medical Museum, *ca.* 1918, for the American troops in World War I. Courtesy of the National Museum of Health and Medicine, Armed Forces Institute of Pathology.

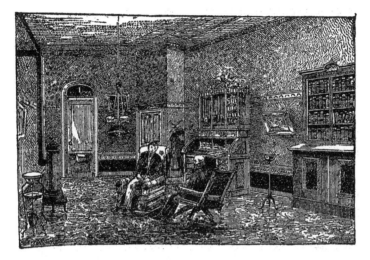

Figure 9.15. Private consultation. *Catalogue, Dr. Baskette's Gallery of Anatomy* (Chicago, n.d. [ca. 1875]). Courtesy of William H. Helfand, New York.

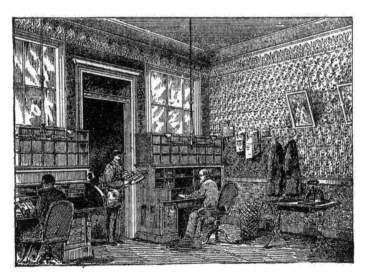

Figure 9.16. Correspondence room. *Catalogue, Dr. Baskette's Gallery of Anatomy* (Chicago, n.d. [ca. 1875]). Courtesy of William H. Helfand, New York.

with lurid and titillating material, sexual topics, crime, scandal, and, above all, venereal disease. As we have seen, this had always been a featured part of the anatomy museum, but after the Civil War physician-proprietors of dubious credentials began systematically mining the territory, operating walk-in and mail-order practices that specialized in treating "private" sexually transmitted diseases and other sexual maladies, in offices alongside or within anatomy museums, here too "for gentlemen only."[47] Much like the medicine show, displays of sexual anatomy and curiosities served as bait to attract male customers—in many cases, museums did not even charge admission. Once inside, patrons would be barraged by fast-talking "professors" and horrific displays of deformed genitals and eroded faces designed to arouse anxieties over spermatorrhea (masturbation), syphilis, gonorrhea, chancroid, impotence, sterility, sexual obsession, and all kinds of "nervous debility." The museum-goer would then be pressured to consult with an on-premises "doctor" (usually for the sum of $5), buy a 25¢ or 50¢ pamphlet, and purchase a patent medicine. The doctor-patient relationship could be maintained on an ongoing basis via correspondence.[48]

On this cultural low ground, the anatomy museum became a particularly inviting target for policers of morality like Comstock.[49] The changing locus of the New York City anatomy museum, from Broadway in the antebellum era to the Bowery in the postbellum era, is symptomatic. The late-nineteenth-century Bowery, a cheap-rent manufacturing and entertainment district of saloons, flophouses, brothels, sweatshops, and dime museums, was a liminal zone, much as Times Square was later to become. On the Bowery, disciplinary anatomy took on a stronger libidinal investment; anatomy came to stand for the very thing it aimed to regulate: desire. The anatomy museum had always been a repository of categories that were excluded from bourgeois identity: the body, disease, sex, crime, freaks, and sadism. With sufficient ambiguity, the anatomy museum could appeal to both a middle- and a lower-class audience. But, shorn of a utilitarian "moral purpose," the anatomy museum became a travesty, "anatomy out of gear," the *New York Herald* called it, an anti-anatomy.[50] And this, detractors claimed, was not merely unproductive, but inflicted actual harm, was a threat to viewers and the larger public.

"A GHASTLY ARRAY": THE POPULAR ANATOMICAL MUSEUM'S THEORY OF SENSATIONALISM

But how? How did anatomical museums, with their representations of the formation and malformation of humanity, affect "the formation of Man"?[51] Museum catalogues and critics alike argued that the viewing of anatomical objects—even a single visit to a museum—shaped the minds and bodies of the viewing public. Such effects were premised on a belief in

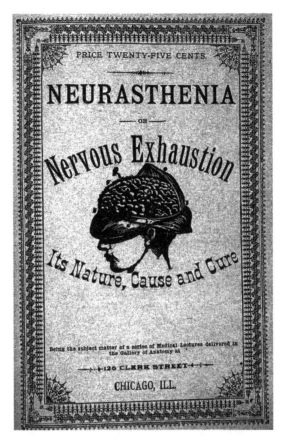

Figure 9.17. *Neurasthenia, or Nervous Exhaustion: Its Nature, Cause and Cure.* Pamphlet bound in *Catalogue, Dr. Baskette's Gallery of Anatomy* (Chicago, n.d. [ca. 1875]). Courtesy of William H. Helfand, New York.

the radical plasticity of human moral (and physical) development. Moral instruction, it was argued, could "mould" children and elevate "the masses"; sensationalist novels and other debased amusements could deform and corrupt them.

If so, then the anatomy museum functioned as a technology for the production of subjectivity. It could produce debased sensations such as sexual arousal, fear, and repulsion (as critics claimed), or "higher," rational, mental, or spiritual "sentiment" (as the museum catalogues claimed): either way "[t]he models must deeply impress the mind"—or body.[52] This power, at its height, activated a kind of disciplinary sublime: viewing the wonders of the body could precipitate a joyous epiphany; viewing the pathologies of the body could induce an anxious moral crisis or horrified revulsion; or spectators might be swept away by sexual arousal or the ghastly pleasures of pathological grotesquery. The objects of the museum acted on the viewer's body. Thus, the newspaper reports commented on the adverse *physical* effects that the anatomical museum displays had on the inspectors and Comstock: "Comstock's moral sense . . . received a severe laceration" when told of the contents of the anatomical museums; the objects "brought the blush of modesty" to Inspector Williams's cheek; Inspector Steers "had his sense of decency torn all to pieces by what he saw."[53] Comstock and the police accused the anatomy museums of purveying "filth" (which degrades the body and physically assaults the senses), while one of the purposes for which Alcott and colleagues developed popular anatomy was to *clean up* the body, to annul its contaminating powers, to textualize and subordinate it. For the moral reformers, there was no legitimate place for bodily desire and sensation; popular anatomy could only find sanction if directed toward the extirpation of desire.

This logic was taken up by the museums as well. As they devolved, they increasingly specialized in scenes of torture, displays of sexual organs, and exhibits of venereal disease. An 1876 catalogue of Philadelphia's European Museum, a large and fairly reputable establishment, boasted as a special attraction an exhibition of "The Inquisition, Their Implements of Torture and Torments, Represented in Life-Size Natural Preparations."[54] Reports of the 1888 New York City raids deplored the "ghastly waxen casts" that portrayed in the most revolting fashion all the most horrifying maladies to which humanity is heir." According to the *Morning Journal*, the windows of the Parisian Museum at 309 Bowery "were filled with a ghastly array of skeletons that sent a cold chill through every passer-by."[55] Inside, the *Sun* reported, were "wax figures and cartoons of a most filthy and suggestive character. There was no apparent purpose in the figures to make them either artistically or anatomically instructive."[56] Some museums were more horrific than others: *The Morning Journal* characterized the European Museum as "a dismal den that makes a specialty of portrayal in wax, fifty examples of human suffering," while the exhibits at the Egyptian Musée "transcended in horror those captured in Kahn's Museum."[57]

"THE COUNTENANCE OF THE EXECUTIONERS": LIBIDINAL DISCIPLINE AND THE DISCIPLINARY LIBIDO

According to the *Star*, the anatomical wax figures confiscated from the Bowery museums amounted to "more than 200 figures or parts of figures, and all were more or less nude and repulsive" (the police publicly esti-

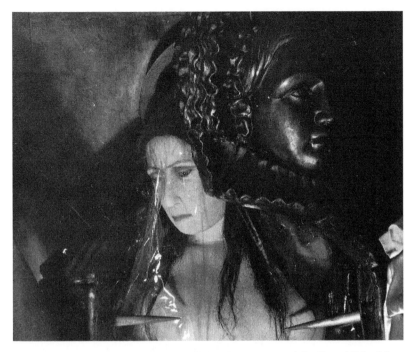

Figure 9.18. The Iron Maiden of Nuremburg, wax, originally exhibited in the European Anatomical, Pathological and Ethnological Museum, Philadelphia. The object is listed in museum catalogues that date back to at least 1876. The photograph was shot in an antique store in the late 1930s or early 1940s. Photo: Sol Mednick. Courtesy of the Atwater Kent Museum and Mrs. Miriam F. Rothman.

mated their value at $37,000). These were eventually destroyed by Comstock and the police in a ritual that was staged at least partly for the press. The tone of the reporting was ironic, smirky, and palpably misogynist. The relish with which the figures were deformed and destroyed served to repackage (to a much broader audience) the very sensationalism and desire that the censors sought to suppress. Thus the *Star* had it that "Comstock smile[d] sweetly while Psyche [was] being decapitated. . . . [T]he way in which the innocents were slaughtered was very suggestive of Indian methods of warfare, and smiles spread over the countenances of the executioners [the police] as they savagely despoiled the features of Diana or the bust of Venus."

Mr. Comstock stood by while the work of destruction was in progress, and only once did his antipathy to nudity get the better of his judgment, when he tore from her soft couch a sleeping damsel with such force as to dislocate one

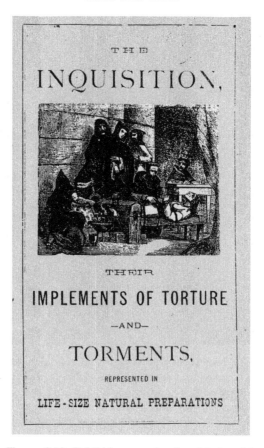

Figure 9.19. Exhibition on the Spanish Inquisi-
tion, in Charles Kreutzberg, *Guide to the European,
Anatomical, Pathological and Ethnological Museum of
Professor Charles Kreutzberg* (Philadelphia, 1876?).
Courtesy of the Atwater Kent Museum.

of her nether extremities. Superintendent Murray dealt the helpless damsel a
terrific blow on the head with an ax, executing a successful decapitation.
Inspector Williams pounded the wax bosom of Psyche with a burglar's ham-
mer and was quite surprised to find that she had no lungs.[58]

Here again, the anatomy museum, Comstock, and the police were on
common ground, sharing a libidinal investment in the very procedures
designed to discipline libido. The museums did so through exhibits of
venereal disease, medieval tortures, and monsters (which according to
the conventional wisdom of the day arose from transgressions of moral/
physiological law, especially sexual transgressions like promiscuity and

masturbation, since the prescriptions of morality and medical science were supposed to be perfectly congruent). The riot of venereal punishments licensed the museums to show the naked body, breasts, and genitals, but also invested representations of venereal disease with a nightmarish sexual glow. The punishment for undisciplined sexual behavior, for insubordinate desire, became identical to desire.

There was then an anatomical gothic. Anatomy and gothic made use of common elements—both featured a nightmarish liminal zone between death and life, both deployed mortuary images. They worked the same tropes: the problem of power, will, and the boundaries of self. (Recall that mesmerism was a staple of the gothic novel and a favorite specialty of antebellum medical performers in both anatomical and nonanatomical museums.) And common to both were *will* and *sensation*: both gothics aimed for a physical impact on the body, evoking fear, disgust, awe, and sexual desire, and the overcoming of the boundaries of the self. As we have seen, the narrative of disembodied will versus bodily power was not confined to the anatomy museum, it was a source of cultural power for physicians, medical colleges, and the medical profession generally. The medical profession performed its gothic through the deployment of physician's skeletons, legends of medical school dissecting-room horrors, graveyard body snatching, and in its own museums. Memoirs and biographies of nineteenth-century anatomy professors often narrated stories of an overweening anatomical will, whose steely mastery of death and the dead body represents a social power analogous (or identical) to the mastery of the scientific, rational haut bourgeoisie over the lower classes.

Take, for example, George E. de Schweinitz's memoir of his teacher Joseph Leidy (1823–91), the eminent Philadelphia anatomist.[59] De Schweinitz portrays Leidy as an intimidating presence, in command of a coterie of fearful but worshipful students and assistants who devotedly guarded the access to his sacred "private room." His depiction of Leidy's man-servant, Nash, could have been lifted straight from the pages of a sensationalist novel:

> It was commonly believed, and no one who knew him ever doubted it, that Nash had been a pirate on the high seas. . . . Over six feet in height, he had a hideous face, covered with a grizzled beard, but his devotion to Leidy was that of a collie dog to its master. Stamping around the laboratory, he was a tower of strength, and neither man nor devil could have entered Leidy's room had Nash forbidden it. . . . Nash was himself a skilful dissector. . . . (62–63)

As a collector of anatomical objects, Leidy was well acquainted with popular anatomical museums: he may even have bid against them for certain items, or disposed of objects by selling to them. Another anecdote hints at the set of social meanings that the popular anatomy museum had for Leidy:

> On [one] occasion a very different type of man came in—a youngish man with his hat on the back of his head, a lighted cigar in his mouth, placed at an angle which is figured in comic papers when they portray some ward politician. This was too much for the prosector, who flew out of his chair and said, "Take off your hat, and take your cigar out of your mouth; throw it away; you are in Dr. Leidy's private room." He was in full retreat, when Dr. Leidy called him back . . . and gently soothed him, questioning him as to who he was, and why he was there. He departed with a pleased grin on his face, and an awkward salutation, neither of them for the prosector. Dr. Leidy turned and said, "My, my, you have bad temper." . . . [H]is assistant . . . in defence . . . replied, "But Dr. Leidy, a disrespectful intrusion like this could not be tolerated." "It may be," he answered, "that he was a specimen worth studying! we might have found out something very valuable. Only yesterday I paid ten cents to go into a museum on Arch Street. I saw five curiosities, two cents apiece. Now this young man was a curiosity, and he did not even cost me two cents."

The elite professor thus revealed himself as a consumer of dime museum grotesqueries, but the larger point is that, for Leidy, the plebeian was himself a pathological curiosity, an object for anatomical study and diversion. A personage of Leidy's standing possesses a magisterial will and intelligence that can easily tolerate and even enjoy the spectacle of proletarian inanity, buffoonery, and bodily deformity. The professor wields the anatomical body, is inured to its effects, and takes his pleasure where he may.

"Too Warm for Their Waxworks"

No one could take seriously the moral claims of the Bowery anatomical museums and they did not insist on them. But one of the anatomical museums closed down by the raids of 9 January 1888 did insist: Kahn's Museum of Anatomy—on Broadway, not the Bowery—according to the *World*, "the most pretentious and respectable" of those raided.[60]

Kahn's was a more substantial and long-lived institution than the others, having been "in existence twenty-six years and never more than a block or so from its present location," with an extensive collection of actual anatomical objects and a large walk-in (and mail-order) medical practice.[61] It charged an admission price of 25¢ or 50¢—the Bowery museums charged only 10¢—and seems to have attracted a more respectable clientele. In 1876, it had even hosted a field trip of students from the Eclectic Medical College of New York, a marginal but respectable institution. (Kahn lectured the "gentlemen" students on "The Value of the Microscope in Examinations of the Urine," instructing them on how to microscopically diagnose diabetes, Bright's disease, and spermatorrhea; he claimed to have examined "urine in every state" under a microscope daily, for over 25 years.)[62]

Of all the museums shut down by Comstock, only Kahn's responded with spirited defiance: museum manager, George M. Livingston, even threatened "to make it warm for Comstock."[63] And only Kahn's had enough resources and legitimacy to mount a legal defense, and attract outside support from a respected professional association: the New York Medico-Legal Society—an elite group whose members included former Civil War surgeon-general William A. Hammond (who helped instigate the creation of the Army Medical Museum), E. A. Spitzka (a well known craniometrist and professor of nervous diseases at the New York Postgraduate Medical College), and other eminent medical men. At the Society's 1888 meeting, a resolution was offered that alluded to Kahn's and that had, according to the *Times*, "a distinctly anti-Comstockian flavor":

> *Whereas*, Certain anatomical museums in the city of New York, some of them established for a number of years, have been summarily invaded, their contents seized, and their managers arrested on the charge that their exhibitions are immoral or "obscene"; and
>
> *Whereas*, The value of proper exhibitions of anatomical exhibitions cannot fail to be recognized as useful for public instruction; and
>
> *Whereas*, We agree with Prof. Agassiz that the "time has come when scientific truth must cease to be the property of the few; when it must be woven into the common life of the world"; and
>
> *Whereas*, There seems serious and wide-spread doubt as to the honesty and sincerity of the persons who instigate such raids as are referred to; and
>
> *Whereas*, There seems to be in the community a superstitious terrorism which prevents fair trials of the persons so summarily arrested.
>
> *[It is] Resolved*, That a committee [of five] be appointed to investigate and to present their conclusions to the Society with all convenient speed, accompanied by such suggestions for the action of the Society as the committee may see fit to recommend.

The resolution was agreed to, but in the end the Society backed down. It deferred further action, supposedly until the committee of five had undertaken its investigation. However, it is unlikely that any investigation was ever carried out. No report was ever published in the Society's journal.[64]

The Medico-Legal Society resolution represents the only known public opposition to the anatomy museum raids. Taking the press as a whole, the reportage of the 1888 campaign ranged from wildly laudatory to mildly approving. There was no hint of dissatisfaction (or pretense of objectivity); the newspapers gleefully milked the story for its entertainment value. The narrative of the suppression of sexual material and nudity was invested with a salacious tone that mocked the museums' claim to anatomical respectability.

Comstock's pretensions were treated more gently but even there the newspapers were playful. A report in the *Star* began: "For several days the habitues of Police Headquarters have noticed the nude head of Anthony Comstock floating around the building." The *Star* gleefully equated Comstock's baldness with nudity, even as the campaigner against representations of naked bodies and sexual literature is depicted as a disembodied head.[65]

And yet Comstock did partly overreach himself. At the trials of the men connected with the Bowery museums, the police easily obtained guilty pleas and convictions, resulting in fines ranging from $50 to $250 and, as mentioned above, destroyed the offending wax figures and anatomical material.[66] The outcome in the Kahn's museum case was different. The court records have not survived, but Comstock's notes describe the trial. They reveal that he failed to convince the court to order the destruction of Kahn's collection (which included "wax figures of females life size, some pregnant & some otherwise & 37 cases of filthy penises"), and failed to gain a conviction on any charge.[67] Kahn's museum withstood the attack, and was still operating in the early twentieth century.[68] But Comstock's campaign had the paradoxical effect of forcing it off lower Broadway and onto the Bowery. Shunted into that suddenly vacant niche, it assumed the more lurid character of the museums it replaced.

"THE ELECTRIC BELLS WERE GAYLY RINGING"

I have argued that, in the nineteenth century, anatomical embodiment (in popular books, medical books, museums, medical schools, public lectures, and performances) was a domestication of the body, a focusing of desire. Anatomy had epistemological authority—the dissector unveiled and mastered the hidden reality of the body, a reality that inevitably inscribed and naturalized social categories, market practices, and political boundaries and procedures. The body became if not a microcosm then a mirror or projection, of nation, class, race, gender, species, history, evolution.

But anatomy, like all discourse, always has an excess of meaning. The anatomical body produced more than any ideology could contain. Desire overflowed its banks, or more precisely, infused them. The edifice built to squelch Eros was made over into its vehicle. And so anatomy quickly became identical to the body: even now "the female anatomy" means colloquially the female body, an emblematic inciter of desire.

Given its ambivalent relation to desire and self, anatomical discourse was readily exploited by entrepreneurs of various kinds, eager to make money but also to build a domain of medical (or in the case of Comstock himself, moral) authority. The anatomical body became the terrain upon which the market, self, class, profession were staked out and fought over. Physicians and anatomy museum proprietors alike explored the opportunities presented by anatomical discourse: at the boundaries of the market. They searched for unoccupied niches and looked to colonize sectors of everyday life. They also looked to displace older institutions—and so for a brief moment in the 1840s the popular anatomical museum was associated with the reform of the medical profession.

The new professionalism that emerged in nineteenth-century America was both an economic and a social strategy. In both respects, professionals sought to carve out sequestered domains that were exempt from the logic and imperatives of capital. But these professional/institutional boundaries were porous and hard to enforce. In nineteenth-century America, anybody could hang a doctor's shingle; anyone with a small amount of start-up money could purchase and exhibit a collection of anatomical objects. Most of those arrested in the 1888 raids were immigrants; none of the lecturers or proprietors arrested, with the exception of Louis J. Kahn (who advertised himself as a medical doctor without specifying where he received his degree), had any plausible claim to even a low degree of medical authority.[69] The attack on anatomy museums then was a policing of social boundaries, an attempt to keep anatomy within its professional sphere, to put it off limits to petty venture capital. The future of the museum was as a secular temple, a repository of sacralized objects, requiring the decorum of hushed spectatorship so familiar to museum-goers today. In contrast, the *Tribune* tells us disparagingly, the police raid on 309 Bowery interrupted "the show . . . in full blast," with "the electric bells . . . gayly ringing within,"[70] while at the European Museum demonstrations of "glassblowers at work" and "Chinese blood testers" (whatever that might be) were in progress.[71]

CONCLUSION: "ANATOMY OUT OF GEAR"

From the above account it is clear that anatomical discourse was available even for the purpose of inverting and travestying bourgeois disciplinary goals and styles. Entrepreneurs responded to public interest in anatomy by offering entertainments and services that provided knowledge about the body, and discursive fodder for the materialization of sexual and social desire, and nearly everything else. The anatomical self was capacious enough to contain a jumble of signifiers. It was both self and other, a discursive field upon which could be projected the anxieties and repres-

sions that defined bourgeois identity: repression of desire, the confinement and organization of the body around boundaries, the need for an
authorizing rationality or utility (outside and above the market) to justify
embodied action on grounds other than the pleasure principle. The dis-
owned body beneath the anatomical template was linked to the sexually
desiring (and desired) female, the working class, criminals, and non-
Europeans, exemplars of the social consequences of undisciplined desire,
analogous to or emblematic of deformity and disease. Within every bourgeois person, beneath the skin, was a body of impulses, sensations, grotesqueries, and desires struggling to trespass or escape its anatomical confines. Like *Frankenstein* and *Dr. Jekyll and Mr. Hyde*, the anatomy museum
played on these contradictions, representing the body as an atavistic, in-
surrectionary core that civilization only partly sheathed. In doing so, it
became a source of the plebeian, antibourgeois self.

This helps to account for the attraction of the anatomical museum,
which, like its public, sought to have it both ways. Anatomical embodiment was a field upon which could be narrated the war of impulse and
confinement. Anatomy simultaneously articulated the emergence of desire and its subordination and erasure. Anatomy became the repository
of the exclusions that defined bourgeois identity (sexual desire, excre-
ment, and other kinds of "filth"). Anatomy domesticated this wasteland,
this savage body, but paradoxically acquired the very significance of its
opposite.

The earliest museums in America, those of Charles Willson Peale and
sons and their contemporaries, aspired to become highly visible public
hegemonic institutions, but by the late 1840s it was well understood that
in America museums could not attract state patronage.[72] In the standard
histories of the museum, the difficulty of institutional establishment in an
egalitarian political culture/republic and capitalist society quickly meant
that entrepreneurs needed to attract the "patronage" of the public (and
so complicated the meaning of that word). This courting of a not very
refined audience meant that museums everywhere, including those pioneered by elite operators like Peale, with moral purposes ranging from
bourgeoisification to nation building, eventually devolved to a distinctly
disreputable group whose strategy was to make a buck by pandering to
coarse appetites.

But the scholarly focus on the Peales has obscured the fact that most
museum proprietors were not of the elite. They appropriated elite forms
like the anatomy museum to legitimate their establishments and broaden
their audiences to include a segment of the public that, if not refined,
aspired to bourgeois status. Such audiences may have wanted to acquire a
"civilized" social identity (and to democratize that identity), but were ambivalent; they also wanted sex and sensation. In the nineteenth century,

the unclothed body was only permitted public representation if furnished with moral claims; pleasure for pleasure's sake was taboo. But, if flesh could be subordinated to the moral purposes of anatomical embodiment, then anatomical embodiment could also be subordinated to the purposes of the flesh. And this was the impasse that was dramatized in the popular anatomical museum.

TABLE 9.1 POPULAR ANATOMICAL MUSEUMS AND EXHIBITIONS IN
AMERICA, 1774–1930

This chronology is far from exhaustive. Many popular anatomical exhibitions and museums were ephemeral, itinerant or too low in social status to leave much documentary evidence. Sources: *Royal Gazette* [NYC], 3–17–1781; Odell, *Annals of the New York Stage*; Orosz, *Curators and Culture*; Catha Grace Rambusch, "Museums and Other Collections in New York City, 1790–1870" (M.A., American civilization, New York University, 1965); William Bentley, diary, 4:441, 3–10–1817; Stewart Holbrook, *Golden Age of Quackery*, 76–84; Ezekiel Porter Belden, *New-York: Past, Present and Future* (New York, 1849), 119; New York, Chicago and Philadelphia city directories; anatomy museum catalogues (collections of William H. Helfand, Francis Countway Library, New York Public Library, New York Academy of Medicine, New-York Historical Society, College of Physicians of Philadelphia, National Library of Medicine).

1774	Philadelphia: Abraham Chovet's anatomical cabinet opens to the public (closes in 1790)
1781	NYC: Dr. Anthony Yeldall gives a lecture at City Hall to "the curious" on "the Nervous System" and "the five senses," illustrated by "a figure . . . prepared in wax shewing where every nerve originates" and "a large eye"
1786	Philadelphia: C. W. Peale's Philadelphia Museum exhibits natural historical, fine art, historical, curiosities
1810	NYC: American Museum, collection of natural historical and human-made oddities, etc.
1816	NYC: New-York Historical Society establishes cabinet of natural history and lecture program
1817	Salem, MA: Public exhibition of anatomical waxworks at P. Stetson's Essex Coffee House; waxworks made by H. Williams of Boston (first American to make anatomical waxes?)
1828	Philadelphia: Academy of Natural Sciences opens its doors to the public, displays eclectic mixture of objects including anatomical objects
1830	NYC: Anatomical figures in wax exhibited at Masonic Hall
1839	Boston: J. C. Warren opens Harvard anatomical museum to thirty or forty women
ca. 1840	NYC: New York Museum (333 Broadway, corner of Anthony St.) features exhibits on natural history and "optical, chemical and other philosophical experiments. . ."
1841	NYC: Barnum buys the American Museum

TABLE 9.1 CONTINUED

1844	NYC: Anatomical Venus exhibited with lectures, National Hall (Canal St., Broadway)
1846	NYC: Anatomical Venus displayed (5–1846) at Barnum's American Museum in a "separate cabinet," extra admission of 25¢; continues for several years
1847	NYC: New York Anatomical Gallery, and Academy of Natural, Medical, and Moral Science (NYAG) (Bowery and Division St.); anatomical lectures (Wooster Beach) and phrenological lectures and examinations (1847–52)
1848	NYC: NYAG (aka Grand Anatomical Museum, Grand National Anatomical Museum, North American and Anatomical Museum) features performances by singers, 4–1848
1849	NYC: NYAG (333 Broadway, previously site of New York Museum)
1850	NYC: NYAG (300 Broadway) features two Anatomical Venuses; Wooster Beach, proprietor
1857	NYC: Reentz's Anatomical Museum ("the Chinese Buildings," 539 Broadway)
1858	Philadelphia: European Anatomical, Pathological, and Ethnological Museum (1858–1922?)
1861	NYC: Parisian Cabinet of Wonders and Anatomy (563 Broadway, Beck and H. J. Jordan) (1861–75) [pamphlets, advertisement, gentlemen only: *Harper's Weekly*, 12–28–1861: 832 and 1–4–1862: 16.]
1863	NYC: Parisian Cabinet changes name to New York Museum of Anatomy (618 Broadway, between Houston and Bleecker) NYC: Some version of Louis J. Kahn's Museum of Anatomy in operation?
1865	San Francisco: L. J. Jordan's Pacific Museum of Anatomy and Natural Science (1865–74)
1867	Washington, DC: Army Medical Museum opens
1869	NYC: Ladies' New York Museum of Anatomy (600 Broadway, later moved to 618½ Broadway) (affil. with H. J. Jordan's NY Museum of Anatomy)
ca. 1869	NYC: Kahn's Museum of Anatomy (745 Broadway at Astor Pl.) (1869–early 20th century)
ca. 1870	Boston: Dr. Hallock & Co.'s Museum of Anatomy and Medical Institute
1870	Boston: Parisian Gallery of Anatomy and Medical Science (Arlington Hall, corner of Washington and Essex Sts.; Robert J. Jourdain, prop.)

TABLE 9.1 CONTINUED

1871	NYC: New York Museum of Anatomy (760 Broadway, P.J. Jordan, prop.)
1871	Philadelphia: Museum of Anatomy, Science and Art in existence (807 Chestnut St.; Drs. Jordan and Davieson, prop.)
1874	NYC: Dr. Kahn's Museum (688 Broadway)
1875	Buffalo: European Anatomical, Pathological, and Ethnological Museum (Charles Kreutzberg, prop.)
1876	Philadelphia: European Anatomical, Pathological, and Ethnological Museum
ca. 1877	Chicago: Dr. Baskette's Gallery of Anatomy (126 Clark St. [with exhibit on Mormons])
ca. 1878	Chicago: Dr. Williams and Co. College of Anatomy (298 State St. [same college as Baskette])
ca. 1880	Coldwater, MI: Dr. Hay's College of Anatomy (Geo. S. Eldred, prop., traveling anatomy museum; 10¢ admission)
1882	NYC: Dr. Kahn's Museum of Anatomy moves to 713 Broadway
1888	NYC: Anthony Comstock and NYC police obtain warrants to close Parisian Museum (309 Bowery), Egyptian Musée (138 Bowery), European Museum (81 Bowery), Kahn's Museum of Anatomy (708 Broadway). Proprietors and employees are arrested and convicted, except for Louis J. Kahn; material confiscated and destroyed
1894	NYC : Kahn's Museum of Anatomy (252 Bowery)
ca. 1900–ca. 1920	Minneapolis and St. Paul (MN); Milwaukee; Omaha; Davenport and Des Moines (IA); Rock Island, Peoria, Moline, Joliet, East St. Louis, Chicago; St. Joseph (MO); Gary, Hammond, Fort Wayne and Indianapolis (IN), all owned by the Reinhardt Brothers
ca. 1905	NYC: Kahn's Museum of Anatomy (312 Bowery, above Houston) (Drs. Kahn and Jordan, prop.)
	NYC: Dr. DiBol College of Anatomy and Gallery of Science, Art, and Mysteries of Man and Woman
1930	Philadelphia: European Museum (708 Chestnut St.) (Drs. LaGrange and Jordan) still in existence
1936	Philadelphia: European Museum no longer listed in the City Directory [source: *Polk's (Boyd's) Philadelphia City Directory 106 (1936)*]

✦ CONCLUSION ✦

Now we are no longer satisfied with the comparatively
rough science which bore the name of human anatomy.

HERMANN VON HELMHOLTZ, "On the Relation of
Natural Science to General Science, Academical
Discourse Delivered at Heidelberg, November 22,
1862," trans. H. W. Eve, in *Popular Lectures on Scientific
Subjects* (London, 1873), 3

"[I]NTEREST . . . IN DISSECTIONS BEGINS TO WANT"

Long before the consolidation of anatomy's triumph in the 1840s and
1850s, the kernel of a new succession was already present. At first, way
back at the dawn of the 1800s, it seemed perhaps like a holding action, a
grudging claim on Edinburghian and Hunterian innovations in anatomy,
or maybe their most exciting potential. In an 1805 lecture at the University of Pennsylvania, Benjamin Rush, the venerable professor of the "institutes of medicine" (a category that combined physiology, pathology, and
therapeutics), cautioned his students that "Simple anatomy is a mass of
dead matter":

> It is physiology which infuses life into it. A knowledge of the structure of the
> body occupies only the memory. Physiology introduces it to the higher and
> more noble faculties of the mind. . . . The anatomist who describes the circulation of the blood, acts the part of a physiologist, as much as he . . . who
> attempts to explain the functions of the brain. In this respect Dr. [John]
> Hunter did honour to our science; for few men ever explained that subject
> . . . , and many others equally physiological, with more perspicuity and eloquence, than that illustrious anatomist.[1]

Anatomy by itself, Rush warned, is too static, too mechanical, too materialist. It lacks the spark of life. Insofar as anatomy is valuable, it must
incorporate physiology (as Rush believed Hunter had done).[2] The two
subjects are inseparable.

Yet, over the course of the nineteenth century, they did separate. And
by the 1870s and 1880s the action was in physiology—and in pathology,
comparative anatomy, and microscopic anatomy, all of which had seceded
from anatomy to become separate fields. A dullness began to afflict the
remainder: after a reign of more than a century, gross anatomy was finally
passé. In his 1870 introductory lecture to the entering class of the Medi-

cal Department of the University of Pennsylvania, D. H. Agnew fretted over the passing of the era: "I should greatly regret to witness a period when the interest of a medical class in dissections begins to want; and yet, I fear, such is the case."[3] Anatomy retained a place in the new medical order of things, but no longer as the main attraction. Students were still required to dissect—actually required to dissect more—and dissection still functioned as an initiation into the cult of medical knowledge. But for ambitious young men practical anatomy served only as a stepping stone. E. W. Holmes, another Philadelphia professor of anatomy, in a paper presented to the Pan-American Medical Congress of 1893, decried the "evident neglect" of the field:

> That anatomical study was the basis of all medical knowledge, that a dissecting room, a supply of bodies, and a corps of teachers were absolutely necessary, have always been axioms. . . . Twenty-five years ago well-equipped physiological and chemical and physical laboratories were uncommon; pathological museums were almost unknown, and practical hygiene and bacteriology were not in existence. To-day the opportunities for research in any one of these would busy a lifetime, but in anatomy we stand only on the basis of the needs of a quarter of a century ago. Formerly, anatomy claimed a good one-seventh of the required studies [and in the late-eighteenth- and early-nineteenth-centuries, one-fourth or one-fifth]; to-day, it but weakly elbows a space with twenty ologies and specialties which have been elevated by their more enthusiastic advocates.[4]

And yet it was not so much that anatomy had declined, but that it had accomplished so much. Anatomy had burst its disciplinary boundaries, divided and redivided. Its progeny—microbiology, zoology, anthropology, health reform, neurology, pathology, gynecology, endocrinology, etc.— were highly productive. In contrast, gross anatomy ceased to generate new theories or major discoveries. Professors of anatomy no longer starred as the leading men of medical science. Instead, they contented themselves with housekeeping, preservative methods and recipes, dissection techniques and technology, the perennial problem of cadaver supply, the pedagogy of entering medical students—and writing and lecturing on the historical, that is to say anatomical, lore of individual institutions and regions, and of medicine as a whole.

To the public, anatomy's decline was in some ways evident and in other ways invisible. But the new physiology and microbiology, in tandem with evolutionary theory, quickly found a mass audience: in the decades after the Civil War, popular and pedagogical writers and lecturers increasingly represented the body in cellular, physiological, pathological, and evolutionary terms. And nearly everywhere, except in the popular anatomy museums, the terms "physiology" and "hygiene" replaced "popular anatomy."

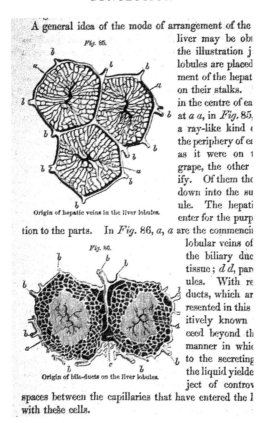

A general idea of the mode of arrangement of the
liver may be ob
the illustration j
lobules are placed
ment of the hepat
on their stalks.
in the centre of ea
at *a a*, in *Fig.* 85,
a ray-like kind (
the periphery of ea
as it were on 1
grape, the other
ify. Of them the
down into the su
ule. The hepati
enter for the purp

Fig. 85.

Origin of hepatic veins in the liver lobules.

tion to the parts. In *Fig.* 86, *a, a* are the commencii
lobular veins of
the biliary duc
tissue; *d d*, par
ules. With re
ducts, which ar
resented in this
itively known
ceed beyond th
manner in whic
to the secreting
the liquid yielde
ject of controv

Fig. 86.

Origin of bile-ducts on the liver lobules.

spaces between the capillaries that have entered the l
with these cells.

Figure 10.1. The cellular structure of the liver. John William Draper, *Human Physiology, Statical and Dynamical; or, The Conditions and Course of the Life of Man* (7th ed., New York, 1870), 160. Courtesy of the National Library of Medicine. After the Civil War, the term *physiology* displaced *popular anatomy* in school textbooks and popular works. The pedagogical iconography of the body increasingly tended to represent the body in cellular terms.

ANATOMY IN THE POSTBELLUM ERA

At the same time, medicine shows, sanitary fairs, anatomical museums, classroom lectures, school textbooks, and popular books and articles continued to present some version of the anatomical body to people of almost every class. Sensationalist narratives of anatomical mayhem, of arrogant dissectors and brutish resurrection men, continued to excite and disturb the public through the penny press, magazines, minstrel shows, and dime novels. This in itself is not surprising: if anatomy no longer occupied center stage, the teaching of anatomy and the dissection of bodies remained a conspicuous feature of American life. After the Civil War, medical schools and students continued to multiply, and the movement to expand, regulate, and reform medical education began to achieve its goals. As a result, entering and advanced medical students alike had to satisfy more rigorous requirements that included an increasing amount of anatomical dissection. Medical schools clamored for dissectable bodies.

States, however, lagged behind in the passage of anatomy laws. Most colleges lacked access to any legal supply of bodies, and so followed the tradition of illicitly procuring their cadavers, an enterprise now greatly facilitated by the growth of rail and shipping networks. Successive waves of scandal rippled throughout the Midwest, Pennsylvania, Maryland, Virginia, and New York. At the highwater mark, the year of 1878, the popular press reported at least twelve body-snatching outrages [see table 10.1]. In the most notorious case, reported in great detail over many days in most of the nation's newspapers, John Scott Harrison, the recently deceased son of President William Henry Harrison (and father of Civil War commander, and President-to-be, Benjamin Harrison), was discovered "with a rope about his neck, by which he was suspended, . . . in the dissecting room" of the Medical College of Ohio in Cincinnati.[5] The 74-year-old former Congressman's body had been stolen from a mausoleum in a respectable cemetery.[6] A follow-up investigation revealed that the college anatomy department had been used as a transshipment hub by a body-snatching gang that packaged bodies for shipment in pickle barrels to other midwestern medical schools.

In this and other cases, the press sounded familiar and contradictory themes: the hubris, complicity, and culpability of the medical profession; the ghoulish inhumanity of lower-class mercenary body snatchers (stereotypically Irish, Scottish, or black) who trafficked in flesh and had the audacity to prey even on the bodies of respectable people; the distress of the survivors and the innocent poor; the legitimate need of anatomists for bodies to dissect; the need for greater penalties for medical grave robbery; the need for laws that would give the bodies of unclaimed paupers to medical schools and end the pillaging of graves and sale of bodies. Resurrection scandals undoubtedly helped sell newspapers to a titillated public, and kept alive old resentments against medical schools and the profession.

But this was outweighed by the growing cultural authority of medical science, in the era of anesthesia, antisepsis, and the new breakthroughs in microbiological medicine. Given the impetus of the new scandals, in most Northern and border states, and Virginia, the medical colleges opportunistically mobilized to push for new anatomy acts or revisions of inade-

TABLE 10.1 NEWSPAPER REPORTS OF BODY-SNATCHING INCIDENTS IN
THE UNITED STATES, 1878

Sources: *New York Times, New York Tribune,* Kaufman and Hanawalt, *Detroit Sunday News.*

Toledo, OH (ca. 1–20): Dr. Henri Le Caron (grad. Detroit Medical College, 1872; aka Dr. Charles O. Morton) arrested, leader of body-snatching gang, along with two others.

Cincinnati (5–30): John Scott Harrison's body discovered at the University of Cincinnati; janitor discloses that "Dr. Morton" used college morgue to hide bodies for shipping to University of Michigan Medical School, in barrels labeled "pickles." Another missing body found there; Dr. William Herdman, demonstrator of anatomy, demands reimbursement of $30 before he will return it.

Cleveland (Willoughby), OH (9–17, 9–23): Body snatchings discovered, resurrectionists arrested along with the dean and members of the faculty of the Homeopathic Medical College; the accused found guilty 6–5–1879, sentenced 7–5.

Detroit (11–2): Body snatching prevented by armed guards.

Keokuk, IA (ca. 11–2): Discovery of two bodies shipped in barrels from Beacon, IA addressed to A. Mackay, a local physician who is attending lectures at the Iowa Medical College; Mackay is arrested.

Fort Wayne, IN (ca. 11–6): Medical college at Fort Wayne refuses to accept body of John Payton, "a wealthy citizen of Roanoke, Ind." brought to the college by a grave robber.

NYC (11–7 et seq.): Body of department-store magnate A. T. Stewart stolen; arrested men had previous record as medical grave robbers and are charged with "feloniously remov[ing] the dead body of a human . . . from the place of its interment for the purpose of dissection," but their real motive is ransom.

Zanesville, OH (11–13): Four graves robbed, physician arrested and convicted, sentenced to maximum ($1000 fine and six months in jail), but pardoned by the governor.

Chicago (11–16): Body-snatching duo arrested; body found at the Chicago Homeopathic College.

Cincinnati (11–18): Body of Betsy Slayton, "a colored woman," discovered missing from the grave.

Cincinnati (12–4): Police arrest five persons, including the widow of notorious body snatcher William Cunningham, for selling the body of a black girl to the Miami Medical College.

Evansville, IN (12–19): An anonymous note sent to the widow, body of Frank M. Murphy ("a respectable painter") found in the dissecting room of Evansville Medical College.

quate laws that were already on the books. The progress of these efforts was in many cases halting, but ultimately successful. In Ohio, for example, the furore over the Harrison case and other incidents in the state in the fall and winter of 1878–79 led to the introduction in the legislature of a bill that provided for an appointed state board to equitably distribute to medical schools unclaimed bodies obtained from state-owned or -supported hospitals, insane asylums, prisons, and poorhouses. The bill died at the end of the session, as had similar bills since at least 1840, but the measure's passage was finally accomplished under the cover of a larger reorganization and rationalization of the state's civil code by a commission appointed by the legislature in 1881.[7] Elsewhere, the old political wisdom also crumbled: it was no longer poison for politicians to support anatomy legislation. For most of the 1880s, body-snatching scandals continued to erupt in the Midwest, Pennsylvania, New York, Maryland, and Virginia. By 1890, nearly every state outside the South had passed or strengthened an anatomy statute, at no discernible political cost to the backers of the legislation.

A test of the political opportunities and liabilities of anatomy came in Massachusetts in 1883, when the maverick Democratic governor and former Civil War general Benjamin Butler charged that the State Almshouse at Tewksbury, a Republican patronage nest, was peddling the bodies of paupers to medical colleges and, even worse, selling their skins to tanners and clothiers to make luxury leather goods. Butler hoped the sensational allegations would fuel his reelection campaign, perhaps even a presidential bid, and personally prosecuted the inquiry. One of the objects introduced into evidence was a slipper allegedly made from the skin of a human breast. But no person was ever indicted in the case. In the face of fierce opposition from the Republican-dominated legislature, the politically contentious investigation was defused and came to an inconclusive close. The affair did little to rouse the working-class and rural electorate against the Republican party, despite ample press coverage. The old general lost his reelection bid by a wide margin, putting an end to his colorful political career.[8]

The power of anatomical narratives perhaps began to fade. In 1884 in Cincinnati a family of three was killed and their bodies sold to the Medical College of Ohio for the sum of $100; in 1886 in Baltimore, an elderly woman was murdered and sold to the University of Maryland Medical School for $15.[9] Although widely reported, neither case achieved the folkloric notoriety accorded the 1828 Burke and Hare murders in Edinburgh; there was no nationwide clamor to punish the medical profession for the only documented instances of burking in America. As in other postbellum scandals, the medical profession in Maryland was able to use the Baltimore murder to push forward a measure that made the state anatomy act more amenable to the colleges. Unlike Robert Knox, the Scottish anatomist whose career was destroyed by the Burke and Hare murders, no American anatomist suffered anything more than a pinprick of embarrassment.

THE DISAPPEARING CADAVER

Even as anatomy declined in the medical curriculum, dissection continued to function as a medical rite of passage, as it still does today. But professors and demonstrators began to police their students more diligently in an effort to discourage dissecting-room, and especially body-snatching, pranks. Such pranks might provoke criminal investigations or newspaper exposés, and fuel the always simmering resentment of "town" against "gown." This had always been a problem: what had changed was the culture of professionalism, which now was being remade around a greater identification with modernity, laboratory science, and industrial technology. And as medicine increasingly affiliated with science, an effort was made to clean up the dissecting room and remake it into a scrupulously hygienic anatomical "laboratory," to get students out of civilian clothes and into lab coats, and to encourage a sober, deliberative attitude in the lab.[10] The movement to improve decorum in the dissecting room and morgue was accompanied by a movement to improve hygiene and the quality of student work. Thus an 1860 manual for students emphasized that "you ought to be able to conduct a post-mortem examination from beginning to end, including every cavity and organ of the body . . . in your best dress suit, with only the cuffs of your coat and shirt-sleeves turned up. This . . . implies a mode of procedure very different from that revolting one which is unfortunately only too often to be witnessed, in which everything about the subject is hacked, mangled and bungled, and everything about the operator bloodied and soiled; the whole affair being a combination of butchery and botchery unparalleled."[11] Arthur Hertzler, looking back from the vantage of the 1930s, saw a vast transformation: the dissecting room he recollected from his medical student days in the 1880s at Northwestern University was a foul, disorganized "mess," and a theater of absurd anatomical hijinks, very unlike the domesticated, sterile anatomy lab of the mid-twentieth century.[12]

This transformation paralleled the conversion effected by the dissection ritual itself. Dissectors increasingly sought to forestall any identification with the body as a person, any identification that would elicit feelings in the anatomical student or the laity, even one so distancing as mockery. In so doing, the tendency was to make the triumph of scientific reason so complete as to minimize and eventually erase the presence of the cadaver, and perhaps even the anatomist, from the iconography of anatomy.

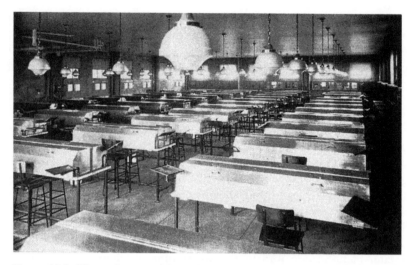

Figure 10.2. The cadaver vanishes. "Anatomical Laboratory." *The Skull (Temple University Medical School Yearbook), 1934*, p. 58. Courtesy of the Library of the College of Physicians of Philadelphia. In twentieth-century medical school yearbooks, the cadaver's presence is often erased in photographs of the anatomy department.

This trajectory was a slow and uneven process, and never fully consummated. Anatomists continued to dissect, and still do (though not all of them); humorous anatomical photos, poems, and cartoons continued to appear in medical school yearbooks, until about the mid-1970s; joking continued to take place in the anatomy lab, as it still does today in an attenuated way.

As we have seen, in other registers and domains, the human body was reduced to the status of "materiel" much earlier. In the mid-nineteenth century, body snatching was a lucrative cottage industry—anatomy departments generally paid between $10 and $35 a body, in an era when the wages of a skilled worker might be $10–$30 a week and a day laborer might make $1 per day or less.[13] Agents in New York exported bodies to schools in New England, the mid-Atlantic states, and the maritime South; agents in Baltimore exported bodies to schools in the upper South and the Midwest. The body in anatomy was a commodity, extracted from the earth or obtained illicitly before burial, an object of exchange whose value fluctuated according to the law of supply and demand. If this served to erase the humanity of the cadaver, it also served as a metaphor for the erasure of the humanity of working people, whose labor was also extracted and reduced to the status of a commodity. The fact that the vast majority of cadavers were working-class secured the connection: The anatomical narrative of body snatching and the body trade was a parable of capitalism.

That parable was an indictment of the market and the inequitable social relations that emanated from it. But the onus could always be redirected. Anatomists disclaimed all responsibility for the actions of their agents and argued that the passage of anatomy acts would end all abuses, secure anatomy's privileged place outside the market, and so terminate the polluting moral and social association between anatomist and purveyor. By the end of the century, when anatomy acts were in effect in almost every state, the point of the anatomical narrative had been precisely reversed: now it was the anatomist who was above the market; the unlettered lower classes were eager to sell themselves. In 1906, Albertus J. Pierce, a down-on-his-luck circus performer, wrote a letter to H. A. Kelly, professor of gynecology at Johns Hopkins, offering his body for sale upon the event of his death. For the entertainment of his colleagues, Kelly printed it in full in the *Johns Hopkins Hospital Bulletin*, with the mispellings retained for comic effect.[14] Pierce, who stuck "huge needles" through his tongue "and one inch from the heart," and swallowed swords, pins, glass, live frogs, and snakes, hoped that his body was anomalous enough to command $100 from the professor, paid in advance. But Kelly dismissed the offer as laughable, a response that betokened an unbridgeable social gulf between the proletariat and medical professoriate. Professional medical identity was premised on the idea that physicians should be disinterested gentlemen, above and outside the market; medicine is a profession and a science, not a trade or a craft; the doctor occupies a privileged position in the social and moral order, untainted by trade. By contrast, Albertus Pierce was tainted not only by his willingness to conduct trade, but by his willingness to become the object of trade.

THE CADAVER'S PERSPECTIVE: DEATH AND THE PERFORMANCE OF CLASS IDENTITY

> The grave is the place where the courted and the
> slighted, the high-minded and the base, the solitary and
> the man of many friends, the envied and the despised,
> the ignorant and the scholar—all lie down together and
> are soon forgotten.
>
> ITEM ON THE FRONT PAGE OF A BLACK
> INDIANAPOLIS WEEKLY, 1902[15]

Here, as in every other aspect of his life, Pierce openly embraced his transgressions; he willfully stepped outside the moral order articulated in conventional funerary practice. In the nineteenth century, I have argued, how one died, and how one's body was treated after death, was a performance that fixed one's moral, aesthetic, and social status. For most poor people, a "decent" burial—placement of the body in a coffin, with some ornamentation; a respectful ceremony; and interment in a bounded plot of land with a marker—was an extraordinary imperative. If you accumulated no other capital in your life, your one bit of savings might go to pay for your burial and the burials of your loved ones. The anatomical encounter, then, was a zero-sum power exchange: the cadaver's loss was the anatomist's gain. An unattended death, death in the poorhouse, followed by burial in a bare pine box in Potter's Field, or by dissection in an anatomical theater or display in an anatomical museum, was a punishment that commented on the life. Whether deserved or undeserved, it was a posthumous torture, a secular hell.

Such ideas, it bears emphasis, were not just the anxiety-ridden superstitions of the poor but were also held by those who lavished large sums of money on fancy coffins and cemeteries and cemetery plots, expensive and fashionable widows' weeds, and private editions of consolatory poetry. The middle and upper classes did not have to worry about whether they could afford decent funerary arrangements, but in the midst of their bereavement they also fretted over the possibility that enemies or predators would blight a funerary performance. George Pullman, the railroad-car magnate who ruthlessly suppressed striking workers, and so became a symbol of the arrogance of the late-nineteenth-century capitalist class, arranged for steel-reinforced concrete to be placed over his grave, to prevent the desecration of his body by embittered ex-employees. Pullman was never accused on this account of being "irrational" or "superstitious."[16] People of all classes, ethnic groups, and educational backgrounds hated the prospect of seeing their bodies, or the bodies of family members, dissected, mutilated, or in any way "disturbed."

This was true also of doctors. When anatomy laws were debated, opponents of the acts proposed that licensed physicians and incoming medical students be required to donate their bodies and the bodies of their kinfolk, rather than the poor. The anatomy lobby always dismissed such proposals on the grounds that the dissection of physicians' bodies would distress family and friends (with the implication that the doctors would gladly accommodate their critics were it not for the highly strung irrational sensibilities of their womenfolk). Following the example of Jeremy Bentham's "auto-icon," J. C. Warren and a few other prominent physicians did make testamentary provisions that their bodies be publicly dissected before a respectful professional assembly and used in the making of anatomical preparations, but such acts remained exceptional.[17] When Dr. George Soresi in 1913 proposed that the Fellows of the New York Academy of Medicine endorse a proposal to require incoming students to pledge their bodies for autopsy as a condition for entry into medical school, not a single hand was raised to second the motion.[18]

What we can conclude from all this is that, from the "cadaver's perspective," opposition to anatomical dissection was not an "irrational" reaction. If critics accused anatomists of malice, they were not far wrong: middle- and upper-class physicians often treated their working-class patients with enormous condescension; elaborate conspiracies to appropriate the bodies of the dead did exist; anatomical students did often treat their subjects with contempt and mockery; and anatomy acts that gave the bodies of paupers to medical schools did create "an invidious distinction between the rich and the poor," as one critic of Connecticut's 1833 act charged.[19] Even charges of necrophilia were not without substance; the anatomical body *did* carry an erotic charge, among anatomists and the public. Similarly, antipathy to anatomical dissection was shared by much of the population, including anatomists, who were by no means eager to lend their own bodies and the bodies of their kin to the task at hand. Insofar as this antipathy was the motivating force behind anatomy rioters and legislative resistance to the progress of medical science, it represented (in H. A. Kelly's words) a "barrier on the road to anatomy." But, at the same time, the cultural power of the anatomist, whether depicted as a disembodied panoptic dissector or an eroticized phallic invader, depended precisely on this reaction: anatomy needed barriers to overcome. Its triumphs over such barriers advertised its moral necessity and epistemological power.

"KNIVES IN THEIR BRAIN": DISSECTION, PROFESSIONALISM, AND THE BOURGEOIS SELF

Given anatomy's prestige as an exemplary science, and the transformation of professional medicine into a popular bourgeois occupation, anatomical dissection provided new emergent academic and scientific professions with a potent rhetoric. The proliferation of medical schools and medical men inevitably resulted in the widespread circulation of anatomical signs—anatomy was put to various uses by middle-class women, working-class men, and anybody else who cared to seize upon it. But it also had particular uses among those who were carving out new disciplines— some of the new professionals came to the social sciences from medicine and had personal experience with the discourse and performance of anatomy. T. S. Lambert, the first president of the American Social Science Association, was a physician who distinguished himself in the 1850s as a popular anatomical author and lecturer. He and his fellow "social scientists," the first group to lay claim to such a title, were not shy about deploying anatomical rhetoric.

Cultural authority clearly was transferable from cadaver to society—
eminent medical professors were at times called on to pronounce publicly on a variety of nonmedical and semimedical questions.[20] But the anatomical trope of disembodied dissector operating on the embodied social
and material world, with its corollary homosocial order, was also deployed
by those who lacked medical credentials. "[T]here is an analogy between
the human body and the body politic, . . . a Social Anatomy, a Social
Psychology, a Social Hygiene, and a Social Surgery and Therapeutics,"
argued Frederick Wines, a Presbyterian minister, president of the Western
Social Science Association and a leading penal reformer, in an 1868 address, "should constitute the four Departments of Social Science."[21] Wines
and his fellow reformers believed that they could use statistical analysis to
perform dissections and postmortems on the body politic and ultimately
make their social science as productive and authoritative as anatomical
medicine.

Many of these professionalizing reformers were attempting to subordinate female philanthropy to social science, just as the physician had earlier subordinated the female midwife. William Graham Sumner, author of
the laissez-faire antihumanitarian 1883 tract, *What the Social Classes Owe to
Each Other*, indicted the sentimental philanthropy of women, and feminized male fellow travelers, in these terms: "The amateur social doctors
are like the amateur physicians—they always begin with the question of
remedies, and they go at this without any knowledge of the anatomy or
physiology of society."[22]

In the period when the ideology of professionalism in America was
being developed, when the notion of "profession" was being expanded
from the traditional three learned professions (theology, law, and medicine) to the sciences and "social sciences," and less lofty occupations like
cemetery management (even magicians, renamed *professional* illusionists),
anatomy was available as a discursive model and an exemplary epistemology. In history, sociology, popular and not so popular science, and all
sorts of reform movements, the trope was almost irresistible: The keen
cut; the destruction of illusionary superstition; the disinterested division
of the subject into parts, with an almost joyful annihilation of obfuscating
boundaries; the conquering disembodied intellect (invariably gendered
male), the genius who lays his subject bare, who opens up a territory for
civilization or field of inquiry for science or social reform.[23] "With the skill
of a surgeon and the keen blade of the scalpel, [Dr. E. B. Foote] dissects
to the bone nearly all our social usages and lays open the rotten places,"
puffed one of Foote's biographers.[24]

The anatomical trope was not merely available for masculinist professionalism, but also for the masculinist bourgeois self. Ralph Waldo Emerson suggests as much in his memoir of life in the 1830s and 1840s: "The

young men," he writes, "were born with knives in their brain, a tendency to introversion, self-dissection, anatomizing of motives."[25] Over the course of the nineteenth century, the anatomical body became a vocabulary of the bourgeois self. Embedded in this vocabulary was the figure of the essential (male) self as a killing, disembodied dissector (depicted metaphorically as an eye, hand, knife, spirit) that operates on the body and the material world. This worked to constitute the dichotomous self as bourgeois, masculine, human, civilized, mind, on the one hand, and animal, savage, primitive, body (and continually subject to eroticization), on the other. The relation of this trope to normative self-making procedures had unpredictable and sometimes contradictory implications. Emerson is a wonderful example, precisely because he takes up the cause of disembodiment to such an exaggerated degree. His young men dissect not only the external world but also themselves, and then so finely that the body disappears—leading not to phallic world conquering but to a disembodying (and to critics effeminating) etherealization. From there it is but a short distance to the compensatory masculinism of Theodore Roosevelt, the Y.M.C.A. movement, and a host of new technologies of embodied self-making devoted to the formation of robust bourgeois manliness. The "homosexual panic," so characteristic of late-nineteenth- and early-twentieth-century psychological and criminological discourse, can then be seen, in part, as a response to the vexing discursive problem that arose from the normative constitution of the bourgeois masculine self as disembodied spirit.

FINALE

> In commencing the annual course of Human Anatomy, I propose to . . . direct . . . your attention . . . to the general structure, essential conditions of existence, and characteristic phenomena of all living beings, of which *man* constitutes the most striking example or highest type in the actual or present state of the earth.
>
> JOSEPH LEIDY, professor of anatomy, to the entering class at the University of Pennsylvania, 1859[26]

There are many loose ends left untied, but we are now at the end of this book. I have shown how anatomical enterprises mobilized networks of anatomists, students, body snatchers, healers, patients, popularizers, and audiences. From another angle, the anatomical enterprise consisted of practices and performances: on paper (the making of articles, engravings, books, and charts); in the graveyard and on the deathbed (the preparation, burial, and exhumation of bodies); in the lecture hall and the dissecting room (the discoursing on and display of bodies, and the cutting open and rending of flesh, bone, and sinew); and, arguably, as the inner performance of the divided bourgeois self. Anatomy extended far beyond the production and reproduction of scientific and technological knowledge about the "human" and "animal" body. Doctors were ideological workers, whose credentials entitled them to comment and intervene on a broad array of social questions ranging far outside their immediate vocation of attending the sick. The authority of medical discourse allowed physicians and reformers to argue that moral, social, and political positions—and categorical entities like negro, woman, criminal, etc.—were "natural" or "normal" or "pathological" and therefore outside the normal contestation of politics and social conflict.

This was not just professional pretension. There was in fact a strong demand for disinterested authority (albeit a demand that physicians worked hard to cultivate and cater to). Thus, in an 1861 libel case in Baltimore, Joseph Leidy, professor of anatomy at the University of Pennsylvania, was asked to render an expert opinion. The defendant had called the plaintiff a "nigger." The case turned on a key question: What, anatomically considered, constitutes a "negro"? Skin color? Hair texture? The shape of the nose? The lips? Brain size? Intelligence? "Facial angle"? Configuration and relative size of the internal organs? Or was it a matter of "blood"? Leidy, the most eminent American anatomist of the day, was called on to resolve whether the plaintiff could legitimately be termed a "negro," by supplying a scientific definition.[27]

The outcome of the case is not known. But in other domains, medical men were asked to offer advice, render opinions, create and administer bureaucracies concerned with sanitation, water supply, human burials, food supply and quality, disease control and prevention, design of schools and classrooms, etc. Such activities dovetailed with the cultural and social aspirations (some said pretensions) of the medical profession—and required, or at least presumed, some notion of the anatomical body and anatomical authority.

Over the course of the nineteenth century, the anatomical body became the regnant idiom of selfhood, with a variety of unanticipated results. However, at the moment of its triumph, perhaps because of its triumph, the anatomical body, and the bourgeois identity which deployed it, suffered a loss of coherence. This was perhaps just the inevitable erosion that afflicted every canon of social identity, exposed to the incessant churning of self-making technologies and practices, but by the late nineteenth century, anatomy was found wanting, disparaged as inadequate to represent the dynamism of the body, or in another way too dynamic, too vulgarly corporeal, easy prey for dime museum proprietors to crassly exploit. The anatomical body was no longer strong enough to carry the weight of modernity, could no longer function as the auto-icon of science and progress. Or was perhaps too heavy, too material in its associations.

But it was not entirely discarded. Rather, the anatomical body became the substrate upon which new technologies of self-making were elaborated: in school instruction and popular health discourse, which emphasized cellular physiology; in psychoanalysis, which offered an imaginary anatomy of subjectivity; in the gland craze of the 1920s, which offered a new hormonal narrative of human subjectivity; in exercise and dietary programs of physical fitness and health; in eugenics and bioengineering; etc. Although the boundaries of medical discourse and practice were, and are, still contested—sex education has never achieved anything close to universal acceptance and antivivisectionism has attracted a new following—the anatomical body in Western societies has no serious competitors. It is so pervasive, in so many different elaborations, as to be nearly invisible. Naturopathic critics, acupuncturists, faith healers, all translate their concepts into anatomical terms and imitate the procedures and rituals of anatomical medicine. The maps we carry of our innards are anatomical and will remain so for the foreseeable future.

That said, there is no resolution. We still construct and negotiate the boundaries of self and other in the changing idioms of the best medical science of Rour time, currently molecular biology and neuroscience. We still struggle over the boundaries of self and other in the idioms of funerary ritual and professional authority, in contests over the study, repatriation, and consecration of archaeological remains, as in the debate over the African-American burial ground in New York City, and perennial arguments about the medicalization of death or the right to physician-assisted suicide. We still negotiate the boundaries of self and market: ongoing controversies about the ownership of products made from body tissues and genes, and about the sale and allocation of organs from cadavers and living donors, attest to that. And we still fantasize about, and play with, the boundaries of self, other, market, and professional authority: witness the recent hoax in which someone put up a kidney for auction on eBay, or the publicity and controversy attending the sculptures of anatomist Gunther von Hagens, whose medium consists of cadavers soaked in his patented preservative "plastination" process.[28]

Beyond all that, it is no longer news that we are now unfurling, or submitting to, a new dispensation. We produce, or compromise, the distinction between Self and Other through technological enhancements that enter and connect our bodies of flesh and blood with proliferating electronic communications grids, computer simulations, and data packs. We no longer know the difference between self, machine, and datum. We are tempted to think that these new conditions call on us to renounce and pleasure the body, to construct and annihilate self, all in the same instant, via the same procedures. Maybe we try to persuade ourselves, or at least fantasize, that the body is not obdurate, that flesh is infinitely malleable, or will be soon. And if that feels strange to us, it also feels familiar: We've been there, done that. The technologies, the sciences, the discourses and practices of Self and Other (or Self *as* Other), have proliferated, but an enduring legacy remains. Our bodies, ourselves, still refer back to cadavers, dissecting physicians, and proliferating texts.

⊰֎ NOTES ֍⊱

Introduction

1. Frantz Fanon, *Black Skin, White Masks* [1952], trans. Charles Lam Markmann (New York, 1967), 116.

2. Rom Harré, *Physical Being: Theory for a Corporeal Psychology* (Oxford, 1991), 14.

3. *Address of Valentine Mott . . . Before the Graduates of 1860 of the University Medical College of New York* (New York, 1860), 13.

4. *Pennsylvania Gazette*, 11-30-1774: 1.

5. See David C. Humphrey, "Dissection and Discrimination: The Social Origins of Cadavers in America, 1760–1915," *Bulletin of the New York Academy of Medicine* 49.9 (1973): 819–27; Steven Robert Wilf, "Anatomy and Punishment in Late Eighteenth-Century New York," *Journal of Social History* 22 (1989): 507–30; Robert L. Blakely and Judith M. Harrington, eds., *Bones in the Basement: Postmortem Racism in 19th-Century Medical Training* (Washington, DC, 1997).

6. Most southern states without anatomy laws had large prison systems, with disproportionately large populations of black prisoners, and made available the bodies of deceased inmates.

7. Raymond Williams, *Keywords: A Vocabulary of Culture and Society* (rev. ed., New York, 1983), 45.

8. *The Physiology of Love: Hints on Courtship* (New York, ca. 1850) [AAS].

9. *An 1855–56 Notebook Toward the Second Edition of Leaves of Grass*, ed. Harold Blodgett (Carbondale, 1959), 8–9 [notebk., pp. 23, 25].

10. Judith Butler, *Bodies That Matter: On the Discursive Limits of "Sex"* (New York, 1993), esp. 12–15.

11. Lenoir, "Was the Last Turn the Right Turn?:" The Semiotic Turn and A. J. Greimas," *Configurations* 2.1 (1994): 122.

12. The ambivalence was not new. According to Katharine Park ("The Criminal and the Saintly Body: Autopsy and Dissection in Renaissance Italy," *Renaissance Quarterly* 47 (1994): 18, in the 1500s, "public concern regarding anatomical practice in Italy, . . . coexisted with . . . enthusiasm for the spectacle of dissection. The reservations of Italian city dwellers . . . concerned not dissection in general but the specific prospect that they or their loved ones might come under the anatomist's knife." My research shows that eighteenth- and nineteenth-century Americans felt equally ambivalent about anatomy.

13. John W. Draper, *University of New-York Medical Department: a Valedictory Lecture, Delivered by Professor Draper* (New York, 1842), 4 [CPP].

Chapter One: "The Mysteries of the Dead Body"

1. Philippe Ariès, *Western Attitudes Toward Death: From the Middle Ages to the Present*, trans. Patricia M. Ranum (Baltimore, 1974), 106.

2. Robert Crowell, *Interment of the Dead, a dictate of natural affection. . . .* (An-

dover, MA, 1818), iii–iv [NYHS]; see also F. C. Waite, "An Episode in Massachusetts in 1818 Related to the Teaching of Anatomy," *New England Journal of Medicine* 220.6 (2-9-1939): 221–27.

3. Sewall was charged, tried, convicted, and fined $800 (his attorney was Daniel Webster), but fled the state and settled in the District of Columbia. He later served as professor of anatomy at Columbian College and became physician to three presidents.

4. *Boston Daily Globe*, 1-26-1885: 1. A skeleton with fibrodysplasia ossificans is on exhibit at the Mütter Museum, College of Physicians, Philadelphia.

5. *Freedom's Journal*, 3-30-1827.

6. James M'Clintock, *Introductory Lecture to the Course on Anatomy and Physiology, in the Vermont Academy of Medicine, delivered April 7, 1841* (Castleton, VT, 1841), 4.

7. F. H. Hamilton, *Introductory Address, and Catalogue of Students attending the Annual Course of Lectures on Anatomy and Surgery* (Auburn, NY, 1837), 4.

8. Robley Dunglison, *An Introductory Lecture to the Course of Institutes of Medicine, &c. Delivered in Jefferson Medical College, November 1, 1841* (Philadelphia, 1841), 12.

9. See, for example, L. F. Edwards, "The Ohio Anatomy Law of 1881, Pt. 1," *Ohio State Medical Journal* 46 (1950): 1190; and A. M. Lassek, *Human Dissection: Its Drama and Struggle* (Springfield, IL, 1958), 126, 257–73 and *passim*.

10. Ruth Richardson, *Death, Dissection, and the Destitute* (London, 1988), ch. 1.

11. *Weekly Magazine of Original Essays* (Philadelphia), 6-1-1798: 144–45, "from a public print, published several years since"; the account is of the Bergen County coroner's inquest of 9-22-1767. The same report is printed in *New-York Journal*, 10-1-1767, along with a similar report from Boston in *New-York Weekly Post-Boy*, 4-11-1768; both are discussed in Sara S. Gronim's, "Natural Bodies: Illness and Healing in British Colonial New York," paper presented to the Seminar on the History of Medicine, New York Academy of Medicine, 10-21-1997. I want to thank Sara Gronim for sharing her research with me, which has informed a good part of the discussion in this section.

12. David C. Humphrey, "Dissection and Discrimination: The Social Origins of Cadavers in America, 1760–1915," *Transactions of the New York Academy of Medicine* 49.9 (1973): 819–27.

13. The phrase "social being" was coined by Robert Hertz, "A Contribution to the Study of the Collective Representation of Death" [*Années Sociologique* 10 (1907)], in *Death and the Right Hand*, trans. R. and C. Needham (Glencoe, IL, 1960), 27–86. See also Thomas Laqueur, "Bodies, Death, and Pauper Funerals," *Representations* 1.1 (1983): 109–31.

14. Charles Lawrence, *History of the Philadelphia Almshouse and Hospitals from the Beginning of the Eighteenth to the Ending of the Nineteenth Century* . . . (Philadelphia, 1905), 160–61, 207–8, 252–53.

15. Crowell, *Interment of the Dead*, 19, 26, 30–31, 34–35.

16. This was not a transhistorical cultural rule. In the Middle Ages, the bodies of saints and monarchs were frequently hacked to bits in order to produce relics for shrines, with no loss of selfhood. Their bodies were powerful enough to retain and even radiate selfhood even in fragmentary form. Still, many versions of Christian theology proposed that redemption was related to bodily integrity and that in heaven the body would be whole again, a cultural presumption that bodily integ-

rity was crucial to the self. The saints were miraculous precisely because they could spiritually transcend attempts to disaggregate their bodies. See Caroline Walker Bynum, *Fragmentation and Redemption* (New York, 1992).

17. The metaphor of eater versus eaten was among the commonest tropes of political rhetoric, as in this 1807 polemic by Abel M. Sargent: "[H]ow often is the poor industrious and honest labourer, reduced to the absolute necessity of yielding up his rights and falling a prey to cruelty and injustice, merely for want of money enough to discharge the fees of those whose interest and livings (like the wolf and raven) depend on the ruin and destruction of others." Qtd. in Nathan O. Hatch, *Democratization of American Christianity* (New Haven, 1989), 76.

18. Richardson, *Death, Dissection, and the Destitute*, 29.

19. Michel Foucault, *The Birth of the Clinic: An Archaeology of Medical Perception*, trans. A. M. Sheridan Smith (New York, 1973), 163.

20. Steven Robert Wilf, "Anatomy and Punishment in Late Eighteenth-Century New York," *Journal of Social History* 22 (1989): 507–130. For incident on shipboard, see 525, n. 16, citing *Pennsylvania Journal and Weekly Advertiser*, 2-22-1786.

21. Crowell, *Interment of the Dead*, 23.

22. Jonathan Sawday, *The Body Emblazoned: Dissection and the Human Body in Renaissance Culture* (New York, 1995).

23. Sara S. Gronim, "Ambiguous Empire: The Knowledge of the Natural World in British Colonial New York" (Ph.D. diss., history, Rutgers University, 1999); see also Herbert Leventhal, *In the Shadow of the Enlightenment: Occultism and Renaissance Science in 18th-Century America* (New York, 1976).

24. Gronim, "Ambiguous Empire."

25. Foucault, *The Birth of the Clinic*, 4, 17: "[T]he best medicine of prerevolutionary France sought to construct Linnaean diagrammatic relationships . . . for disease," a "scheme . . . which abstracts disease from the body. . . . "

26. See Charles Rosenberg, "The Therapeutic Revolution: Medicine, Meaning, and Social Change in Nineteenth-Century America," in Rosenberg, *Explaining Epidemics and Other Essays in the History of Medicine* (Cambridge, 1992); and John Harley Warner, *The Therapeutic Perspective: Medical Practice, Knowledge, and Identity in America, 1820–1885* (Cambridge, 1986).

27. F. Gonzalez-Crussi, *The Day of the Dead and Other Mortal Reflections* (New York, 1993), 4–5, argues that "death is essentially . . . unthinkable, and beyond all possibility of description. . . . it must elude discourse: . . . the tendency to evade naming this reality must be universal." The cultural power of Vesalian anatomy stems in part from its determination to systematically represent the dead body, to make it thinkable.

28. Cotton Mather, *Addresses to Old Men* (Boston, 1690), qtd. in Gordon E. Geddes, *Welcome Joy: Death in Puritan New England* (Ann Arbor, 1981), 28. The passage is a paraphrase of William Harvey.

29. Nehemiah Walter, *The Body of Death Anatomized . . . delivered . . . in Boston, 12 d. 7 m. 1706 . . .* (2d ed., Boston, 1736) [MHS], A3, 1–2.

30. Angelina Grimké, *Appeal to the Christian Women of the South* (New York, 1836), 28, 33, qtd. in Karen Sánchez-Eppler, *Touching Liberty: Abolition, Feminism, and the Politics of the Body* (Berkeley, 1993), 2.

31. Gerda Lerner, *The Grimké Sisters from South Carolina: Rebels Against Slavery*

(Boston, 1967), 22, 68–74; Catherine Birney, *Sarah and Angelina Grimké: The First Women Advocates of Abolition and Woman's Rights* [1885] (rpt. Westport, CT), 11. Grimké spent a transitional year (1827) as a Presbyterian.

32. Hatch, *Democratization of American Christianity*; quote is on 158.

33. According to David D. Hall, *Worlds of Wonder, Days of Judgment: Popular Religious Belief in Early New England* (Cambridge, MA, 1990), 16, mid-seventeenth-century Boston's churches could accommodate no more than a third of the adult population. What the other two-thirds did on any given Sunday, and how closely they identified with Calvinism, is unknown.

34. Andrew Marvell, "A Dialogue Between the Soul and Body" (1681), in M. E. Abrams et al., *The Norton Anthology of English Literature* (New York, 1968), 1: 985–86.

35. Norbert Elias, *The History of Manners: The Civilizing Process, Vol. 1* [1939], trans. Edmund Jephcott (New York, 1978), is the classic work.

36. Richard Bushman, *The Refinement of America: Persons, Houses, Cities* (New York, 1992); John Kasson, *Rudeness and Civility: Manners in Nineteenth-Century Urban America* (New York, 1990); Stuart Blumin, *The Emergence of the Middle Class: Social Experience in the American City, 1760–1900* (Cambridge, 1989).

37. Poe "The Magnetizer; or, Ready for Any Body," *Broadway Journal,* 9-6-1845: 133–34.

38. Blackwell, *Pioneer Work in Opening the Medical Profession to Women* (London, 1895), 27–28.

39. See Martin Pernick, *A Calculus of Suffering: Pain, Professionalism, and Anesthesia in Nineteenth-Century America* (New York, 1985), esp. ch. 7.

40. See G. J. Barker-Benfield, *The Culture of Sensibility: Sex and Society in Eighteenth-Century Britain* (Chicago, 1992).

41. Esther Schor, *Bearing the Dead: The British Culture of Mourning from the Enlightenment to Victoria* (Princeton, 1994), 5–6, 20.

42. Adam Smith, *Theory of Moral Sentiment* (London, 1759), I.i.1.1.13.

43. "The Buried Alive," *Freedom's Journal,* 8-17-1827; rpt. from *Edinburgh Review.*

44. David Cressy, "Death and the Social Order: The Funerary Preferences of Elizabethan Gentlemen," *Continuity and Change* 5 (1989): 99–119.

45. David Stannard, *The Puritan Way of Death: A Study in Religion, Culture, and Social Change* (New York, 1977), 110–15; Geddes, *Welcome Joy,* ch. 6; James J. Farrell, *Inventing the American Way of Death, 1830–1920* (Philadelphia, 1980); David Charles Sloane, *The Last Great Necessity: Cemeteries in American History* (Baltimore, 1991).

46. Harriet Martineau, *Retrospect of Western Travel* (London, 1838; rpt. New York, 1969), 3: 273.

47. Isabella Lucy Bird, *The Englishwoman in America* [1856] (Madison, 1966), 376.

48. *New York Times,* 3-30-1866: 2.

49. Alexander H. Stevens, *A Plea of Humanity in behalf of Medical Education: The Annual Address Delivered before the New-York State Medical Society. . . .* (Albany, NY, 1849), 5 [HS].

50. This anesthesia regimen is undermined by the taboo on opiate-derived or synthetic narcotics which, critics allege, leads to the undertreatment of pain.

51. Cf. Ronald Dworkin, Thomas Nagel, Robert Nozick, John Rawls, Thomas Scanlon, and Judith Jarvis Thomson, "Assisted Suicide: The Philosophers' Brief [amicus curiae, *State of Washington et al. v. Glucksberg et al.* and *Vacco et al. v. Quill et al.*, U.S. Supreme Court, 1-8-1997]," *New York Review of Books*, 1-27-1997: 41–47, who argue that "Most of us see death—whatever we think will follow it—as the final act of life's drama, and we want that last act to reflect our own convictions, those we have tried to live by, not the convictions of others forced on us in our most vulnerable moment." (44) If so, the ban on suicide, and the routinization of terminal medical treatment, are obstacles to the staging of a meaningful death. Physician-assisted suicide becomes a ritual affirmation of liberal political philosophy, an affirmation of individual freedom and "choice" (albeit with the imprimatur of liberal academic and medical authority), a contribution to the progress of reason over unreason. In this way, death regains the status of the moral conclusion of the life narrative. But this paradoxically requires opposition (in the form of the state, the regnant professional medical ethic, and the Catholic church). See Ivan Illich, *Medical Nemesis: The Expropriation of Health* (New York, 1976), who argues for a dignified acceptance of death, against the authority and routinized procedures of the state and professional medicine.

52. *New York Tribune*, 11-25-1850: 5.

53. Taylor, *Sources of the Self: The Making of Modern Identity* (Cambridge, MA, 1989), 288–89.

54. "Influence of death," *The American Museum, or, Universal Magazine* 8 (1790): 227–29.

55. Hiram Mattison, *Popular Amusements: An Appeal to Methodists, in regard to the evils of Card-Playing, Billiards, Dancing, Theatre-Going, etc.* (New York, 1867), 74.

56. Elliot, *New England's Chattels: or, Life in the Northern Poor-House* (New York, 1858), quote is from 181.

57. Association for the Benefit of Colored Orphans, *Annual Reports* (New York, 1837–50).

58. Harriot K. Hunt, *Glances and Glimpses; or Fifty Years Social, including Twenty Years Professional Life* (Boston, 1856), 62–73.

59. William Andrus Alcott, *Forty Years in the Wilderness of Pills and Powders; or, the Cogitations and Confessions of an Aged Physician* (Boston, 1859), 49.

60. Elliot, *New England's Chattels*, 473.

61. Martineau, *Retrospect of Western Travel*, 3: 272.

62. S. J. Kleinberg, "Death and the Working Class," *Journal of Popular Culture* 11.1 (1977): 193–209.

63. Henry G. Dunnel, "Annual Report of the Interments in the City and County of New York, showing their Age, Sex, Colour and Places of Nativity, for the year 1837 . . . " *American Journal of the Medical Sciences* 13 (1838): 242; New York City, Board of Aldermen, *Report on Deaths in the City of New-York*, #63, 2-10-1845: 826; New York City, Board of Assistant Aldermen, *Annual Report of the City Inspector of the Number of Deaths and Interments in the City and County of New York, for the Year 1847*, #21, 3-27-1848: 94.

64. Edward L. Bell, "The Historical Archaeology of Mortuary Behavior: Coffin Hardware from Uxbridge, Massachusetts," *Historical Archaeology* 24 (1990): 54–78. Bell argues that the differential distribution of cheap coffin ornamentation does

not reflect differential social status, but rather the spotty market availability of such products.

65. *Documents of the Board of Aldermen of the City of New York* 14 (5-1847 to 5-1848): 213–16 (doc. no. 14, 10-25-1847), 226.

66. Qtd. in David Cannadine, "War and Death, Grief and Mourning in Modern Britain," in Joachim Whaley, ed., *Mirrors of Mortality: Studies in the Social History of Death* (New York, 1981), 189.

67. Such distinctions in some places were reinforced by state and municipal policy. According to Frederick Hoffman, *Pauper Burials and the Interment of the Dead in Large Cities* (Newark, NJ, 1919), 15, in the year 1918 the city of Atlanta provided $15 for an adult white pauper's burial, but only $8 for a black pauper.

68. Ibid., 107.

69. *New York World*, 2-2-1896: 31; Kenneth Jackson and Camilo José Vergara, *Silent Cities: The Evolution of the American Cemetery* (Princeton, 1989).

70. At the same time, the bourgeois expenditure on death received its own critique. Beginning in the 1850s and accelerating in the 1870s and 1880s, *Harper's Monthly* and other middle-class journals show periodically published articles criticizing funerary rituals as an unproductive, immodest, and irrational use of resources; as an alternative many of these articles proposed cremation. The critique of the vulgarization of death reached an apogee of sorts in the twentieth century with Jessica Mitford's *The American Way of Death* (New York, 1963).

71. *Harper's New Monthly Magazine* 57 (1878): 305.

72. S. J. Kleinberg, "Death and the Working Class."

73. *New York Times*, 1-10-1884: 1

74. Crowell, *Interment of the Dead*, 40.

75. See C. B. Macpherson, *The Political Theory of Possessive Individualism: From Hobbes to Locke* (New York, 1962); and also Gillian Brown, *Domestic Individualism: Imagining Self in Nineteenth-Century America* (Berkeley, 1990).

76. Elliot, *New England's Chattels*, 35.

77. A. B. Winfield, *Sermon at the Interment of the Bodies of John G. Van Nest, Mrs. Sarah Van Nest, Mrs. Sarah Van Nest, G. W. Van Nest, Their Son, and Mrs. Phebe Wykoff, who were murdered . . . by a colored man named William Freeman. . . .* (Auburn, NY, 1846), 3–4 [NYHS].

78. Elizabeth Keckley, *Behind the Scenes, or, Thirty Years a Slave, and Four Years in the White House* (New York, 1868), 24.

79. Robley Dunglison, *The Medical Student; or, Aids to the Study of Medicine. . . .* (Philadelphia, 1837), 192.

80. Jay Ruby, *Secure the Shadow: Death and Photography in America* (Cambridge, 1995), 47, 110.

81. "Human Petrefaction," *Buffalo Morning Express*, 3-9-1854: 1.

82. Milton P. Braman, Danvers, MA, to J. C. Warren, 10-13-1830 [J. C. Warren Papers, MHS].

83. Azel Backus, *An Inaugural Discourse, delivered in the Village of Clinton, December 3, 1812 by the Rev. Azel Backus . . . on the day of his Induction into the office of the President of Hamilton College* (Utica, 1812), 11.

84. Against this popular stereotype, prominent medical figures took pains to assure the public of their own and the profession's religious rectitude. The medi-

cal discourse of the period is filled with disavowals of freethinking materialism, and avowals of religious orthodoxy. Most physicians publicly adhered to the dominant religious beliefs, and many seem to have had deep religious commitments.

85. *The American Museum, or, Universal Magazine* 8 (1790): 227–29.

86. Elliot, *New England's Chattels*, 299.

87. George Lakoff and Mark Johnson, *Metaphors We Live By* (Chicago, 1980).

CHAPTER TWO: "A GENUINE ZEAL"

1. Francis Hopkinson, *An Oration, Which Might Have Been Delivered to the Students in Anatomy, on the Late Rupture Between the Two Schools in this City* (Philadelphia, 1789). For the dispute between the College of Philadelphia and University of Pennsylvania, see George W. Corner, *Two Centuries of Medicine: A History of the School of Medicine, University of Pennsylvania* (Philadelphia, 1965), 35–43.

2. Joseph Carson, *A History of the Medical Department of the University of Pennsylvania, from its Foundation in 1765, with Sketches of the Lives of Deceased Professors* (Philadelphia, 1869), 81, 217; Jules C. Ladenheim, "The Doctor's Mob," *Journal of the History of Medicine* 5 (1950): 23–53; Claude Heaton, "Body Snatching in New York City," *New York State Journal of Medicine* 43 (1943): 1861–65; Steven Robert Wilf, "Anatomy and Punishment in Late Eighteenth-Century New York," *Journal of Social History* 22 (1989): 507–30; Jonathan Harris, "The Rise of Medical Science in New York 1720–1820" (Ph.D. diss., history, New York University, 1971), 99.

3. The name likely refers to the browning of the skin that occurs when the cadaver begins to undergo an advanced state of deterioration, but it may also be an allusion to its racial identity.

4. *Two Introductory Lectures . . . to his Last Course of Anatomical Lectures. . . .* (London, 1784), 73.

5. See Kenneth M. Ludmerer, *Learning to Heal: The Development of American Medical Education* (New York, 1985); William G. Rothstein, *American Physicians in the Nineteenth Century: From Sects to Science* (Baltimore, 1972); idem, *American Medical Schools and the Practice of Medicine: A History* (Oxford, 1987); Richard H. Shryock, *Medicine and Society in America, 1660–1860* (New York, 1960); idem, *Medicine in America: Historical Essays* (Baltimore, 1966); and Paul Starr, *The Social Transformation of American Medicine* (New York, 1982).

6. U.S. Department of Commerce, *Historical Statistics of the United States* (Washington, 1975), 1: 76 (B 275–90). The estimated U.S. resident population went from 7,224,000 in 1810 to 31,513,000 in 1860; ibid., 1: 8 (A 6–8).

7. Caldwell, *Thoughts on the Impolicy of Multiplying Schools of Medicine* (Lexington, KY, 1834), 21 [NYAM].

8. *Historical Statistics of the United States*, 1: 76 (B 275–90); this includes alternative practitioners who had undergone formal medical training.

9. J. C. Warren, London, to John Warren, Boston, 8-18-1800 [J. C. Warren Papers, MHS].

10. Emily Jane Cohen, "Enlightenment and the Dirty Philosopher," *Configurations* 5 (1997): 371. See also Barbara M. Stafford, *Body Criticism: Imaging the Unseen in Enlightenment Art and Medicine* (Cambridge, MA, 1991), 47–129.

11. See Adrian Wilson, *The Making of Man-Midwifery: Childbirth in England, 1660–*

1770 (Cambridge, MA, 1995); and Irvine Loudon, "The Making of Man-Midwifery" (rev. of Wilson), *Bulletin of the History of Medicine* 70 (1996): 507–15.

12. Corner, *Two Centuries of Medicine,* 6–7.

13. Shryock, *Development of Modern Medicine,* 62. This needs some qualification; surgery had a long craft tradition, but also an academic tradition that dates back to the Middle Ages, if not earlier.

14. John Morgan, *A Discourse upon the institution of Medical Schools in America; Delivered . . . May 30 and 31, 1765. . . .* (Philadelphia, 1765), xxiii.

15. Hopkinson, *An Oration,* iii, 7.

16. See John Harley Warner, *Against the Spirit of System: The French Impulse in Nineteenth-Century American Medicine* (Princeton, 1998).

17. See Russell C. Maulitz, *Morbid Appearances: The Anatomy of Pathology in the Early Nineteenth Century* (Cambridge, MA, 1987); Michel Foucault, *The Birth of the Clinic: An Archaeology of Medical Perception,* trans. A. M. Sheridan Smith (New York, 1973); and Stanley Joel Reiser, *Medicine and the Reign of Technology* (Cambridge, 1978), ch. 3, "Visual technology and the anatomization of the living." The quote is from P. M. Latham, "Lectures on Subjects Connected with Clinical Medicine," *London Medical Gazette* 17 (1835–36): 280, in Reiser, 31. In fact, Laënnec objected to the materialist implications of pathological anatomy, and hoped that his work on living patients would be a corrective to the pathologist's fixation on the cadaver; he argued that certain diseases, such as asthma, only manifested themselves as invisible lesions of the vital principle, not as visible lesions that could be seen in post-mortem dissection. But, from a distance, contemporaries regarded him as a founder of pathological anatomy rather than a critic. See Jacalyn Duffin, *To See with a Better Eye: A Life of R. T. H. Laennec* (Princeton, 1998).

18. Thomas F. Harrington, *The Harvard Medical School: A History, Narrative, and Documentary* (New York, 1905), 1: 303–4.

19. James Alfred Spalding, *Dr. Lyman Spalding: the Originator of the United States Pharmacopeia* (Boston, 1916), 149–50.

20. John Harley Warner, "Remembering Paris: Memory and the American Disciples of French Medicine in the Nineteenth Century," *Bulletin of the History of Medicine* 65 (1991): 301–25, and *Against the Spirit of System: The French Impulse in Nineteenth-Century American Medicine* (Princeton, 1998).

21. Leidy, *Lecture Introductory to the Course on Anatomy in the University of Pennsylvania for the Session 1858–59* (Philadelphia, 1859), 7.

22. Henry William Ducachet, *Tribute to the Memory of Jacob Dyckman, M.D., Late Health Commissioner of the City of New-York. . . .* (New York, 1823), 18–19 [HS].

23. Jefferson, Monticello, 1812, to Crawford, in H. A. Washington, ed., *The Writings of Thomas Jefferson* (Washington, 1853–54), 6: 32.

24. See Cohen, "Enlightenment and the Dirty Philosopher," 369–424.

25. W. Bruce Fye, *The Development of American Physiology: Scientific Medicine in the Nineteenth Century* (Baltimore, 1987), 55–56.

26. James M'Clintock, *Introductory Lecture to the Course on Anatomy and Physiology, in the Vermont Academy of Medicine, delivered April 7, 1841* (Castleton, VT, 1841), 10 [NYAM]. For science and medical identity, see John Harley Warner, "Science, Healing, and the Physician's Identity: A Problem of Professional Character in Nineteenth-Century America," *Clio Medica* 22 (1991): 65–88.

27. Mary Elizabeth Wieting, *Prominent Incidents in the Life of Dr. John M. Wieting* (New York, 1889), 6.

28. See John Harley Warner, "Ideals of Science and Their Discontents in Late Nineteenth-Century American Medicine," *Isis* 82 (1991): 454–78.

29. Steven J. Harris, "Long-Distance Corporations, Big Sciences, and the Geography of Knowledge," *Configurations* 6 (1998): 269–304, argues that anatomy was a "small science" as opposed to larger long-distance collective scientific enterprises (disciplines like "geography," or institutional networks like the Society of Jesus or Dutch East India Company). But eighteenth- and early-nineteenth-century anatomy (and medicine as a whole), while not a unitary entity, had a kind of nodular loosely hierarchical shape that operated over transoceanic distances. For example, J. C. Warren of Boston studied anatomy with Sir Astley Cooper in London, and the two maintained a collegial or client-patron relationship over decades that was embedded in a much larger network.

30. Lester King, *Transformations in American Medicine* (Baltimore, 1991), ch. 9; Martin Pernick, *A Calculus of Suffering* (New York, 1985), 95–102, 114–15, 142–47 and *passim.*

31. See Fye, *Development of American Physiology*, 59–63.

32. Robley Dunglison, *The Medical Student; or, Aids to the Study of Medicine. . . .* (Philadelphia, 1837), 169.

33. Massachusetts Medical Society, *Address to the Community on the Necessity of Legalizing the Study of Anatomy* (Boston, 1829), 27.

34. [George Bancroft], rev. of Massachusetts Medical Society, *Address to the Community*, in *North American Review* 32.70 (1–1831): 67.

35. G. W. Corner, "The Role of Anatomy in Medical Education," *Journal of Medical Education* 33 (1958): 2; Martin S. Pernick, *Calculus of Suffering*, 4. Austin Flint Jr., "The First Century of the Republic: Medical and Sanitary Progress," *Harper's Monthly* 53 (6–1876): 70–84, also praised vaccination, the stethoscope, the thermometer, the ophthalmoscope, and the development, improvement, and multiplication of scientific medical institutions such as colleges, journals, and medical societies.

36. Edward Jenner's technique of smallpox vaccination, and John Snow's research linking cholera outbreaks with particular drinking water supplies, were celebrated medical accomplishments that clearly saved lives. Both, while not inherently anatomical in nature, were the work of anatomically trained physicians (Jenner was John Hunter's protegé).

37. Dunglison, *Medical Student*, 168.

38. Late-twentieth-century historians are tempted to find anatomical medicine wanting on different grounds: the new operations of the late eighteenth and early nineteenth century were performed rapidly, without anesthesia or asepsis, and were therefore liable to induce shock or infection. Prior to the twentieth century, no clear correlation can be made between life expectancy and advances in anatomical knowledge and surgical technique. Cf. Pernick, *Calculus of Suffering*, 7, 249–62 (tables summarizing data), who argues that the introduction of anesthesia led to an increase in surgical operations that were "mostly necessary, not experimental," with a death rate that was fairly low when all factors are taken into account.

39. Pernick, *Calculus of Suffering,* 242.

40. Mircea Eliade, *Shamanism: Archaic Techniques of Ecstasy* [1951] (Princeton, 1964).

41. Simon Baatz, "'A Very Diffused Disposition': Dissecting Schools in Philadelphia, 1823–1825," *Pennsylvania Magazine of History and Biography* 108 (1984): 203–17, qtd. from 212–14 [edited text, "Communication from the Medical Faculty to the Trustees on Introducing the Dissections into the Common Course of Study for Graduates in Medicine, 1824," Medical Faculty Papers, General Archives, University of Pennsylvania]. See also William Barlow and David O. Powell, "A Dedicated Medical Student: Solomon Mordecai, 1819–1822," *Journal of the Early Republic* 7 (1987): 377–97.

42. Barlow and Powell, "Dedicated Medical Student," 390–97.

43. Heber Chase, *The Medical Student's Guide; . . . a compendious view of the Collegiate and Clinical Medical Schools, the Courses of Private Lectures, the Hospitals and the Almshouses . . . of Philadelphia* (Philadelphia, 1842) [CPP].

44. Jacalyn Duffin, *Langstaff: A Nineteenth-Century Medical Life* (Toronto, 1993), 17–19.

45. John Warren and Aaron Dexter, "Memorial & Petition for the Removal of Med. Lect. to Boston," 2-20-1810 [John Warren Papers, MHS].

46. See, for example, John F. Sanford, *Introductory Lecture, Delivered in the College of Physicians and Surgeons of the Upper Mississippi, Session of 1849–50* (Davenport, MS, 1849), 8.

47. Martha Ballard, diary, 2–1801, 4.4, qtd. in Laurel Thatcher Ulrich, *A Midwife's Tale: The Life of Martha Ballard, Based on Her Diary, 1785–1812* (New York, 1990), 236.

48. Ulrich, *Midwife's Tale,* ch. 7. See also A. Wilson, *Making of Man-Midwifery;* and Loudon, "The Making of Man-Midwifery."

49. The timing of the transition varied from locale to locale and class to class. In America, the movement of doctors into midwifery began among the elite in Boston, Charleston, and Philadelphia in the 1750s and 1760s, with New York lagging; see Philip Cash, "The Professionalization of Boston Medicine," in Frederick S. Allis, Jr., et al., *Medicine in Colonial Massachusetts, 1620–1820* (Boston, 1980), 75–76, 91.

50. Ulrich, *Midwife's Tale,* 250–51. There is little eighteenth- or nineteenth-century evidence for the superiority of man-midwives over female midwives in terms of lower infant or maternal mortality rates. Ibid., 175–79, shows that Benjamin Page, the callow new physician in town, was less skilled and prudent than Ballard.

51. For the exclusion of women from dissecting, and scientific activity generally, see Londa Schiebinger, *The Mind Has No Sex? Women in the Origins of Modern Science* (Cambridge, MA, 1989).

52. See Susan Shifrin, "'The Worst Are Women Doctors': Nineteenth-Century Attitudes Toward the Appearance and Professionalism of Women Physicians," *Transactions & Studies of the College of Physicians of Philadelphia,* ser. 5, 16 (12–1994): 47–65, esp. 51 and 56.

53. *Remarks on the Employment of Females as Practitioners in Midwifery, by a Physician* (Boston, 1820), 7. Ulrich, *Midwife's Tale,* 401, n. 24, suggests the author may have been Walter Channing, professor of midwifery at Harvard; Regina Markell Mor-

antz, ed., *In Her Own Words: Oral Histories of Women Physicians* (New Haven, 1982), 8–9, 36, n. 12, suggests the author was John Ware, a younger professor.

54. Richard L. Bushman, *The Refinement of America: Persons, Houses, Cities* (New York, 1992).

55. Wilson, *Making of Man-Midwifery*, 191.

56. Dan King, *Quackery Unmasked: or a Consideration of the Most Prominent Empirical Schemes of the Present Time* (Boston, 1858), 262–63.

57. Alexander H. Stephens, *A Plea of Humanity in behalf of Medical Education: The Annual Address Delivered before the New-York State Medical Society. . . .* (Albany, 1849), 7 [NYHS].

58. William A. Alcott, *Forty Years in the Wilderness of Pills and Powders; or, the Cogitations and Confessions of an Aged Physician* (Boston, 1859), 3. For more on Alcott, see chaps. 1 above and 6 below.

59. Warner, *Against the Spirit of System*.

60. See, for example, Ludmerer, *Learning to Heal*; Shryock, *Medicine and Society in America* and *Medicine in America*; and Starr, *Social Transformation of American Medicine*.

61. [E. H. Dixon], "An M.D., or a Modern Doctor of Medicine; Pursuit of Practice under Difficulties," *Scalpel* 10 (10–1858): 407–8.

62. [E. H. Dixon], "Scenes in a Medical Student's Life: Resurrectionizing," *Scalpel* 7 (1855): 93–100.

63. Whitfield J. Bell, Jr., "Nathan Smith Davis: An Autobiographical Letter, Previously Unpublished," *Journal of the American Medical Association* 224.7 (5-14-1973): 1014–16 [N. S. Davis, Chicago, to Joseph M. Toner, Washington, DC, 3-25-1875, Toner Papers, Library of Congress].

64. Smith to James Jackson, Jr., 2-21-1834, qtd. in Warner, "Remembering Paris," 310.

65. W. J. McKnight, *The Pioneer Doctor: "Who Skinned the Nigger" or the Origin and Enactment of Pennsylvania's State Anatomical Law* (n.p., n.d.; rpt. *Brookville Republican*, 3-1-1915).

66. See, for example, Charles Stephen Gurr, "Social Leadership and the Medical Profession in Antebellum Georgia" (Ph.D. diss., University of Georgia, 1973).

67. Massachusetts Medical Society, *Address to the Community, on the Necessity of Legalizing the Study of Anatomy* (Boston, 1829), 3.

68. See G. C. Sanchez, "John Collins Warren," in M. Kaufman et al., eds., *Dictionary of American Medical Biography* (Westport, CT, 1984), 2: 779; J. C. Warren journals [J. C. Warren Papers, MHS]; Edward Warren, *The Life of John Collins Warren, M.D.* (Boston, 1860), 2 vols.

69. J. W. Draper, *University of New-York Medical Department: a Valedictory Lecture* (New York, 1842), 11–12.

70. Daniel Drake, *An Introductory Lecture, On the Means of Promoting the Intellectual Improvement of the Students and Physicians of the Valley of the Mississippi. . . .* (Louisville, KY, 1844), 20.

CHAPTER THREE: "ANATOMY IS THE CHARM"

1. G. W. Corner, *Anatomy* (New York, 1930), 1.

2. Jerome Van Crowninshield Smith, Boston, to J. C. Warren, 5-16-1825; see also Smith to Warren, 1-31-1825 [J. C. Warren Papers, MHS].

3. D. H. Agnew, *Lecture Introductory to the One Hundred and Fifth Course of Instruction in the Medical Department of the University of Pennsylvania, delivered Monday, October 10, 1870* (Philadelphia, 1870), 25. I want to thank Susan Wells for alerting me to this passage.

4. Robley Dunglison, *The Medical Student; or, Aids to the Study of Medicine. . . .* (Philadelphia, 1837), 147.

5. The term "cultural poetics" is borrowed from Stephen Greenblatt, *Renaissance Self-Fashioning: From More to Shakespeare* (Chicago, 1980), 4–5. It suggests that eighteenth- and nineteenth-century anatomy can be regarded as a poetic idiom, performed and interpreted by a historically specific set of actors and historically specific audiences. The historian's role is to provisionally decode the poetics, to propose a historically specific reading or readings (what Greenblatt calls "the interpretive constructions the members of a society apply to their own experiences"), much as the literary critic decodes poems and other texts. The term "cultural poetics" also suggests that the historian can usefully apply technical concepts derived from poetics and rhetoric: synecdoche, trope, etc.

6. Morgan, *A Discourse upon the Institution of Medical Schools in America. . . .* (Philadelphia, 1765), 6–7.

7. John F. Sanford, *Introductory Lecture, Delivered in the College of Physicians and Surgeons of the Upper Mississippi, Session of 1849–50* (Davenport, MI, 1849), 8.

8. Daniel Drake, *An Introductory Lecture, On the Means of Promoting the Intellectual Improvement of the Students and Physicians of the Valley of the Mississippi, Delivered in the Medical Institute of Louisville, November 4th, 1844* (Louisville, 1844), 4.

9. F. H. Hamilton, *Introductory Address, and Catalogue of Students attending the Annual Course of Lectures on Anatomy and Surgery* (Auburn, NY, 1837), 12.

10. Qtd. in Michel Foucault, *The Birth of the Clinic: An Archaeology of Medical Perception,* trans. A. M. Sheridan Smith (New York, 1973), 146.

11. John D. Godman, *Introductory Lecture to the Course of Anatomy and Physiology, in Rutgers Medical College, New-York, Delivered, November 11, 1826* (New York, 1826), 27, 29 [NYAM].

12. W. W. Keen, *A Sketch of the Early History of Practical Anatomy: the Introductory Address to the Course of Lectures on Anatomy at the Philadelphia School of Anatomy. . . .* (Philadelphia, 1870), 3. The trope of the anatomist's interrogation of the dead body was often deployed in the writings of the Parisian school and its admirers. It can be traced further back to Francis Bacon, who favored extended metaphors in which the new science forcibly interrogated and even raped a recalcitrant but ultimately yielding female Nature; see Carolyn Merchant, *The Death of Nature: Women, Ecology, and the Scientific Revolution* (San Francisco, 1983).

13. This mimetic component predated romanticism and persisted into the twentieth century. In his 1765 address, Morgan asked his students to "place before your eyes the illustrious examples of great men, who, by pushing their researches into the bosom of nature, have extended the bounds of useful science. Tread in their steps. . . . " [55] Similarly, Corner, in a 1958 address, emphasized that "A microscopic section of the pancreas will tell . . . even the youthful student [that he] can make a significant discovery, as did Langerhans. The surface of the brain recalls the name of Sylvius, and section of the cerebellum speaks of Purkinje, Golgi, and Cajal." [7] As in geographical discovery and conquest, anatomical dis-

coveries were often embedded in the proprietarial names of the parts, "the Fallopian tubes," "the Eustachian tubes," "the crescents of Gianuzzi," etc.

14. See, for example, E. M. Hartwell, "The Present Legal Status of the Study of Human Anatomy in the United States," *Annals of the Anatomical and Surgical Society* 3 (7–1881): 8.

15. Robley Dunglison, *The Medical Student*, 150.

16. George Eliot, *Middlemarch* [1871–72] (London, 1959), 1: 128

17. Today, while dissection no longer occupies a central place in the medical curriculum, for beginning students it still functions as a symbolically laden rite of passage (and, some now argue, little else). See Frederic W. Hafferty, *Into the Valley: Death and the Socialization of Medical Students* (New Haven, 1991).

18. Qtd. in Howard M. Feinstein, *Becoming William James* (Ithaca, 1984), 167. James spoke from experience; a few decades earlier, he had been an anatomy student.

19. J. Marion Sims, *The Story of My Life* (New York, 1884), 128–29. Thanks to Jenna Johnson for bringing this to my attention.

20. See Alain Corbin, *The Foul and the Fragrant: Odor and the French Social Imagination* [1982], trans. Miriam Kochan (Cambridge, MA, 1986).

21. For nineteenth-century views on this subject, see Jacob Bigelow, *Remarks on the Dangers and Duties of Sepulture: or, Security for the Living, with Respect and Repose for the Dead* (Boston, 1823); Felix Pascalis, *An Exposition of the Dangers of Interment in Cities* (New York, 1823); Stephen Wickes, *Sepulture: Its History, Methods and Sanitary Requisites* (Philadelphia, 1884).

22. T. Southwood Smith, "The Use of the Dead to the Living," *Westminster Review* 2 (1824): 92 n.

23. Bigelow, *Remarks on the Dangers and Duties of Sepulture*, 31–32. The dissecting room is still a biohazard; see William Bachop, "Minimizing Risks and Maximizing Benefits Educational Abuses."

24. [Dixon], "Scenes in a Medical Student's Life—Resurrectionizing," *The Scalpel* 7 (1855): 95.

25. Cf., letter, Brett Levinson, a medical student at the University of Maryland, Baltimore, to *New York Times*, 1-19-99: D5, which revives this theme, and endorses some form of counterbalancing humanizing training: "We take human anatomy concurrently with a class on medicine and literature, which is designed to impress upon us the humanistic nature of our profession despite our dehumanizing hours in the anatomy lab."

26. Qtd. in J. O. G., "Religio Medicorum," letter to *Boston Medical and Surgical Journal*, 7-19-1854: 503.

27. Francis Hopkinson, *An Oration, Which Might Have Been Delivered to the Students in Anatomy of the Late Rupture Between the Two Schools in this City* (Philadelphia, 1879), 9.

28. Solomon Mordecai to Ellen Mordecai, 11-20-1819, 1–29 and 2-26-1820, qtd. in W. Barlow and D. O. Powell, "A Dedicated Medical Student: Solomon Mordecai, 1819–1822," *Journal of the Early Republic* 7 (1987): 387.

29. See Philip Sohm, "Gendered Style in Italian Art Criticism from Michelangelo to Malvasia," *Renaissance Quarterly* 48 (1995): 759–808. (Michelangelo and other artists dissected, but Sohm confines his discussion to painting.)

30. "Medical Education," *New York Medical Inquirer* 1 (1830): 130.

31. Cf. Elisha North, *Outlines of the Science of Life* ("A Vindication of the Rights of Anatomists"), 145: "the study of anatomy . . . may sometimes occasion hallucination or delusion, in the brain of a very zealous medical student; and a state of hallucination in the brain of an anatomist may sometimes be made to appear like a state of horrid inhumanity, to the . . . brains of a court and jury. . . ."

32. Arthur E. Hertzler, *The Horse and Buggy Doctor* (New York, 1938), 43.

33. William Eustis, Boston, to John Warren, Salem, 11-17-1773 [John Warren Papers, MHS]; Jonathan Norwood, Falmouth, MA, to John Warren, 6-5-1775 [John Warren Papers, MHS]; *Boston News Letter*, 10-21-1773; Albert Matthews, "Notes on Early Autopsies and Anatomical Lectures," *Publications of the Colonial Society of Massachusetts* 19 (1916–17): 273–90, esp. 286–88. Eustis's later political career included terms as Governor of Massachusetts and Secretary of War under James Madison.

34. Eve Kosofsky Sedgwick, *Between Men: English Literature and Male Homosocial Desire* (New York, 1985), 1–2: "'Homosocial' is a word [that] . . . describes social bonds between persons of the same sex; it is a neologism, obviously formed by analogy with 'homosexual,' and just as obviously meant to be distinguished from 'homosexual.' In fact, it is applied to such activities as 'male bonding,' which may, as in our society, be characterized by intense homophobia, fear and hatred of homosexuality. To draw the 'homosocial' back into the orbit of 'desire,' . . . is to hypothesize the potential unbrokenness of a continuum between homosocial and homosexual." Homosociality takes specific forms; it always serves to construct and enforce boundaries between men and women, but can also do so between hetero- and homosexual men, rich and poor, particular groups of young men, young and old men, profession and laity, and, of particular interest to Sedgwick, the sexual and the nonsexual, "what *counts* as sexuality."

35. Samuel Craddock, Jr., Geneva, NY, to D. E. Craddock, Weedsport, NY, 10-25-1847, Williams and Craddock Family Papers, Cornell University, Dept. of Manuscripts and University Archives.

36. Bachop, "Educational Abuses," 29, argues that present-day first-year anatomical instruction functions as a kind of hazing.

37. "Editor's Table," *Harper's New Monthly Magazine* 8 (April 1854): 692.

38. "Medical Education in New York," *Harper's New Monthly Magazine* 65 (10–1882): 672. According to Hertzler, *Horse and Buggy Doctor*, 44, at Northwestern University in the 1880s, anatomical lectures "were given in amphitheaters in which the seats were arranged in an angle of about forty-five degrees. The students amused themselves by 'passing up' their fellows. . . . Two students sitting just back of the victim selected would pass their hands under his arms and raise him up. Then another pair of students in the seat above assumed the burden. By these successive efforts the victim soon found himself at the topmost row. . . . The members of the class not so engaged supplied the music, rendering . . . such tunes as 'There is a hole in the bottom of the sea' or 'The girl I left behind me.' "

39. James S. Terry, "Dissecting Room Portraits: Decoding an Underground Genre," *History of Photography* 7.2 (1983): 96–98; James Edmonson and Steven De-Genaro, curators, "Haunting Images: Photography, Dissection, and American Medical Students," Exhibition, Dittrick Medical History Center, Cleveland, Fall

1998; "Group of Three Students at Dissecting Table with Cadaver, c.1844," in Joel Peter Witkin and Stanley Burns, *Masterpieces of Medical Photography: Selections from the Burns Archive* (Pasadena, 1987). The development of medical school yearbooks and comic postcards in the 1880s and 1890s provided a venue for such photographic subjects (made possible by improvements in print technology, especially the development of photographic screening). As student body snatching was progressively curtailed and then suppressed, it became safe to celebrate and display anatomical high jinks in semipublic media such as published reminiscences and yearbooks.

40. Hertzler, *Horse and Buggy Doctor*, 43.

41. Valentine Mott, *Reminiscences of Medical Teaching and Teachers in New York: An Address Introductory to a Course of Lectures at the College of Physicians and Surgeons . . .* (New York, 1850), 12–13.

42. Minutes of the Faculty, Transylvania University Medical Department, ms. vol., 10-25-1822, qtd. in John H. Ellis, *Medicine in Kentucky* (Lexington, KY, 1977), 12, 84, n. 8.

43. S. W. Francis, *Biographical Sketches of Distinguished Living New York Physicians* (New York, 1867), 99–100.

44. "The Negro Steaks (A Chapter from the Diary of a N.Y. Physician)" ["from the N.Y. Transcript"], *Thomsonian Manual* 1 (1835): 181–82.

45. O. W. Holmes, Sr., *Medical Essays, 1842–1882* (Cambridge, MA, 1891), 278–79.

46. See Ludmilla Jordanova, *Sexual Visions: Images of Science and Medicine Between the Eighteenth and Twentieth Centuries* (Madison, 1989).

47. McKnight, *The Pioneer Doctor.*

48. Spencer, *Poem on the Hubbardton Raid*, 26 [NYHS].

49. See Shifrin, "'The Worst Are Women Doctors,'" esp. 51 and 56.

50. King, *Quackery Unmasked.*

51. See Susan Wells, *Out of the Dead House: 19th-Century Women Physicians and the Practice of Medicine* (Madison, WI, 2001); Regina Morantz-Sanchez, *Sympathy & Science: Women Physicians in American Medicine* (New York, 1985).

52. *The Gilded Age: A Tale of To-Day* (New York, 1873; rpt. New York, 1915), ch. 15, esp. 1: 153.

53. Elizabeth Blackwell, *Pioneer Work in Opening the Medical Profession to Women* (London, 1895), 27–28, 35. I want to thank Susan Wells for sharing her research on Blackwell with me and helping me to think about the position of the female dissector. Also Wells, *Out of the Dead House.*

54. See, for example, Ladies' Medical Academy, *First Annual Report* (Boston, 1860) [MHS]; Ann Preston, *Valedictory Address to the Graduating Class of the Female Medical College of Pennsylvania, for the Session of 1857–58* (Philadelphia, 1858) [CPP].

55. Qtd. in Ruth J. Abram, ed., *"Send Us a Lady Physician": Woman Doctors in America, 1835–1920* (New York, 1985), 143.

56. Pauline Stitt, oral history, in Regina Markell Morantz, Cynthia Stodola Pomerleau, and Carol Hansen Fenichel, eds., *In Her Own Words: Oral Histories of Women Physicians* (New Haven, 1982), 110.

57. Horace Walpole, *Anecdotes of Painting in England; with Some Account of the*

Principal Artists; and Incidental Notes on Other Arts; Collected by the Late George Vertue (1762; London, 1786), 3: 195.

58. *Pennsylvania Chronicle, and Universal Advertiser*, 3-2-1767: 594.

59. *New-England Weekly Journal*, 11-18-1734.

60. Henry K. Brooke, compil., *Tragedies on the Land, Containing an Authentic Account of the Most Awful Murders that have been committed in this country; with a report of the trial, judge's charge, and the execution of the criminals, from the year 1823 to 1840, inclusive* (Philadelphia, 1847), 19–25, 81; *New York Gazette*, 11-24-1823.

61. *New York Herald*, 2-27-1836.

62. *Mutiny and Murder; Confession of Charles Gibbs* . . . (Providence, 1831), 24 [NYHS]; *Catalogue of the Grand Anatomical Museum, or National Academy of Natural, Anatomical and Pathological Science* (New York, 1854), 64 [FC]; *Catalogue: Dr. Baskette's Gallery of Anatomy* (Chicago, n.d. [ca. 1875]), 737 [collection of William Helfand]. For a description of the hanging, Gibbs's dissection, and the transformation of his skull into an anatomical object "put it in a case, with a label" (with the disclaimer that the story is "strictly true"), see George Lippard, *The Quaker City* (Philadelphia, 1845), 432–34.

63. *New York Sun*, 2-26-1836: 2; *New York Herald*, 2-27-1836: 1, 3-1-1836: 2, 3-2-1836: 1. See also Benjamin Reiss, "P. T. Barnum, Joice Heth and Antebellum Spectacles of Race," *American Quarterly* 51 (1999): 78–107.

64. *Providence Gazette, and Country Journal*, 4-24-1773: 642.

65. William H. Holcombe, *How I Became a Homoeopath* (Philadelphia, 1866), 3 [AAS].

66. See James Edmonson, "The Medical Period Room," *Caduceus* 3.4 (Winter 1987): 27–43.

67. D. W. Cathell, *The Physician Himself and What He Should Add to the Strictly Scientific* (Baltimore, 1882), 11. Two years later, in the 4th edition (1884), 11, Cathell reversed field, advising physicians to "keep from sight . . . repulsive objects, [such] as catheters, specula, obstetric forceps, . . . amputating knives, skeletons, jars of amputated extremities, tumors, and the unripe fruit of the uterus."

68. Mary Shelley, while underplaying the role of electricity in animating her monster, acknowledged Aldini as a source; Martin S. Pernick, "Back From the Grave: Recurring Controversies Over Defining and Diagnosing Death in History," in Richard M. Zaner, ed., *Death: Beyond Whole-Brain Criteria* (Dordrecht, 1988), 23. In his later career, Ure was an apologist for the industrial revolution; in *Capital, vol. 1*, Marx calls him "the Pindar of the automatic factory."

69. See Steven Earl Forry, "The Hideous Progenies of Richard Brinsley Peake: *Frankenstein* on the Stage, 1823 to 1826," *Theatre Research International* 11 (1986): 13–31; Donald F. Glut, *The Frankenstein Catalogue* (Jefferson, NC, 1984); and Tim Marshall, *Murdering to Dissect: Grave-Robbing, Frankenstein and the Anatomy Literature* (Manchester, U.K., 1995).

70. "Galvanism," *New York Mirror and Ladies Literary Gazette*, 4-10-1824: 294–95; and F. C. Hollick, *Neuropathy* (Philadelphia, 1847), 186–89. Pernick, "Back from the Grave," 17–74, shows that advances in resuscitation techniques (artificial respiration, electroresuscitation) worked to increase medical authority in the dying process. The 1790s saw the printing of medical works on techniques for resuscitating the drowned or critically injured, and the founding of "humane" societies to

promote such knowledge; John Warren, the Harvard anatomist, was president of the Massachusetts Humane Society.

71. "Execution and Dissection of Manuel Fernandez alias Richard C. Jackson," *New York Sun*, 11-20-1835: 2. "Report of a Series of Experiments made by the Medical Faculty of Lancaster, on the body of Henry Cobler Moselmann, Executed in the Jail Yard of Lancaster County, Pa., on the twentieth of December, 1839," *American Journal of the Medical Sciences* 26 (May 1840; rpt. Philadelphia, 1840). For a similar experiment in Baltimore, see *The Confession of Adam Horn* (Baltimore, 1843) [Historical Society of Pennsylvania]; "Body of Horn Galvanized," *Baltimore Republic and Daily Argus*, 1-13-1844. Thanks to Michael Zakim, Tel Aviv University, and Gretchen Worden, director, Mütter Museum, Philadelphia, for providing me with this material.

72. "Editor's Table," *Harper's New Monthly Magazine* 8 (April 1854): 690.

73. "Radical Cure for Body-Snatching," letter to *Chicago Inter-Ocean*, 11-23-1878: 8.

74. See, for example, S. L. Clark, "Medical Education from the Ground Up or Our Late Resurrection Men," *Journal of Medical Education* 37 (1962): 1291–96, which describes an illicit network to provide bodies for Vanderbilt University that lasted into the mid-1920s.

CHAPTER FOUR: "A TRAFFIC OF DEAD BODIES"

1. The term "bioethics" came into use in the 1970s, as a product of the post-World-War-II and Vietnam-War era reassessment of medical ethics.

2. *Proceedings of the National Medical Conventions, Held in New York, May, 1846 and in Philadelphia, May, 1847* (Philadelphia, 1847), 106 (ch. 3, II.1).

3. J. G. Coffin, *A Discourse on Medical Education and on the Medical Profession* (Boston, 1822), 39–40.

4. A. M. Lassek, *Human Dissection: Its Drama and Struggle* (Springfield, IL, 1958), 182–83.

5. Albert Matthews, "Notes on Early Autopsies and Anatomical Lectures," *Publications of the Colonial Society of Massachusetts* 19 (1916–17): 276.

6. Matthews, "Notes on Early Autopsies," 279, from *Boston News Letter*, 3-30-1733.

7. *Boston News Letter*, 3-28-1734; Matthews, "Notes on Early Autopsies," 279.

8. Edward M. Hartwell, *The Study of Human Anatomy, Historically and Legally Considered: A Paper Read at the Meeting of the American Social Science Association, September 9, 1880* (Boston, 1881), 13.

9. Lassek, *Human Dissection*, 183; F. C. Waite, "The Development of Anatomical Laws in the States of New England," *New England Journal of Medicine* 233 (1945): 716–26; Hartwell, *Study of Human Anatomy*, 15–16.

10. F. C. Waite, "An Episode in Massachusetts in 1818 Related to the Teaching of Anatomy," *New England Journal of Medicine* 220 (1939): 222 and "The Development of Anatomical Laws in New England."

11. Linden Edwards, "The Ohio Anatomy Law of 1881," *Ohio Medical Journal* 46 (1950): 1191.

12. Martin Kaufman and Leslie L. Hanawalt, "Body Snatching in the Midwest," *Michigan History* 55 (Spring 1970): 25.

13. Matthews, "Notes on Early Autopsies," 276–77, from Sewall's diary, 1: 21.

14. Clossy, New York to Samuel Cleghorn, Dublin, 8-1-1764, in Byron Stookey, "Samuel Clossy, A.B., M.D., F.R.C.P. of Ireland: First Professor of Anatomy, King's College (Columbia), New York," *Bulletin of the History of Medicine* 38 (1964): 153–67; John B. Blake, "Anatomy," in Ronald Numbers, ed., *The Education of American Physicians: Historical Essays* (Berkeley, 1980), 31; Claude Heaton, "Body Snatching in New York City," *New York State Journal of Medicine* 43 (1943): 1861–62. Most historians, following David Hosack's nineteenth-century account, credit John Bard and Peter Middleton with priority, a 1750 dissection of Hermanus Carroll, who is said to have been convicted of murder and hanged. Spencer Turkel, letter, 11-25-1998, points out that the Bard family papers and John Middleton's essay on the history of medicine in New York lack any corroborating mention of the dissection, and municipal records and contemporary newspapers make no mention of the hanging. Professor Turkel suggests that the Bard family may have falsely claimed priority for reasons of medical politics. I want to thank him for alerting me to these and other discrepancies in the standard histories of anatomy in New York City, and for his generosity in sharing his research with me.

15. In the nineteenth century, autopsy did acquire some of dissection's stigma, especially in poor and immigrant communities.

16. Matthews, "Notes on Early Autopsies," 280, quoting *New England Journal*, 2-10-1736.

17. *The Narrative of Whiting Sweeting, Who was Executed at Albany, the 26th of August, 1792* (Albany, 1794), 11, 19 [Brown University Library].

18. Ibid., 45.

19. Ibid., 59.

20. Heaton, "Body Snatching in New York City," 1861, from *New York Gazette*, 11-28-1763.

21. *Greenleaf's New York Journal and Patriotic Register*, 3-3-1792, qtd. in Steven Robert Wilf, "Anatomy and Punishment in Late Eighteenth-Century New York," *Journal of Social History* 22 (1989): 510.

22. Joseph Carson, *A History of the Medical Department of the University of Pennsylvania, from its Foundation in 1765. . . .* (Philadelphia, 1869), 81, 217; *Pennsylvania Gazette*, 10-31-1765. About five years later, Shippen issued a similar announcement, *Pennsylvania Gazette*, 1-11-1770.

23. Dirk Hoerder, *Crowd Action in Revolutionary Massachusetts 1765–1780* (New York, 1977), 52; Wilf, "Anatomy and Punishment," 509; the riot occurred ca. 2-25-1771.

24. Ira Rosenwaike, *Population History of New York City* (Syracuse, 1972), 18.

25. Wilf, "Anatomy and Punishment," 511.

26. Jules C. Ladenheim, "The Doctor's Mob," *Journal of the History of Medicine and Allied Sciences* 5 (1950): 23–53; Heaton, "Body Snatching in New York City," 1861–65.

27. Turkel letter, 11-25-1998, citing petition, *Daily Advertiser*, 2-14-1787 and letter, *Daily Advertiser*, 2-16-1788; petition to the Common Council in "Petitions 1700–1795," Records of the City Clerk, New York, qtd. in I. N. Stokes, *The Iconography of Manhattan Island* (New York, 1928), 6: 46; Wilf, "Anatomy and Punishment," 511.

Turkel points out that Stokes erroneously gives the date of the petition as 2-4-1788 and that some historians have conflated the petition and the letter.

28. *Daily Advertiser*, 2-16-1788, qtd. in Ladenheim, "Doctors' Mob," 27.

29. *Daily Advertiser*, 2-22-1788, cited in Turkel letter, 11-25-1998; John Shrady, ed., *The College of Physicians and Surgeons, New York. . . . A History* (New York, 1903), 1: 25–26. Turkel has examined burial sites from this period and has found evidence—empty and disturbed graves—indicating that grave robbery was widespread "and included essentially all churchyards and burying grounds throughout the city, both for blacks and whites."

30. *Daily Advertiser*, 2-28-1788, qtd. in Ladenheim, "Doctors' Mob," 26–28.

31. *New York Packet*, 4-25-1788, in Ralph G. Victor, "An Indictment for Grave Robbing at the Time of the 'Doctors' Riot,' 1788," *Annals of Medical History*, 3d ser., 2 (1940): 368.

32. *Massachusetts Sentinel*, 4-23-1788; *Boston Gazette*, 5-5-1788; qtd. in Ladenheim, "Doctors' Mob," 29–30. The conflicting accounts are hard to sort out. The closest contemporary report is the letter of William Heth, New York, to Edmund Randolph, 4-16-1788, in Whitfield J. Bell, "Doctors' Riot, New York, 1788," *Bulletin of the New York Academy of Medicine* 47 (1971): 1502: "as some people were strolling by the hospital, they discovered *a something* hanging up at one of the windows, which excited their curiosity, and making use of a stick to satisfy that curiosity, part of a mans arm or leg tumbled out upon them."

33. William Heth, New York, to Edmund Randolph, 4-16-1788, in Bell, "Doctors' Riot," 1502.

34. Ladenheim, "Doctors' Mob," 30–36; Wilf, "Anatomy and Punishment," 513.

35. Wilf, "Anatomy and Punishment," 514–16.

36. In 1790, Congress passed an "Act for the Punishment of Certain Crimes" that gave federal judges the right to include dissection as an additional penalty for murder committed at sea, in a military garrison, or other federal domain. The same year, the New Jersey legislature passed an "Act for the Punishment of Crimes" that gave courts discretion to impose a sentence of dissection on convicted murderers. Neither law referred to the benefit of anatomical science; dissection was purely added punishment. See Wilf, "Anatomy and Punishment," 516.

37. *Greenleaf's New York Journal and Patriotic Register*, 5-3-1792, in Wilf, "Anatomy and Punishment," 514.

38. My account of the John Young case follows Wilf, "Anatomy and Punishment," 517–22.

39. This was so despite Jefferson's admiration for anatomy.

40. Margaretta V. Faugeres, *The Ghost of John Young the Homicide. . . .* (New York, 1797).

41. *Report of a Committee of the Regents of the University Appointed to Visit the College of Physicians and Surgeons in the City of New-York, . . . to the Regents, January 12, 1826* (Albany, NY, 1826), 18–20.

42. *Report of a Committee of the Regents . . . January 12, 1826*, 18–20.

43. P&S Faculty, *Response to the Report of the Regents* [2-18-1826] (New York, 1826) [HS]. The words are taken directly from the British surgeon Thomas Southwood Smith.

44. Minutes of the College of Physician & Surgeons, New York, 1-18-1814 [HS].

45. New York State, Laws, 42 sess., chap. 217, 4-3-1819, V, 279, in Jonathan Harris, "The Rise of Medical Science in New York 1720–1820" (Ph.D. diss, New York University, 1971), 127–28; *Journals of the Senate of the State of New York* [2-14-1820], 126.

46. W. E. Horner, Philadelphia, to J. C. Warren, Boston, 11-30-1824 [J. C. Warren Papers, MHS].

47. *Wayne County Sentinel*, 9-30-1824; Richard L. Bushman, *Joseph Smith and the Beginnings of Mormonism* (Urbana, 1984), 64–65. The nearest medical school was hundreds of miles away in Fairfield, but local physicians and apprentices may have been robbing graves in order to obtain anatomical subjects.

48. N. P. Wiley to I. B. Van Schaick, New York, 1-14-1820? [NYAM].

49. U.S. Dept. of Commerce, *Historical Statistics of the United States* (Washington, 1975), 163 (D 715).

50. Parmelee (var. spelling, Parmeli, Permelee, Parmalee) was indicted ca. 5-19-1824 in the Court of Sessions; [T. Southwood Smith], "*Uses of the Dead to the Living: From the Westminster Review. . . .* " (Albany, NY, 1827), 88–89; *New York Evening Post*, 5-20-1824. For Parmalee's business activities, see *New York Herald*, 1-21-1848; N.Y. State Senate #43, 2-10-1851 and 2-14-1852; *Albany Argus*, 2-16-1852: 2.

51. W. E. Horner, Philadelphia, to J. C. Warren, Boston, 11-30-1824 [J. C. Warren Papers, MHS].

52. Revere, New York, to J. C. Warren, 11-6-1827; Revere, New York, to J. C. Warren, 12-14-1827; Revere, New York, to J. C. Warren, 3-6-1828 [J. C. Warren Papers, MHS]; Revere also suggested that Warren contact Dr. Amos Turnbull in Baltimore. The Reveres and Warrens were part of a tightly interwoven network, the Boston-area Revolutionary elite: Warren's uncle, Joseph Warren, the Revolutionary War hero, dispatched Paul Revere on his midnight ride; John Revere's brother was named Joseph Warren Revere; John Warren (Joseph Warren's brother and J. C. Warren's father), Harvard's first professor of anatomy, employed Paul Revere to engrave the tickets that certified completion of the course of anatomy.

53. Godman, New York, to J. C. Warren, Boston, 6-7-1828; Godman to Warren, Saratoga Springs, NY, 6-?-1828; Godman, Philadelphia, to Warren, Boston, 9-29-1828 [J. C. Warren Papers, MHS].

54. James Henderson, New York, to J. C. Warren, 12-23-1828 [J. C. Warren Papers, MHS].

55. Godman, New York, NY, to J. C. Warren, Boston, 1-1-1829 [J. C. Warren Papers, MHS]; in Patsy A. Gerstner, "A Note on Body Snatching in the United States," *Bulletin of the Cleveland Medical Library Association* 18 (7–1971): 64–65. A few months later, Warren tried to rig up a regular supply of bodies from the Boston workhouse, but the resident physician refused direct help: "I could not render you the aid you desire without violating written obligations which I was . . . required to sign on entering upon the duties of the Medical department of the House of Industry . . . [and] without subjecting myself . . . to the liability of being discovered, and . . . placing at hazard my character and reputation—Should I lose these I lose every hope of success in my profession in this place—I have not

the influence of wealth & of friends to aid and to urge me forward. . . . All that I can promise you, therefore, in regard to the obtaining of subjects, is that I will throw no obstacles in your way in obtaining them—and should there be any procured from the institution . . . ; I wish not to know anything of, or to be questioned concerning them"; John D. Fisher, Hayward Plain, to J. C. Warren, 9-30-1829 [J. C. Warren Papers, MHS].

56. Letter of F. S. Beattie to W. E. Horner, 11-16-1830, in James Webster, *Facts Concerning Anatomical Instruction in Philadelphia* (Philadelphia, 1832), 11.

57. [E. H. Dixon], "Scenes in a Medical Student's Life: Resurrectionizing," *Scalpel* 7 (1855): 93–100.

58. Webster, *Facts Concerning Anatomical Instruction.* In the mid-1830s, the University of Pennsylvania, like Harvard, began importing bodies from New York to cover shortages.

59. House of Commons, Sess. 1–29 to 7-28-1828, vol. 7, "Report from the Select Committee on Anatomy," 68–69; and Russell Maulitz, *Morbid Appearances: The Anatomy of Pathology in the Early 19th Century* (Cambridge, 1987), 142. Pattison testified that bodies could be had for $1.50 in France, $3 in the United States, and $40 in Great Britain, but his figure for the United States should not be taken at face value: prices in Baltimore, where he had taught, were atypically low for the United States, and the British anatomy lobby had a vested interest in exaggerating its own hardships and minimizing the hardships of others.

60. P&S Faculty, *Response to the Report of the Regents* [2-18-1826], 150–51 [HS].

61. William Rowley, *On the Absolute Necessity of Encouraging, instead of Preventing or Embarrassing the Study of Anatomy* . . . (London, 1796) was earlier, but does not seem to have been widely known.

62. See Ruth Richardson, *Death, Dissection and the Destitute* (London, 1988).

63. Ruth Richardson and Brian Hurwitz, "Jeremy Bentham's Self Image: An Exemplary Bequest for Dissection," *British Medical Journal* 295 (7-18-1987): 195–98; Tim Marshall, *Murdering to Dissect: Grave-robbing,* Frankenstein *and the Anatomy Literature* (Manchester, U.K., 1995), 19–20. The auto-icon was well known in America; see, for example, *National Era,* 2-18-1847, a report on Margaret Fuller's visit to the auto-icon and Southwood Smith. Following Bentham's example, J. C. Warren made a testamentary provision for his body to be publicly dissected, and for his skeleton to be displayed in the anatomical museum at Harvard.

64. T. Southwood Smith, "The Use of the Dead to the Living" [rev. of Wm. Mackenzie, *An Appeal to the Public and to the Legislature, on the Necessity of affording Dead Bodies to the Schools of Anatomy,* Glasgow, 1824], *Westminster Review* 2 (7–1824): 59–97, rpt. Boston (1826) and Albany, NY (1827).

65. The discursive formation of the "public" has a crucial place in utilitarian discourse. The repeated invocation of the rights, anxieties, and perturbation of the "public" produces a reified entity that ostensibly stands for society as a whole, but which continually defines itself in campaigns against the customs, privileges, and habits of the aristocracy and the working classes, who are thus implicitly excluded from membership in the category.

66. J. C. Warren Journal, 3-11-1846 [MHS].

67. Dewey, *Introductory Lecture Delivered to the Medical Class of the Berkshire Medical Institution; August 5, 1847* (Pittsfield, MA, 1847), 25–26.

68. Rural schools replied that they had sufficient numbers of subjects and that residence in large cities endangered the morals of students. The relative merits of rural vs. urban schools was a frequent topic of medical discourse in this era. See, for example, Dewey, *Introductory Lecture*, 25–26.

69. J. S. Buckingham, *America, Historical, Statistic and Descriptive* (London, 1841), 1: 159–60.

70. University of New-York, Medical Department, *Annual Announcement of Lectures, Session of 1841–42* (New York, 1841) [NYU].

71. University of Pennsylvania Medical Dept., Dept. of Anatomy, Accts. of the Anatomical Chair, 10-1-1839 to 6-6-1853 [CPP] (hereafter, "Penn Anatomy Accts.").

72. Hartwell, *Study of Human Anatomy*, 29. The poorhouse superintendent who refused to implement the 1831 anatomy act died in 1847. After that, Hartwell reports, Harvard was amply supplied with cadavers "in consequence of the influx of Irish paupers, and the great mortality among them."

73. Cyrus Weeks, New York, to J. C. Warren, 1-24-1837. Weeks supplied Warren with bodies up until 1848 and also supplied the University of Pennsylvania; Penn Anatomy Accts.

74. J. C. Warren Journals, 10-8-1843; Samuel Parkman, Boston, to Warren, New York, 10-1-1843 [J. C. Warren Papers, MHS].

75. C[yrus]W[eeks], New York, to Warren, Boston, 10-15-1843. Weeks, New York, to Warren, Boston, 1-24-1837; Weeks, New York, to Warren, Boston, 10-5-1848 [J. C. Warren Papers, MHS].

76. J. C. Warren Journals, 10-8-1843 [MHS].

77. Alexander Hosack, New York, to J. C. Warren, 1-20-1844 [J. C. Warren Papers, MHS].

78. James Webster et al., *To the Medical Profession of the City of New-York* (New York, 1846), 1–2 [CPP].

79. Webster, *To the Medical Profession*, 3. Andrew Boardman, *An Essay on the Means of Improving Medical Education and Elevating Medical Character* (Philadelphia, 1840), 6, exposed Geneva's failings in the 1839–40 session: "Promise of the Circular. That the Anatomical class should have a full supply of subjects for dissection. Fulfilment. Not a single subject was provided for dissection during the whole session, though students deposited money for them at the rate of $40 a subject at the commencement of the term. Nor was there more than a single subject, . . . a very poor one, used for demonstration during the entire anatomical course. . . ." In subsequent years, this shortage of cadavers may very well have been rectified by the importation of bodies from New York City: Elizabeth Blackwell, who studied anatomy at Geneva under Webster in 1848–49, makes no mention of a cadaver shortage in her memoirs.

80. *Documents of the Board of Aldermen of the City of New York* 14 (5–1847 to 5–1848): 213–16 (#14, 10-25-1847) [NYMA]. Elizabeth Blackmar, personal communication, suggests that in the late 1840s, after burials were banned in Manhattan and Potter's Field moved to Ward's Island, the relocated burial grounds may have been harder to guard and easier to plunder.

81. J. W. Draper, *An Appeal to the People of the State of New-York, to Legalise the Dissection of the Dead* (New York, 1853), 10.

82. F. A. Conkling, speech to the Assembly, 2-28-1854, *New York Tribune*, 3-1-1854: 3.

83. E. R. Peaslee, *The Moral Character of the Medical Profession: An Address introductory . . . in the New York Medical College, Session of 1852–53* (New York, 1852), 11.

84. Amy Bridges, *A City in the Republic: Antebellum New York and the Origins of Machine Politics* (Ithaca, 1984), 65–70.

85. The *New York Times* and *New York Tribune* were passionate supporters. See also *Buffalo Morning Express* (3-31-1854: 2), *Brooklyn Eagle* (1-16-1854: 2; 1-27-1854: 2), *Albany Evening Journal* (3-3-1854: 2, Thurlow Weed's paper), and *Albany Atlas*.

86. *Promotion of Medical Science. Remarks of Mr. F. A. Conkling, on the Bill for the Promotion of Medical Science. In Assembly, February 28, 1854* (Albany, 1854); *New York Herald*, 3-3-1854: 7. (Conkling was the brother of future Republican boss Roscoe Conkling.)

87. *The Brooklyn Daily Eagle*, 1-16-1854: 2, assailed the sacralization of the dead body in stronger terms: "It is a strange kind of repugnance that exists against permitting a student to cut up a human body, that must in a very short time become a mass of loathsome putridity, and resolve into utter nothingness, dissected by the most hateful reptiles that burrow in the ground."

88. Conkling, *Promotion of Medical Science*, 9–10, 13.

89. Germain to the Assembly, 2-28-1854, in *Buffalo Morning Express*, 3-7-1854: 2.

90. *New York Times*, 3-9-1854: 4.

91. The only physician of note to publicly denounce the bill was Dr. William Turner of New York City, a former Board of Health commissioner and an exponent of an alternative medical theory called chrono-thermalism; *People's Medical Journal, and Home Doctor* 1–2 (1853–54): 2, but Assemblyman Levi Harris (Whig-Chenango), speech, 2-28-1854, in *Albany Evening Atlas*, 3-1-1854: 2, argued that privately "country physicians are very generally opposed to this bill." This resistance may have been on other than moral grounds. Assemblyman Abram Lozier (Whig-Livingston) opposed the bill because it was limited to cities over 30,000 in population (there were then six in New York State), and gave physicians residing in large cities "a monopoly of this traffic" (*Albany Evening Journal*, 3-7-1854: 3).

92. *Freeman's Journal*, 2-11-1854; *Assembly Journal* (1-25-1854): 160–61; S. W. Francis, *Biographical Sketches of Distinguished Living New York Physicians* (New York, 1867), 25–28; Board of Supervisors of Kings County, Resolution, 1-26-1854; the vote was 16 to 3.

93. *Documents of the Assembly of the State of New York, 77th Sess., 1854, Vol. 1* (Albany, 1854), 31: 2.

94. *New York Herald*, 3-18-1854: 8; the parade took place on 3-17-1854.

95. *Freeman's Journal*, 2-25-54: 4. Hughes's absence conveniently allowed him to abstain from the debate; he was then making overtures to the Whigs, with whom he had previously fought over the teaching of the Protestant Bible in public schools.

96. Assembly debate, 3-17-1854, in *New York Herald*, 3-18-1854: 1; *Albany Argus*, 3-18-1854: 2.

97. Joseph Cook in Assembly debate, 3-11-1854; *Albany Evening Journal*, 3-17-1854: 2.

98. *Albany Evening Journal*, 3-1-1854: 2.

99. *Buffalo Morning Express*, 3-2-1854: 2; *Albany Evening Atlas*, 2-28-1854: 2; both reporting on Assembly debate of 2-25-1854.

100. *New York Herald*, 3-18-1854: 1, reporting Assembly debate of 3-17-1854.

101. Francis W. Palmer (Whig-Chautauqua), in Assembly debate of 2-28-1854, *Albany Evening Journal*, 3-1-1854: 2

102. S. H. Elliot, *New England's Chattels; or Life in the Northern Poor-House* (New York, 1858), 396.

103. *Harper's New Monthly Magazine* 8 (4–1854): 690–93.

104. The editorialist similarly objected to "the enlargement of the places of trade and business; when the narrow house [the grave] is to be disturbed to make room for wider thoroughfares" (692).

105. For other body-snatching incidents in New York, see *New York Times*, 10-22-1877: 2; 4-24-1879: 2; *Medical Record* 23.14 (4-7-1883): 381 and 24.20 (11-17-1883): 548.

106. David Charles Sloane, *The Last Great Necessity: Cemeteries in American History* (Baltimore, 1991), 84.

107. Frederick L. Hoffman, *Pauper Burials and the Interment of the Dead in Large Cities* (Newark, NJ, 1919), 11–12. Working-class demand for decent burials spurred some New Jersey manufacturers to form the Prudential Friendly Society in 1875 (subsequently renamed Prudential Insurance Company of America). The mass marketing of commercial death insurance—one of the great success stories of nineteenth-century capitalism—resulted in a decline in pauper burials in American cities from 171 per 100,000 in 1880–84 to 78 per 100,000 in 1915–18, while making Prudential and Metropolitan Life two of the largest companies in the world.

108. Frederick L. Hoffman, *History of the Prudential Insurance Company of America (Industrial Insurance), 1875–1900* (n.p., 1900), 4: "only those . . . familiar with the life and the labor of the industrial masses can fully grasp the deeper meaning of the abhorrence of a pauper burial . . . in the potter's field. . . . "

Chapter Five: "Indebted to the Dissecting Knife"

1. *American Journal of Homeopathy* 2 (1852): 234–35.

2. *Albany Argus*, 2-24-1852: 2, rpt. from *Cleveland Plain Dealer*, including an "Address to the Public," by C. D. Williams.

3. *Albany Argus*, 2-24-1852: 2.

4. See, for example, Linden F. Edwards, "Body Snatching in Ohio During the Nineteenth Century," *Ohio State Archaeological and Historical Quarterly* 59 (1954): 334–35.

5. Roy Porter, *Health for Sale: Quackery in England 1660–1850* (Manchester, U.K., 1989), 143, distinguishes between *quackery* and *alternative medicine*, contending that "quackery did not . . . create alternative understandings of health and disease: it battened on to those already existing." I would argue that, given the range of disagreement among regulars, and between regulars and alternative sects, the dialectics of medical belief in antebellum America cannot support Porter's distinction. In addition to the range of therapeutic practices, there were canons of social standing and affiliation: manners, competence, credentials, professional propriety, etc. A slippage, ignorance, or violation of any of these might result in the

application of the pejorative *quack*, a term promiscuously employed by combatants in all sorts of medical controversies and members of all camps. Whether the term stuck depended on a host of factors: some groups/persons had larger networks, and more power to enforce standards. This chapter shows that alternative sects, despite their differences from the regulars (who accused them of quackery), also battened on to existing beliefs, in this case the anatomical body.

6. "Thomsonism," in *Thomson's Almanac for the Year 1844* (Boston, n.d. [1843]), 14; rpt. from *Philadelphia Botanic Sentinel*.

7. Samuel Thomson, *Address to the People of the United States* (n.p. [Boston?], 1817); *The Secrets of the Noted Empyric Samuel Thompson, Comprehending the Theory of Disease and Mode of Practice* (n.p., 1818); *An Earnest Appeal to the Public, Showing the Misery Caused by the Fashionable Mode of Practice of the Doctors at the Present Day* (n.p., 1824); and *Learned Quackery Exposed* (Boston, 1824).

8. *Learned Quackery Exposed* (1824), 1; the quote is from a poem Thomson wrote in Newburyport jail in 1809. Thomson's support for female midwifery has obscured his masculinism. He condemned the regulars as an effeminating and effeminate gentry that pandered to a female clientele.

9. Thomson, *Address to the People of the United States*, 1.

10. In fact, this was not true. Contemporary Parisian medicine (something that Thomson was not well informed about) called for the anatomization of the living. See S. J. Reiser, *Medicine and the Reign of Technology* (Cambridge, 1978), ch. 3; and Russell Maulitz, *Morbid Appearances* (Cambridge, 1987).

11. Samuel Thomson, *Learned Quackery Exposed; or Theory According to Art, as Exemplified in the Practice of the Fashionable Doctors of the Present Day* (Boston, 1836), 45.

12. *Medical Reformer* 1.2 (New York, 2-1-1823): 27. The *Medical Reformer* had no formal tie to Thomson, but championed his agenda: botanical remedies, opposition to metallic medicines, blood-letting, and state licensing of regular medicine. (The first official Thomsonian journal, the *Thomsonian Recorder*, began publication in 1832.) Articles attributed to Thomson appear in *Medical Reformer* 1.1 (1-1-1823): 21; and 1.5 (5-1-1823): 111, 117–20. The editor's identity is unknown; I refer to him as the "Reformer," as he refers to himself in the journal. I want to thank Michael Flannery, Alex Berman, and Michael G. Kenny for sharing with me their knowledge of Thomsonianism.

13. Ibid., 31, 46.

14. See John Harley Warner, *Therapeutic Perspective: Medical Practice, Knowledge, and Identity in America, 1820–1885* (Cambridge, 1986), ch. 6.

15. *Medical Reformer* 1.2 (1823): 24.

16. *Medical Reformer* 1.1 (1823): 30.

17. See Joan Burbick, *Healing the Republic: The Language of Health and the Culture of Nationalism in Nineteenth-Century America* (New York, 1994), ch. 1.

18. *Medical Reformer* 1.2 (1823): 26.

19. *Medical Reformer* 1.2 (1823): 47–48. Michael G. Kenny, email message, 3-1-1996, suggests that the passage comes from a Boston newspaper edited by Elias Smith, an evangelical preacher and, at the time, a close ally of Thomson. In 1822, Smith charged, correctly, that physicians were robbing graves to supply Harvard's dissecting tables; Kenny, *The Perfect Law of Liberty: Elias Smith and the Providential History of America* (Washington, 1994), 218.

20. Cf. contemporary Britain, where anatomy was identified with middle-class

reformers who sought to overthrow the prerogatives enjoyed by the medical and land-owning gentry; see Adrian Desmond, *The Politics of Evolution: Morphology, Medicine and Reform in Radical London* (Chicago, 1989).

21. *Documents of the New York State Assembly, #235* (3-28-1828): *Report of the comitia minora of the select committee on the petition of John Thomson and others relative to the Thomsonian practice of physic. . . .* [rpt., *Journal of the Assembly . . . 51st Session . . .* Appendix F] (Albany, 1828), 3–4. Of course, such charges do not realistically capture the social, moral, and intellectual distinction between botanics and regulars. The regulars were not immune from market culture and the demands of the market economy: they sold remedies wholesale and retail, competed for patients' dollars, conspired to fix prices and monopolize trade, wrote books and gave lectures for cash remuneration, etc. Many regular doctors had only the barest rudiments of medical education, and limited training in anatomy and dissection; many could not plausibly claim the status of learned gentleman. But the medical professoriate and individual physicians of a variety of social origins shared a vested interest in asserting, prescribing, and enforcing the genteel identity of orthodox medicine.

22. Alex Berman, "Neo-Thomsonianism in the United States," *Journal of the History of Medicine* 11 (1956): 133–52; John S. Haller, Jr., *Medical Protestants: The Eclectics in American Medicine, 1825–1939* (Carbondale, 1994), 62–78. "Neo-Thomsonianism" is Berman's term for second- and third-generation Thomsonians who adopted some aspects of regular practice.

23. Haller, *Medical Protestants*, 78; Alexander Wilder, "Eclectic Medicine in the Eastern States," *Transactions, National Eclectic Medical Association* 20 (1892–93): 478; and Uri Lloyd, "A Review of the Principal Events in American Medicine," *Eclectic Medical Journal* 86 (1926): 262–69.

24. John Wesley, *Primitive Physick* (1747), qtd. in Wooster Beach, *The American Practice Condensed, or the Family Physician* (10th ed., New York, 1847), viii.

25. *Catalogue of the New York Anatomical Gallery, and Academy of Natural, Medical and Moral Science* (New York, 1847); W[ooster] Beach, *A Treatise on Anatomy, Physiology, and Health, designed for students, schools, and popular use* (New York, 1847); *The American Practice of Medicine. . . .* (New York, 1836, and many editions thereafter); see also *The Improved System of Midwifery. . . .* (New York, 1847), which had finely engraved anatomical illustrations (unlike the crude engravings in the 1836 edition).

26. Janet Farrell Brodie, *Contraception and Abortion in Nineteenth-Century America* (Ithaca, 1994), 146.

27. "Copious Extract from an Introductory Lecture on Anatomy by Mr. Abernethy . . . ," *Thomsonian Recorder* 1 (1833): 274–78; for extracts from Paley's *Natural Theology*, see *Thomsonian Recorder* 2 (1834): 7–8, 145–46, and *passim*; W[ilson] T[homson], "Logical Deductions from Anatomical Facts," *Thomsonian Recorder* 1 (1833): 293–97, rpt. in *Southern Botanico-Medical Journal* 1.2 (Forsyth, GA, 1841): 32–34.

28. Wilson Thomson, "Lecture Delivered at Lebanon, Ohio . . . ," *Thomsonian Recorder* 2.7 (1-4-1834): 98–99.

29. *The Midwife's Practical Directory; or, the Woman's Confidential Friend* (2d ed., Columbus, OH, 1838), 60, qtd. in Brodie, *Contraception and Abortion*, 146.

30. *Thomsonian Manual* 2 (1836): 8, 133–34; see also *Thomson's Almanac for the Year 1844* (Boston, [1843]), 2.

31. See Stephen Nissenbaum, *Sex, Diet, and Debility in Jacksonian America* (Westport, 1980); Martha H. Verbrugge, *Able-Bodied Womanhood: Personal Health and Social Change in Nineteenth-Century Boston* (New York, 1988); Lamar Riley Murphy, *Enter the Physician: The Transformation of Domestic Medicine, 1760–1860* (Tuscaloosa, 1991), ch. 4–5; Charles Rosenberg, "Catechisms of Health: The Body in the Prebellum Classroom," *Bulletin of the History of Medicine* 69 (1995): 175–97.

32. *Boston Thomsonian Manual and Lady's Companion* 5 (1838–39).

33. *Thomson's Almanac for the Year 1844* (Boston, [1843]).

34. Rpt. in *Thomsonian Manual and Lady's Companion* 5.10 (1839): 159.

35. *Journal of Medical Reform* 1.1 (1854): 47–48; 1.2 (1854): 55, 84; 1.4 (1854): 85.

36. *Journal of Medical Reform* 1.5 (1854): 127.

37. Samuel Hahnemann, *Organon of Homœopathic Medicine* [1810] (1st Amer. ed. from Brit. trans. of 4th German ed.; Allentown, PA, 1836), 26 n. All other quotes in this section are from H. L. Coulter, *Divided Legacy: The Conflict between Homœopathy and the American Medical Association* (Richmond, CA, 1973), 12–14, except where an American edition of Hahnemann is cited.

38. *Lesser Writings of Samuel Hahnemann*, ed. and trans. R. E. Dudgeon (New York, 1852), 714, n. 1; see also Hahnemann, *Chronic Diseases, Their Peculiar Nature and Their Homœopathic Cure* [1828; 2d enlarged German ed., 1835], Louis H. Tafel, ed. (Philadelphia, 1904), 11.

39. *Lesser Writings*, 422.

40. Ibid., 491–93; see also Hahnemann, *Organon of Homœopathic Medicine* (1st Amer. ed.), §13.

41. Dan King, *Quackery Unmasked: or a Consideration of the Most Prominent Empirical Schemes of the Present Time* (Boston, 1858), 115.

42. See Warner, *Therapeutic Perspective*, ch. 4; Martin Kaufman, *Homeopathy in America: The Rise and Fall of a Medical Heresy* (Baltimore, 1971), 113–24.

43. Hering, "Introductory Remarks," in Hahnemann, *Organon of Homœopathic Medicine* (3d Amer. ed., New York, 1849), 3–4. Cf. D. White, *Homoeopathic Advocate and Guide to Health* 1.1 (Keene, NH, 4-1-1851): 1, who argued that homeopathy and regular medicine had greater epistemological affinities before the emergence of Parisian pathological anatomy.

44. Naomi Rogers, "The Proper Place of Homeopathy: Hahneman Medical College and Hospital in an Age of Scientific Medicine," *Pennsylvania Magazine of History and Biography* 108 (1984): 182–85, discusses an 1867 controversy at the Hahnemann Medical College of Philadelphia over the establishment of a chair in Pathology and Diagnostics. But homeopaths there still taught and practiced surgery despite the philosophical obstacles their doctrine opposed to surgery (and, also anatomy).

45. *Cleave's Biographical Cyclopædia of Homœopathic Physicians and Surgeons* (Philadelphia, 1873), vi; see also B. F. Joslin, *Principles of Homœopathy* (New York, 1850), 8–9.

46. Worthington Hooker, *Lessons From the History of Medical Delusions* (New York, 1850), 54. King, *Quackery Unmasked*, charged that homeopathy appealed to women

("many females . . . if we may believe them, are kept alive from day to day by the constant use of homœopathic attenuations," 125), and to feminized bourgeois men, hypochondriacs who "are constantly suffering or anticipating pains in the head, or side, or somewhere else . . . and are ever making use of some genteel remedy. Some of these exquisites would be ashamed to acknowledge themselves quite well, as that would be thought extremely vulgar; and since this class of patients must be furnished with something adapted to their fastidious appetites, the more the articles which they use are attenuated, the better. Can any one believe that these fashionable effeminates are the descendants of the Anglo-Saxons who first colonized America?" (314). The other constituency for homeopathy was people of German origin or descent.

47. D. White, *Homœopathic Advocate and Guide to Health* 1.1 (4-1-1851): 73 [AAS]. White contrasts "the man of intelligence" with "the vulgar and uncultivated" who "go in for the grosser material."

48. W. T. Helmuth, *Surgery and its Adaptation into Homeopathic Practice* (Philadelphia, 1855), shows that homeopathic surgical training was identical to regular training and derived from nonhomeopathic sources, even if Helmuth also discusses homeopathic treatments that may replace conventional surgical treatment. Cf. Joslin, *Principles of Homœopathy*, 104–05, who argues that while "[t]here will always be cases requiring mechanical [i.e., surgical] treatment, . . . Homœopathia, in its present state, could obviate by far the greater part of surgery; and . . . is destined to obviate nearly the whole." For an example of a homeopathic college textbook, see *Announcement of the Homeopathic Medical Department of the State University of Iowa* (Iowa City, 1877) which recommends "Gray, Quain, Holden, Wilson" as anatomical textbooks, and "Flint, Dalton" as physiological textbooks, all of them standard works.

49. Samuel Dickson, *The Principles of the Chrono-Thermal System of Medicine, with the Fallacies of the Faculty. . . . Introduction and Notes by William Turner, M.D.* (13th ed., New York, 1850), 33.

50. V[air] Clirehugh ["Hair Cutter, Corner of Broadway and Fulton Street"], *A Treatise on the Anatomy and Physiology of the Skin and Hair. . . .* (New York, ca. 1838–42) [AAS]. Charles Haswell, *Reminiscences of New York by an Octogenarian, 1816–1860* (New York, 1896), ch. 3, remarks that the "absurdities of . . . 'anatomical' hair-cutting and boot-making" were unknown in 1816.

51. Sherwood's earliest publication, "A Case of Spina Bifida Cured by Surgical Operation," was in the respectably orthodox *New York Medical Repository*, n.s. 1 (1813): 28–30. Testimonial of J. B. Cook, 10-30-1840, *Motive Power of Organic Life and Magnetic Phenomena . . .* (New York, 1841), 157, reported that "Dr. S. is a regularly educated physician." Sherwood probably did not graduate from a medical college; he received an honorary medical degree from the regular New York State Medical Society in 1829. His turn to magnetism, electrotherapy, and medical heterodoxy came in the 1830s.

52. *New or Electric Symptoms of Chronic Diseases, or Chronic Tubercula of the Organs and Limbs . . . and Their Natural or Electric Remedies* (Cincinnati, 1836); *Electro-Galvanic Symptoms, and Electro-Magnetic Remedies, in Chronic Diseases of the Class Hypertrophy, or Chronic Enlargements of the Organs and Limbs, including All Forms of Scrofula, with Illustrative Diagrams and Cases* (3d ed. rev., New York, 1837); *Motive Power of*

Organic Life, and Magnetic Phenomena of Terrestrial and Planetary Motions, with the Application of the Ever-Active and All-Pervading Agency of Magnetism, to the Nature, Symptoms, and Treatment of Chronic Diseases (New York, 1841); *The Motive Power of the Human System, with the Symptoms and Treatment of Chronic Disease* (New York, 1841). See also *U.S. 25th Cong. 2d Sess. Committee of Naval Affairs*, "Rpt. . . . on the memorial of Henry Hall Sherwood . . . claiming . . . new and important discoveries in magnetism generally and more particularly in the magnetism of the earth and representing that he is the inventor of . . . the geometer. . . ." [American Philosophical Society, 996] (Washington, DC, 1838).

53. Orson Fowler, *Love and Parentage* (New York, 1851), 25. For animal magnetism in America, see Robert C. Fuller, *Mesmerism and the American Cure of Souls* (Philadelphia, 1982), esp. 16–47. For eighteenth- and early-nineteenth-century animal magnetism and *elan vital*, see Robert Darnton, *Mesmerism and the End of the Enlightenment in France* (Cambridge, MA, 1968).

54. Fuller, *Mesmerism and the Cure of Souls*, 30 [citing "A Practical Magnetizer," *The History and Philosophy of Animal Magnetism* . . . (Boston, 1843), ch. 2], and 69–70.

55. Reynolds, *Whitman's America*, 212, quoting Whitman, *Notebooks and Unpublished Prose Manuscripts*, ed. E. F. Grier (New York, 1984), 1: 304 [n.d. given].

56. *The New-York Dissector: A Quarterly Journal of Medicine, Surgery, Magnetism, Mesmerism and the Collateral Sciences* 1–4 (1844–47) [CPP]. The *Dissector* reprinted many of its articles from British and French medical journals. Two well-known nonmedical authors to be found in its pages are Harriet Martineau (letters on mesmerism [2: 74–87]) and Edgar Allan Poe ("Mesmeric Revelation," one of Poe's hoaxes, here treated as fact [1: 185–89]).

57. Unlike Sherwood, Wakley never endorsed animal magnetism. *The Dissector* lasted only four years, never coming close to attaining *The Lancet's* commercial success, scientific credibility, and large medical readership. Other American medical journals also emulated *The Lancet:* the reform-minded but orthodox *American Lancet* in the 1830s and *The Scalpel* in the 1840s and 1850s, which far outdid *The Dissector* in sarcasm, literary quality, and scientific credibility.

58. William Fishbough, intro., in Andrew Jackson Davis, *The Principles of Nature, Her Divine Revelations, and a Voice to Mankind* (35th ed., Boston, 1847), xii–xiii.

59. Rev. Gibson Smith [and Andrew Jackson Davis], *Lectures on Clairmativeness: or, Human Magnetism, with an Appendix* (New York, 1845), 19–20.

60. *Dissector* 4 (1847): 153–54.

61. *The Harbinger of Health; Containing Medical Prescriptions for the Human Body and Mind* [New York, 1861] (19th ed., Rochester, NY, 1909), 55; *The Great Harmonia; Being a Philosophical Revelation of the Natural, Spiritual, and Celestial Universe* (Boston, 1850), vol. 1, subtitled "The Physician." Davis first made his anatomical claims in Smith [and Davis], *Lectures on Clairmativeness.*

62. For Sherwood on quackery, see *Dissector* 4 (1847): 224.

63. *Dissector* 2 (1845): 108; for Sherwood on pathological anatomy and auscultation, see 1 (1844): 8, 91 and 4 (1847): 55–56; on P. C. A. Louis's "numerical method," see 1 (1844): 84–86.

64. For more on the anatomical self and physiological law, see chap. 6 below.

65. "Progression," *Homoeopathic Advocate and Guide to Health* 1.1 (4-1-1851): 8

[AAS]. The analogy was common; see, for example, A. J. Davis, *Harbinger of Health*, 410: "Every ganglionic center is a telegraphic station. It receives impressions and transmits the signs of disturbances from part to part."

66. Sherwood, *Motive Power of Organic Life* (2d ed., 1844), 73.

67. F. H. Hamilton, *Introductory Address, and Catalogue of Students attending the Annual Course of Lectures on Anatomy and Surgery* (Auburn, NY, 1837), 4. Along with lobelia (an herb with purgative effects), as remedies, Thomsonians favored large doses of cayenne pepper and exposure to steam.

68. Hamilton, *Introductory Address*, 5–6.

69. Ibid., 12.

70. Waterman Sweet, *Views of Anatomy and the Practice of Natural Bonesetting by a mechanical process different from all book knowledge* (Schenectady, 1844), 21: "I use lineaments and embrocations, and reduce the joints to their proper places, and put drafts on the feet or hands, made of rye meal mixed with hot vinegar— mustard sprinkled on burdock or horse-radish leaves, five or six thicknesses, wilted and put in hot vinegar and bound on the sole of the foot; these draw out soreness or prevent pain, . . . I am called, and examine and find . . . dislocation is the cause of the lameness, which I endeavor to relax and put in order."

71. Robert J. T. Joy, "The Natural Bonesetters with Special Reference to the Sweet Family of Rhode Island," *Bulletin of the History of Medicine* 28 (1954): 416–39. See also Joseph Comstock, "On the Study of Living Anatomy," *Boston Medical and Surgical Journal* 49 (1-18-1854): 500–2; Martha McPartland, "The Bonesetter Sweets of South County, Rhode Island," *Yankee* (1–1968): 80–102; and Walter I. Wardwell, *Chiropractic: History and Evolution of a New Profession* (St. Louis, 1992), 23–24.

72. *Providence Journal*, 2-16-1830, quoted in Joy, "Natural Bonesetters," 425.

73. Sweet, *Views of Anatomy*, 21.

74. Waterman Sweet, *An Essay on the Science of Bone Setting . . . In which the author undertakes to prove, that surgery and anatomy are intuitive sciences, and which can be understood, only by those who have a talent for the profession, and are endowed by nature with the sufficient ability to discharge the duties of one of the most complicated sciences known to man* (Providence [RI], 1829), back matter, testimonials (7 of 17 mentioned having consulted surgeons or physicians before turning to Sweet); Sweet, *Views of Anatomy*.

75. Comstock, "On the Study of Living Anatomy," reports that the Sweet family effected many cures, and attempts to reconcile bonesetting with orthodox treatment and theory.

76. Parsons, *The Importance of the Sciences of Anatomy and Physiology as a Branch of General Education; . . . an Introduction to a Course of Lectures to the Upper Classes of Brown University* (Cambridge, 1826), 12–13.

77. Sweet, *Essay on the Science of Bone Setting*, 12.

78. For the changing usage of the word *science*, see Sydney Ross, "*Scientist:* The Story of a Word," *Annals of Science* 18 (1962): 65–84.

79. The earliest tract on bonesetting, published in 1656, was *The Compleat Bone-Setter, . . . the Method of Curing Broken Bones and Strains and Dislocated Joynts, together with Ruptures, commonly called Broken Bellyes. . . . Revised, Englished, and Enlarged by R[obert] Turner* (2d ed., London, 1665). It is unknown whether any Sweets knew of

or consulted this work, but no nineteenth-century American could be innocent of the written word. Sweet, a devout Baptist, must have known the Bible.

80. Sweet, *Essay on the Science of Bone Setting*, 6.

81. F. C. Hollick, "Something Which Should Be Generally Taught," *The People's Medical Journal* 2.10 (1854): 56. Wooster Beach, *The American Practice Condensed* (New York, 1860), 550–51, praised bonesetting in his 1836 edition as one of the therapies that could be employed by eclectic practitioners and, since he never deleted material, kept doing so in later editions, even as they grew larger by incorporating anatomical and physiological material.

82. Wardwell, *Chiropractic*, 24.

CHAPTER SIX: "THE HOUSE I LIVE IN"

1. Rev. of Amariah Brigham, *Remarks on the Influence of Mental Cultivation and Mental Excitement upon Health* (2d ed., Boston, 1833), in *Annals of Phrenology* 2 (1835): 488, rpt. from *Edinburgh Phrenological Journal* 45 (1833?).

2. Samuel A. Edgerly, diary, 1-27-1860: 92–93 [NYPL].

3. Coventry, *Address to the Graduates of the Medical Institution of Geneva College, delivered January 25th, 1842* (Utica, 1842), 7.

4. Coventry, *Address to the Graduates*, 13–15.

5. Thomas Beddoes, *Hygëia: or Essays Moral and Medical, on the Causes Affecting the Personal State of our Middling and Affluent Classes* (London, 1802–3), 2: vi: 48, 91, qtd. in Roy Porter, *Doctor of Society: Thomas Beddoes and the Sick Trade in Late-Enlightenment England* (London, 1992), 76–77; Jan Golinski, *Science as Public Culture: Chemistry and Enlightenment in Britain, 1760–1820* (Cambridge, 1992), ch. 6.

6. Another prescient effort at popular anatomy was William Burke, *A Popular Compendium of Anatomy; or A concise and clear description of the human body and physiology. . . .* (London, 1805; 2d ed., 1813), illustrated with five plates.

7. Paley did not originate the idea of natural theology. Robert Boyle's *Disquisition About the Final Causes of Natural Things* (London, 1688), aimed at countering the religious enthusiasm of the 1640s, probably served as Paley's model.

8. Paley, *Natural Theology; or Evidence of the Existence and Attributes of the Deity, Collected from the Appearance of Nature* (London, 1802); published in various abridgments and revisions in Boston, 1810–12, 1827, 1829, 1831, 1836, 1854, 1863; New York, 1814, 1824, 1842–52; and Philadelphia, 1831, 1836, 1840, 1841, 1845, 1857. Editions with lithographed plates start appearing in the late 1820s; many of the post-1836 editions are illustrated by woodcuts. Some editions were stereotyped, which indicates larger print runs. For Whitman's review, see David S. Reynolds, *Walt Whitman's America: A Cultural Biography* (New York, 1995), 241–43. Excerpts from *Natural Theology* were published in *Thomsonian Recorder* 2 (1834): 7–8, 145–46.

9. See, for example, J. V. C. Smith, *Mind and Matter; or, familiar conversations on the body and soul* (Boston, 1833); S. G. Goodrich, *Peter Parley's Farewell* (Boston, 1839), 65–70; Sophia White, *Dialogues, Essays, and Stories for the use of children* (Boston, 1859), 90–98. The *Bridgewater Treatises* were perhaps the most influential reworkings of natural theology. Written in Britain in the 1820s and 1830s to combat an assault on hereditary privilege emanating from radical anatomy schools and

literary and philosophical societies, they were read in the United States without reference to the contentious cultural politics that gave birth to them.

10. Alexander Ramsay, *Prospectus of Fifteen Lectures on the Animal and Intellectual Economy of Man*. . . . (New York, 1816), 3, 6; *Announcement and Prospectus of Lectures of Alexander Ramsay* (New York, 1817); *Farewell Discourse* (Montreal, 1818, 1820?) [NYAM]; *Address and Anatomical Prospectus* (Concord, 1819). James Alfred Spalding, *Dr. Lyman Spalding: the Originator of the United States Pharmacopeia* (Boston, 1916), 149. Ramsay (1754?-1824) studied with Alexander Monro II in Edinburgh and Matthew Baillie in London; Dumas Malone, ed. *Dictionary of American Biography* (New York, 1935), 15: 337.

11. U.S. Department of Commerce, *Historical Statistics of the United States* (Washington, 1975), 1: 163–65 (Series D 705–738). The approximate figures given are for the antebellum era.

12. Granville Sharp Pattison, *Syllabus of a Popular Course of Lectures on General Anatomy and Physiology, as illustrative of the natural history of man* (Philadelphia, 1819).

13. Usher Parsons, *The Importance of the Sciences of Anatomy and Physiology as a Branch of General Education; . . . an Introduction to a Course of Lectures to the upper classes of Brown University* (Cambridge, 1826), 11–12.

14. John L. Kirkland, Cambridge, to J. C. Warren, Boston, 3-28-1814 [J. C. Warren Papers, MHS].

15. Ramsay, *Prospectus of Fifteen Lectures*, 3.

16. See F. L. M. Pattison, *Granville Sharp Pattison: Anatomist and Antagonist, 1791–1851* (Tuscaloosa, 1987).

17. Ramsay, *Address and Anatomical Prospectus*, 14

18. W. T. Berry and H. E. Poole, *Annals of Printing* (Toronto, 1966); Philip Gaskell, *A New Introduction to Bibliography* (New York, 1972). The steam press, invented in 1811, emerged as a significant factor in print production in America in the 1830s. Other significant technological innovations in print invented or introduced in the 1820s and 1830s include cloth book covers; stereotyped printing plates; chromolithography; and improvements in wood and steel engraving, binding, and papermaking.

19. Jeffries Wyman, Richmond, VA, to Elizabeth A. Wyman, Boston, 1-31-1846 [FC].

20. *Address to the Community; on the Necessity of Legalizing the Study of Anatomy* (Boston, 1829), 21–23; rpt. in *New-York Medical Inquirer* 1.5–1.6 (1830); and Medical Society of Maine, *Address to the Community on the Necessity of Legalizing the Study of Anatomy* (Brunswick, ME, 1832) [MHS].

21. Nelson Sizer, *Forty Years in Phrenology* (New York, 1891), 200–1; Robert C. Fuller, *Mesmerism and the American Cure of Souls* (Philadelphia, 1982), 16–30, 69–70.

22. For studies of phrenology, see John Dunn Davies, *Phrenology, Fad and Science: A 19th-Century American Crusade* (New Haven, 1955); Madeleine B. Stern, *Heads & Headlines: The Phrenological Fowlers* (Norman, 1971); Arthur Wrobel, "Orthodoxy and Respectability in Nineteenth-Century Phrenology," *Journal of Popular Culture* 9 (1975): 38–50; idem, "Phrenology as Political Science," in Wrobel, ed., *Pseudo-*

Science and Society in Nineteenth-Century America (Lexington, KY, 1987); Roger Cooter, *The Cultural Meaning of Popular Science: Phrenology and the Organization of Consent in Nineteenth-Century Britain* (Cambridge, 1984); Reynolds, *Walt Whitman's America*; Charles Colbert, *A Measure of Perfection: Phrenology and the Fine Arts in America* (Chapel Hill, 1997).

23. Rev. of Brigham, in *Annals of Phrenology* 2 (1835): 488.

24. Cooter, *Cultural Meaning of Popular Science*, 109.

25. Sizer, *Forty Years in Phrenology*, 97, 385.

26. *Christian Examiner* 17 (1834): 254, qtd. in Davies, *Phrenology, Fad and Science*, 68. Over time, the equation of phrenology with anatomy became increasingly problematic. Even early on, many anatomists expressed reservations about phrenology. After experiments by physiologists Pierre Flourens (1845) and Paul Broca (1861) established that the sites in the brain affecting the ability to reproduce and to speak did not correspond to the phrenological regions identified by Gall and his successors, phrenology was left with few credible scientific supporters; Davies, *Phrenology, Fad and Science*, 142.

27. *Library of Health* 1 (1837): 130; Alcott also recommends Paley's *Natural Theology* and "the more scientific works of Dr. Oliver and Dr. [Robley] Dunglison."

28. William A. Alcott, *The House I Live In* (Boston, 1832–34); George Hayward, *Outlines of Human Physiology: Designed for the Use of the Higher Classes in Common Schools* (Boston; 1834); J. V. C. Smith, *The Class Book of Anatomy, explanatory of the first principles of Human Organization, as the basis of Physical Education, Designed for Schools* (Boston, 1834).

29. For nineteenth-century American instructional literature on the body, see Charles E. Rosenberg, "Catechisms of Health: The Body in the Prebellum Classroom," *Bulletin of the History of Medicine* 69 (1995): 175–97.

30. The two men were also connected by William's marriage to their mutual cousin Phoebe Bronson. Bronson Alcott, a well known transcendentalist thinker, was Louisa May Alcott's father.

31. William A. Alcott, *Forty Years in the Wilderness of Pills and Powders; or, the Cogitations and Confessions of an Aged Physician* (Boston, 1859), 3.

32. *National Cyclopaedia of Biography* 12: 60; James Whorton, "William Andrus Alcott," in M. Kaufman et al., eds., *Dictionary of American Medical Biography* (Westport, CT, 1984), 1: 10; R. M. Lewis, "William Andrus Alcott," in *Burrage and Kelley, Dictionary of American Medical Biography*, 10.

33. *Juvenile Rambler; Designed for Families and Schools* 1–2 (Boston, 1832–33) was a weekly dedicated to the moral and intellectual "improvement of youth." Its circulation is unknown; subscriptions were $1 per year. Each issue had sections on history, geography, natural history, biography, proverbs, poetry, and, from November 1832 on, anatomy.

34. "The House I Live In," *Juvenile Rambler* 2.19 (5-8-1833): 72, continuing in almost every issue thereafter.

35. *The House I Live In . . . Pt. 1: the Human Frame* (Boston, 1834); *The House I Live In . . .* (Boston, 1836). By 1839, the book had gone through seven stereotyped editions (which had larger runs than regular editions), and by 1847 thirteen editions; a new revised edition came out in 1854. It remained in print in the

United States until at least 1857, the year John P. Jewett, publisher of *Uncle Tom's Cabin*, put out *The Laws of Health; or the Sequel to "The House I Live In"* (Boston, 1857).

36. *House I Live In*, 1836, v (all quotations cited hereafter are from this edition). The full biblical passage praises God: "I will praise thee; for I am fearfully *and* wonderfully made: marvellous *are* thy works; and *that* my soul knowest right well" (King James Bible).

37. In the Bible, the body is compared to a temple (fallen man = the destruction of the Second Temple): "Know ye not that ye are the temple of God, and that the Spirit of God dwelleth in you? If any man defile the temple of God, him shall God destroy; for the temple of God is holy, which temple ye are" (I Corinthians 3:16–17).

38. Richard L. Bushman, *The Refinement of America: Persons, Houses, Cities* (New York, 1992), 255–57.

39. Alcott, "The Manikin," *Teacher of Health* 1 (1843): 167.

40. "The Science of Human Life," *Moral Reformer & Teacher of the Human Condition* 2 (1836): 5.

41. James C. Whorton, "'Christian Physiology': William Alcott's Prescription for the Millennium," *Bulletin of the History of Medicine* 49 (1975): 475–76, n. 35, citing *Moral Reformer* 1 (1835): 77; *Library of Health* 1 (1837): 160–62. Alcott defined slavery broadly and also opposed the domestic enslavement of women [*Library of Health* 4 (1840): 345–46; *Moral Reformer* 2 (1836): 212–15; *Library of Health* 1 (1837): 380–82; *The Young Husband*, 339], and the economic enslavement of laborers [*Moral Reformer* 1 (1835): 91, 335; *Library of Health* 6 (1842): 168–82]. His larger stance on slavery was connected to his mission to redeem "the slavery of a being made originally in the image of God, but now . . . subjected to appetite, lust, and passion" (Whorton, "Christian Physiology," 476).

42. *The House I Live In*, 134–35. Alcott here belatedly entered the debate between Samuel Stanhope Smith and John Augustine Smith; see S. S. Smith, *An Essay on the Causes of the Variety of Complexion and Figure in the Human Species* (New Brunswick, NJ, 1810; rpt. Cambridge, MA, 1965), ed. Winthrop Jordan, xxxix–xl, 177. He may also have been influenced by James Cowles Prichard, *Researches in the Physical History of Mankind* (2d ed., London, 1826), 1: 160, 233; William Lawrence, *Lectures on the Physiology, Zoology and the Natural History of Man, delivered at the Royal College of Surgeons* (Salem, MA, 1828), 236–66. For a preliminary discussion of anatomical universalism, see Nancy Leys Stepan, *The Idea of Race in Science: Great Britain, 1800–1960* (London, 1982), ch. 1, 2.

43. *The House I Live In*, 44, 88, 237–39. In later works, Alcott argues that the difference between the sexes is symmetrical: man is physically superior, woman spiritually superior.

44. Ibid., 107. The doorway skeleton appears in only some editions; other editions feature a skeleton gesturing welcome, with no background.

45. *Library of Health* 3 (1839): 95, qtd. in Whorton, "Christian Physiology," 476.

46. "Teaching Anatomy to the Indians," *Library of Health* 1 (1837): 103.

47. "The Study of Physiology," *Library of Health* 1 (1837): 47.

48. Qtd. in Alcott, "Physiological Vice" [an address to the Boston Physiological Society], *Library of Health* 1 (1837): 160.

49. John M. Keagy, qtd. in Alcott, *Teacher of Health and the Laws of Human Constitution* 1 (1843): 69.

50. Qtd. in Alcott, "The Science of Human Life," *Moral Reformer* 2 (1836): 7. Ely (1789–1861) edited the *Philadelphian*, an evangelical newspaper, and was professor of theology at Marion College.

51. "Teaching Anatomy to the Indians," *Library of Health* 1 (1837): 103; "Physiological Vice," 161.

52. Advocates of anatomical instruction similarly argued that belief in supernatural agencies obstructed the progress of medical knowledge; see Austin Flint, Sr., *The Reciprocal Duties and Obligations of the Medical Profession and the Public.* . . . (Chicago, 1844), 18.

53. "Sandwich Island Anatomy," *Graham's Journal* 3.10 (5-11-1838): 163, rpt. *Boston Medical and Surgical Journal*; the title of the work referred to is *Anatomia: He Palapala ia E Hoike Ai I Ke Ano O Ko Ke Kanaka Kinn. Ua Kakania ma ka olelo Hawaii, I mea e ao ai I na haumana o ke Kula Nui, ma Lahainaluna* ("Anatomy. A work showing the structure of the Human System. Compiled in the Hawaiian Language, for the benefit of the members of the Seminary at Lahainaluna").

54. *The House I Live In . . . (Lu Kuiy' Khan' dha 'aim' e' 'a Kron' ca)*, trans. Stella Kneeland Bennett (Tavoy-Rangoon, Burma, 1843–84).

55. *Anatomy, Physiology, and Hygiene (in Sgau Karen)*, trans. and adapt. Mrs. J. G. Binney, from the rev. ed. [with 150 engravings; 1st ed. of 1000] (Rangoon, 1872). This was preceded by *Anatomy, Physiology, and Hygiene* (Madras, 1857) [NLM], in the Tamil language, "printed for the American Missions in Ceylon and South India."

56. Alcott, *Forty Years in the Wilderness*, 1–2.

57. For popular medical discourse in this period, see Janet Farrell Brodie, *Contraception and Abortion in 19th-Century America* (Ithaca, 1994); Lamar Riley Murphy, *Enter the Physician: The Transformation of Domestic Medicine, 1760–1860* (Tuscaloosa, 1991); Stephen Nissenbaum, *Sex, Diet, and Debility in Jacksonian America: Sylvester Graham and Health Reform* (Westport, 1980); Martha H. Verbrugge, "The Social Meaning of Personal Health: The Ladies' Physiological Institute of Boston and Vicinity in the Mid-19th Century," in Susan Reverby and David Rosner, eds., *Health Care in America: Essays in Social History* (Philadelphia, 1979); Verbrugge, *Able-Bodied Womanhood: Personal Health and Social Change in 19th-Century Boston* (New York, 1988).

58. "The Science of Human Life," *Moral Reformer* 2 (1836): 6. Smith (1800–1879) founded and edited the *Boston Medical Intelligencer*, the first weekly medical journal in the United States (1823), later known as the *Boston Medical & Surgical Journal*. He also edited a weekly paper, wrote natural histories, travelogues, and other nonmedical works, served as port physician of Boston (1829–1849) and in the Massachusetts legislature (1837, 1848), and as mayor of Boston (1854); Robert M. Green, "J. V. C. Smith," in W. L. Burrage and H. A. Kelley, *Dictionary of American Medical Biography* [1928] (rpt. Boston: Milford House, 1971), 1128–29.

59. Nissenbaum, *Sex, Diet, and Debility*, 20.

60. See Alcott, "Uses of the Manikin," *Teacher of Health* 1 (1843): 45–48.

61. *Botanico-Medical Investigator and Journal of Health* 1 (5-1-1843): 1–3 (Mann); 7 (Allen).

62. "The Work Progressing," *Library of Health* 1 (1837): 103.

63. T[homas] S[cott] Lambert, *Hygienic Physiology* (Portland, ME and New York, 1852), 15–18; idem, *Pictorial Anatomy* (Portland, ME, 1851), iv.

64. New York State Education Department, *Fifteenth Annual Report* (Albany, 1919), 172, in Harold M. Childs, "A History of the School Health Education Program in New York State" (Doc. Educ. diss., Syracuse University, 1961), 16–17.

65. Calvin Cutter, *The Physiological Family Physician, designed for Families and Individuals* (West Brookfield, MA, 1845); *First Book on Anatomy and Physiology* (Boston, 1847); *Anatomy and Physiology, designed for Academies and Families* (Boston, 1847); and many editions and revisions thereafter.

66. *Boston Medical and Surgical Journal*, 9-27-1848: 185.

67. Zabdiel Boylston Adams (1829–1902), "Interesting reminiscences of a long professional life," typescript, 3-6-1894 [FC].

68. J. C. Warren journal, 12-22-1838 [J. C. Warren Papers, MHS]; "A Knowledge of Anatomy and Physiology Should Be Accessible to All," *Graham's Journal* 3.5 (3-2-1839): 84.

69. J. C. Warren to ?, 6-25-1842 [J. C. Warren Papers, MHS].

70. Regina Markell Morantz, "Nineteenth-Century Health Reform and Women: A Program of Self-Help," in Guenter B. Risse, Ronald L. Numbers, and Judith Walzer Leavitt, eds., *Medicine Without Doctors: Home Health Care in American History* (New York, 1977), 77.

71. Mary Gove, "Lectures to Ladies on Anatomy and Physiology," *Graham's Journal* 2.21 (1838): 325–30; 2.22 (10-28-1838): 338–42 (using some of the same illustrations as J. V. C. Smith, *Class Book of Anatomy*; Hayward, *Outlines of Human Physiology*; and *The House I Live In*); *Boston Morning Post*, qtd. in *Graham's Journal* 3.5 (3-2-1839): 84; "Important Lectures to Females," editorial, *Advocate of Moral Reform* 1 (3–1839): 44.

72. Morantz, "Nineteenth-Century Health Reform and Women," 78; Verbrugge, "Social Meaning of Personal Health," 45–66; idem, *Able-Bodied Womanhood*.

73. Catharine Beecher, *A Treatise on Domestic Economy, for the use of Young Ladies at Home* (Boston, 1841; rev. 2d ed., 1843). See also Beecher, *Physiology and Calisthenics, for Schools and Families* (New York, 1856); and Beecher and H. B. Stowe, *American Woman's Home, or Principles of Domestic Science* [New York, 1869] (Hartford, 1975). Thanks to Ben Mutschler for bringing Beecher to my attention.

74. Mrs. Jane Taylor, *Primary Lessons in Physiology: for Children* (1839; rev. ed., New York, 1848); *Wouldst Know Thyself, the Outlines of Human Physiology* (New York, ca. 1858) [AAS].

75. See Joan Burbick, *Healing the Republic: The Language of Health and the Culture of Nationalism in Nineteenth-Century America* (Cambridge, 1994), 86–95.

76. Susan Wells, *Out of the Dead House: 19th-Century Women Physicians and the Practice of Medicine* (Madison, 2000), argues that, in taking up anatomy, women simultaneously challenged and reinforced prevailing bourgeois ideas of woman's sphere. Anatomy could be seen as a nongendered or even female activity, and was especially linked to female reading practices. See also Regina Morantz-Sanchez, *Sympathy & Science: Women Physicians in American Medicine* (New York, 1985).

77. For the antebellum lecture circuit, see Donald A. Scott, "The Popular Lecture and the Creation of a Public in Mid-nineteenth-Century America," *Journal of*

American History 66 (1980): 791–809; Paul Theerman, "Dionysius Lardner's American Tour: A Case Study in Antebellum American Interest in Science, Technology, and Nature," in Theerman and K. Hunger Parshall, eds., *Experiencing Nature* (Amsterdam, 1997), 211–36.

78. Mary Elizabeth Wieting, *Prominent Incidents in the Life of Dr. John M. Wieting. . . .* (New York, 1889), 1–12, 213–15; Brodie, *Contraception and Abortion*, 111.

79. Cooter, *Cultural Meaning of Popular Science*, 370, n. 108, 379, n. 32; George Holyoake, *Sixty Years of an Agitator's Life* (London, 1892; 3d ed., 1906), 1: 47–49, 60–68, 255.

80. Harry J. Carman, *Social and Economic History of the United States* (Boston, 1934), 2: 136–37. In 1845 postal rates were reduced and simplified; a further reduction followed in 1851. Between 1790 and 1860, the geographical range of postal service expanded from 89 post offices in 1791 to 27,977 in 1859; in the same period, service miles went from 846,468 to 86,308,402.

81. Brodie, *Contraception and Abortion*, 197–201; F. C. Hollick, *Outlines of Anatomy and Physiology for Popular Use* (Philadelphia, 1847); *The Origin of Life: A Popular Treatise on the Philosophy and Physiology of Reproduction . . . with a full description of the Male and Female Organs* (10th stereotype ed.; original ed., New York, 1845), 14; *Neuropathy . . .* (Philadelphia, 1847); *The Marriage Guide . . .* (New York, 1850; rpt. New York, 1974); *The American Class-Book of Anatomy and Physiology . . .* (New York, 1853). See also *Practical Facts in the Medical Application of Galvanism and Electro-Magnetism* (New York, 1848) [AAS].

82. Hollick typically reprinted reviews of his lectures and testimonials in the front and backmatter of his books. From these one can piece together his itineraries for some years. In New York, Philadelphia, and some other cities, he lectured for long and repeated runs.

83. *Boston Post*, 2-28-1848; rpt. in Hollick, *The Marriage Guide*, 422.

84. Brodie, *Contraception and Abortion*, for example, does not discuss the relation between sexology and popular anatomy. She does, however, show that sexological books and lectures reached up into the ranks of the middle and upper-middle classes for their audience.

85. *Origin of Life*, xi.

86. *Boston Times*, 2-23-1848; rpt. in *Marriage Guide*, 423.

87. *Boston Courier*, 6-3-1844; rpt. in *Origin of Life*, xlvi–xlvii.

88. *Origin of Life*, xxiii.

89. Ibid., xvi.

90. See, for example, *A Popular Treatise on Venereal Diseases, in All Their Forms* (New York, 1852).

91. *People's Medical Journal & Home Doctor* 1.1 (7–1853): 8–10; it ran from 7–1853 to 12–1854.

92. Hollick, *An Inquiry into the Rights, Duties, and Destinies, of the Different Varieties of the Human Race, with a view to a proper consideration of the subjects of slavery, abolition, amalgamation, and aboriginal rights* (New York, 1843), argued that the northern and British working classes were treated worse than southern slaves. He condemned bourgeois abolitionists who hypocritically denounced slavery while condoning and committing worse offenses against working people in their own homes, shops, and factories.

93. *Baltimore Republican*, 3-30-1846; *Philadelphia Daily Keystone*, 4-21-1846; *Philadelphia Spirit of the Times*, 4-21-1846; in Hollick, *Origin of Life*, xlv–xlvx.

94. Verbrugge, "Social Meaning of Personal Health," 56.

95. *Origin of Life*, viii–x.

96. Michel Foucault, *The History of Sexuality, Volume I: An Introduction* [1976], trans. Robert Hurley (New York, 1990).

97. Marianne Finch, *An Englishwoman's Experience in America* (London, 1853; rpt., New York, 1969), 85–86.

98. Edgerly diary, 92–93.

99. Samuel Dickson, *Principles of the Chrono-Thermal System of Medicine.* . . . (13th ed., New York, 1850), 33, 142.

100. Charles W. Taylor, *Sources of the Self: The Making of Modern Identity* (Cambridge, MA, 1989), 35.

101. Ibid., 111.

102. Ibid., 173–75. Note that Taylor's "we" both queries and enforces the "modern self."

CHAPTER SEVEN: "THE FOUL ALTAR OF A DISSECTING TABLE"

1. *American Journal of Medical Reform* 1.1 (5–1851): 1–2.

2. Samuel A. Edgerly, New York City, diary, 1859–1860 [NYPL].

3. S. W. Clark, *From the Ridiculous to the Sublime* (Chicago, 1875), 31.

4. *The Gypsy Dream Book and Fortune Teller, with Napoleon's Oraculum* (New York, n.d. [ca. 1850]).

5. "The Philosophy of Composition" (1846), qtd. in Elisabeth Bronfen, *Over Her Dead Body: Death, Femininity, and the Aesthetic* (New York, 1992).

6. J. H. Robinson, *Marietta, or the Two Students: A Tale of the Dissecting Room and Body Snatching* (Boston, 1846); George Lippard, *The Quaker City; or the Monks of Monk Hall* (Philadelphia, 1845).

7. The phrase "narrative of sexual danger" comes from Judith Walkowitz, *City of Dreadful Delight: Narratives of Sexual Danger in Late-Victorian London* (Chicago, 1992).

8. Taylor Stoehr, *Hawthorne's Mad Scientist: Pseudoscience and Social Science in Nineteenth-Century Life and Letters* (Hamden, CT, 1978), 118, reminds us that, outside the genre of sensationalism, mid-nineteenth-century American novels often idealized the physician, "concentrating on his eligibility as a husband for spirited but impoverished heroines." And yet, Stoehr shows, Hawthorne's fiction is full of memorable mad scientist-physicians, though none is precisely an anatomist. See also William Leach, *True Love and Perfect Union: The Feminist Reform of Sex and Society* (New York, 1980), 172.

9. Some of Hovey's published novels credit him as an M.D., but there is no evidence to show that he graduated from Harvard or any place else.

10. *Silver-Knife, or the Hunter of the Rocky Mountains; A Romance of the Wild West* (Boston, 1850) also incorporates a short anatomical narrative: the hero's hurried departure from an Eastern city after being implicated in a body-snatching scandal as a young medical student.

11. The above distinctions are intended to emphasize antebellum cultural expectations and beliefs about literary genres, an ideal typology that was never abso-

lute in practice. Sensationalist fiction shared certain narrative and rhetorical elements with high romanticism and philosophical fiction. Hawthorne's prose, for example, worked on his readers' bodies, while even the crudest novel made claims to have morally beneficial effects. Readers assessed the rhetoric, authorial voice, style, quality of paper, binding, and illustrations, etc.—and the balance between pleasurable effects, moral rhetoric, and aesthetic niceties—to see whether such claims had credibility.

12. Bette London, "Mary Shelley, *Frankenstein,* and the Spectacle of Masculinity," *Publications of the Modern Language Association of America* 108.2 (1993): 263–64, argues that Shelley's catalogue of the monster's "beauties" is a parody of Petrarch. *Marietta,* obviously, is greatly indebted to *Frankenstein.*

13. Frederick Clayton Waite, "Grave Robbing in New England," *Bulletin of the Medical Library Association* 33 (1945): 290–91, 294, nn. 38–39. Waite found a similar tale in G. T. Ridlon, Sr., *Saco Valley Settlements and Families, Historical, Biographical, Traditional, and Legendary* (Portland, ME, 1895), 387–88.

14. J[edediah] Vincent Huntington, *Rosemary, or Life and Death* (New York, 1860).

15. See Gayle Rubin, "The Traffic in Women: Notes on the 'Political Economy' of Sex," in Rayna R. Reiter, ed., *Toward an Anthropology of Women* (New York, 1975).

16. David S. Reynolds, *George Lippard* (Boston, 1982); idem, ed., *George Lippard, Prophet of Protest: Writings of an American Radical* (New York, 1983); George Lippard, *The Quaker City . . .* , ed. D. S. Reynolds (Amherst, 1995), vii–xli; Michael Denning, *Mechanic Accents: Dime Novels and Working-Class Culture in America* (New York, 1987), 85–117 (*Godey's* quote, 87). According to Reynolds, *Beneath the American Renaissance: The Subversive Imagination in the Age of Emerson and Melville* (New York, 1988), 204–9, *The Quaker City* sold 60,000 copies as a book in 1845 and averaged 30,000 per year for the next five years. Lippard, *Quaker City* (1845), 2, boasted that his book was "more attacked, and more read, than any work of American fiction ever published." See also "Pen, Press, and Pencil," *Potter's American Monthly* 12 (1878): 350–51; Julia Curtis, "Philadelphia in an Uproar: *The Monks of Monk Hall,* 1844," *Theatre History Studies* 5 (1985): 41–47.

17. *The Quaker City* [newspaper], 3–31–1849: 3; all citations of *The Quaker City* below refer to the Philadelphia, 1845 edition, except where otherwise noted.

18. See Lippard, *The Quaker City; The Nazarene, or, the Last of the Washingtons, a Revelation of Philadelphia, New York, and Washington, in the Year 1844* (Philadelphia, 1846); *The Monk of Wissahikon* (Wissahikon, PA, 1848); *The Empire City, or, New York By Night and Day, Its Aristocracy and Its Dollars* [1850] (Philadelphia, 1864); *New York: Its Upper Ten and Lower Million* (Cincinnati, 1853); Denning, *Mechanic Accents,* 85–117, argues that *The Quaker City's* "sinusoidal structure" (in my reading, shapelessness) is not "premature modernism," but "replicates the narrative structure" of the antebellum newspaper (90).

19. *Quaker City,* 42.

20. Ibid., 38.

21. Reynolds, intro., in Lippard, *The Quaker City* (1995), xiv.

22. See Michel Foucault, *The Birth of the Clinic: An Archaeology of Medical Perception,* trans. A. M. Sheridan Smith (New York, 1973), 90.

23. Lippard's details here are accurate. According to Charles Lawrence, *History*

of the Philadelphia Almshouses and Hospitals (Philadelphia, 1905), 161–64, in the 1840s bodies were illegally culled from the almshouse to supply Philadelphia's dissecting tables.

24. For an extended discussion, see Elisabeth Bronfen, *Over Her Dead Body: Death, Femininity and the Aesthetic* (New York, 1992).

25. *Life of the Notorious Kidnapper, George F. Alberti. . . .* (Philadelphia, 1851) [NYHS]; L. F. Edwards, "Cinci's 'Old Cunny': A Notorious Purveyor of Human Flesh," *Ohio Medical Journal* 50 (1954): 466–69.

26. *Albany Evening Journal*, 3-17-1854: 2.

CHAPTER EIGHT: THE EDUCATION OF SAMUEL TUBBS

1. George Worthington Adams, *Doctors in Blue: The Medical History of the Union Army in the Civil War* (New York, 1952), 4, 9; James H. Cassedy, *Medicine in America: A Short History* (Baltimore, 1991), 64–65; Kenneth M. Ludmerer, *Learning to Heal: The Development of American Medical Education* (New York, 1985), 9–11, 15–16; Richard Shryock, *Medicine in America: Historical Essays* (Baltimore, 1966), 101.

2. John M. Keagy, qtd. in William A. Alcott, "Physiological Vice," *The Teacher of Health and the Laws of Human Constitution* 1 (1843): 69.

3. Popular authors tended not to differentiate much between anatomy and physiology, seeing them as interrelated fields concerned with natural knowledge and laws governing the human body; the phrase "physiological anatomy" was often employed. At the same time, in popular discourse the word "physiology" became identified with the healthy body, the binary opposite of "pathology"; Arnold I. Davidson, "How to Do the History of Psychiatry: A Reading of Freud's *Three Essays on the Theory of Sexuality*," *Critical Inquiry* 18 (1987): 266–67; Toby A. Appel, "Physiology in American Women's Colleges: The Rise and Decline of a Female Subculture," *Isis* 85 (1994): 29. In the 1870s and 1880s, three overlapping groups of people called themselves "physiologists": health reformers like Foote; professors of physiology; and, after the rise of "German" laboratory medicine and the educational reforms of the 1870s and 1880s, laboratory researchers attached to universities (i.e., scientific physiologists). The last group laid claim to the highest degree of epistemological authority and in the twentieth century took exclusive title to the name "physiologist."

4. Edward Bliss Foote, *Science in Story: Sammy Tubbs, the Boy Doctor, and "Sponsie," the Troublesome Monkey* (New York, 1874–75), illustrations by H. L. Stephens: v. 1, "The Boy Tubbs: The Bones, Cartilages and Muscles"; v. 2, "The Student Tubbs: Circulation & Absorption: Arteries, Lymphatics, Veins, Lacteal Capillaries, Radicles, Villi"; v. 3, "The Practitioner Tubbs: Digestive, Nutritive, Respiratory, and Vegetative Systems"; v. 4, "The Lecturer Tubbs: Brain and Nerves, Cerebral Physiology"; v. 5, "The Gymnast Tubbs: Elimination and Reproduction, a Book for Private Reading." The fifth volume, copyrighted in 1874, came out in early 1875. Foote kept the set in print in flexible cloth, hardcover, and deluxe hardcover editions—and as separate volumes, a five-volume set, and a four-volume set (omitting the fifth) until at least 1895. For this book I use a combination of 1874–75, 1876, and 1887 editions, which are identical in content and pagination, except for a few pages in volume 5 (the significance of which is noted below).

5. See Anita Clair Fellman and Michael Fellman, *Making Sense of Self: Medical Advice Literature in Late 19th-Century America* (Philadelphia, 1981); William Leach, *True Love and Perfect Union: The Feminist Reform of Sex and Society* (New York, 1980); Martha Verbrugge, *Able-Bodied Womanhood: Personal Health and Social Change in Nineteenth-Century Boston* (New York, 1988); Barbara Goldsmith, *Other Powers: The Age of Suffrage, Spiritualism and the Scandalous Victoria Woodhull* (New York, 1998).

6. Foote claimed to have applied for a patent on the womb veil (*Medical Common Sense* [New York, 1864], 380), but the patent office has no record of this. German gynecologist Friedrich A. Wilde devised a cervical rubber cap or diaphragm in 1838; Vincent J. Cirillo, "Edward Foote's *Medical Common Sense:* An Early American Comment on Birth Control," *Journal of the History of Medicine and Allied Sciences* 25 (1970): 344. Whether Foote knew of Wilde is unclear.

7. *National Cyclopædia of American Biography* (New York, 1893), 3: 68; *Dr. Foote's Health Monthly* 1.5 (8–1876): supp., 1–2. For scholarship on Foote, see Hal D. Sears, *The Sex Radicals: Free Love in High Victorian America* (Lawrence, 1977), 147, 183–203; Janet Farrell Brodie, *Contraception and Abortion in 19th-Century America* (Ithaca, 1994), 181, 202, 232, 237–41, 281–82, who focuses on Foote's career as "the most successful self-publisher of those involved in reform or reproductive control in the 19th century" (240); Vincent J. Cirillo, "Edward Bliss Foote: Pioneer American Advocate of Birth Control," *Bulletin of the History of Medicine* 47 (1973): 471–79 and "Edward Foote's *Medical Common Sense,*" 341–45; Linda Gordon, *Woman's Body, Woman's Right* (New York, 1974), 167–69, 173–75, 179; James Reed, *From Private Vice to Public Virtue: The Birth Control Movement and American Society Since 1830* (New York, 1978), 16–17; and Leach, *True Love,* 94–98.

8. An 1861 R. G. Dun & Co. credit report described Foote as a "splendid specimen of the genus humbug," doing a "first-rate business" through extensive advertising of mail-order products; Brodie, *Contraception and Abortion,* 240.

9. Qtd. in Gordon, *Woman's Body, Woman's Right,* 168–69 and Sears, *Sex Radicals,* 186, from an undated *New York Independent* article rpt. in *Plain Home Talk* (New York, 1870), 933–34.

10. Foote claimed his monthly had 20,000 subscribers in 1876 (its first year), reported printing over 150,000 copies in 1880 (over 12,000 per month), and claimed to be planning 200,000 in 1881; *Foote's Health Monthly* 1.7 (1876): supp., 8; and 6.3 (1881): 8. The sales figure of 750,000 books as of 1893 (*National Cyclopædia of American Biography,* 3: 68; probably furnished by Foote) is perhaps an overstatement; Brodie, *Contraception and Abortion,* 202, cites an 1887 letter from Foote to Elizur Wright that puts *Plain Home Talk* sales at 250,000, while in contemporary advertisements Foote claimed 500,000—but by any measure his books sold well. Sales figures for other popular medical books are hard to come by, but *Uncle Tom's Cabin* sold 500,000 copies between 1852 and 1857, while Mrs. Henry Wood's *East Lynne* sold 1,000,000 copies between 1861 and 1887; John Tebbel, *The Media in America* (New York, 1974), 138, 270. Foote aimed for a mass audience; he advertised *Plain Home Talk* as "the cheapest book in the English or German language," at $1.50 for a cloth edition; *Foote's Health Monthly* 4.12 (1879): 4. His monthly sold for 10¢ an issue, $1 for a year's subscription, reduced to 5¢ per issue and 50¢ per annum in 1880.

11. Gordon, *Woman's Body, Woman's Right,* 168, asserts that in the 1850s Foote

was "still . . . a follower of traditional medicine," while in later years he turned toward more orthodox and respectable ideas, but this is problematic. Foote's advocacy of Thomsonian-influenced herbalism, animal magnetism, electrotherapy, positivist science, and anatomical medicine was consistent throughout his career, and these should all be characterized as modern rather than traditional. Gordon remarks that Foote's "early sympathies with spiritualism and phrenology gave way later in his life to liberal Unitarianism and evolutionism," but for Foote these things entailed no contradiction; well into the 1880s, he enthusiastically recommended phrenology, and saw no conflict between phrenology and evolutionary theory. His flirtation with "liberal Unitarianism," under Theodore Parker's influence, began in the antebellum era, at the same time that Foote was embracing phrenology and defending spiritualism; Samuel P. Putnam, *Four Hundred Years of Freethought* (New York, 1894), qtd. in T. B. Wakeman, *In Memory of Edward Bliss Foote, M.D.: A "Beloved Physician," of the New, Scientific, Human, Social "Agnostic" Faith. . . .* (New York, 1907), 51. Foote's later religious transformation, in the 1880s, was from unitarianism to agnosticism. Gordon, 169–70, is also on shaky ground in asserting that in later life Foote and his son, Edward Bond Foote, "won the respect of the established [medical] profession." While both men were respected by freethinkers and other cultural radicals, neither ever gained much acceptance by the regulars; they were never listed, for example, in the *Medical Register of New York, New Jersey and Connecticut.* Edward Bond Foote graduated with distinction from the very orthodox New York College of Physicians and Surgeons, but also studied at the Eclectic Medical College of New York (*Medical Eclectic* 2.6 (11-15-1876): 255). He considered himself an "eclectic, with preference for hygienic practice, but a believer in the utility of medicine" and "an advocate of . . . [the] abrogation of all restrictive laws that rule out undiplomaed 'healers' "— heresy for a regular physician. He was also an anti-vaccinationist and called for limits on vivisection; Putnam, *Four Hundred Years*, 732. Students from the College of Physicians and Surgeons so disliked his medical politics that they disrupted a lecture he tried to deliver at the New York Liberal Club; *Foote's Health Monthly* 2.12 (1877): 8–12.

12. Putnam, *Four Hundred Years*, 726–31 (qtd. in Wakeman, *In Memory*, 50–51); D. M. Bennett, *The World's Sages, Thinkers and Reformers* (2d. ed., New York, 1876), 968; *The Biographical History of Westchester County* (Chicago, 1899), 1: 112. Foote almost certainly provided the information for these accounts.

13. The frontispiece of *Medical Common Sense* (Boston, 1858), Foote's first medical publication, describes him as a "medical and electrical therapeutist at Saratoga Springs," a spa town. Foote got his M.D. in 1860 from Penn Medical University, an irregular school devoted to chrono-thermal and eclectic medicine. By the late 1870s it had devolved into a diploma mill and was forced to close in 1881; Harold J. Abrahams, *Extinct Medical Schools of Nineteenth-Century Philadelphia* (Philadelphia, 1966), 176–223.

14. Brodie, *Contraception and Abortion*, 347 nn. 140–41.

15. Bennett, *World's Sages*, 970.

16. Sears, *Sex Radicals*, 167. George E. MacDonald states that D. M. Bennett, T. C. Leland, Stephen Pearl Andrews, and T. B. Wakeman "could scarcely have kept the field without his assistance, . . . when they needed funds for printing and

hall rent, he supplied them" (in Wakeman, *In Memory*, 20). Putnam, *Four Hundred Years* (qtd. in Wakeman, *In Memory*, 53–54), says Foote contributed to legal bills and fines incurred by Susan B. Anthony and C. B. Reynolds (who was prosecuted under a blasphemy statute in New Jersey) and aided freethinkers Ezra Heywood and Moses Harman.

17. It was not so much phrenology that was suspect—despite many detractors within the medical profession, phrenology still had respectable lay supporters like Henry Ward Beecher—but rather the enthusiasm and style of his phrenology. In this form, phrenology in the 1870s retained its connection with the world of reformist and radical cultural politics. For sarcognomy, see John S. Haller, *Medical Protestants: The Eclectics in American Medicine, 1825–1939* (Carbondale, 1994), 111–13.

18. Wakeman, *In Memory*, 12; George E. Macdonald, *Fifty Years of Freethought: The Story of the Truthseeker* (New York, 1929), 2:83.

19. Foote condemned alcohol and tobacco, but opposed prohibition as an illiberal measure.

20. Wakeman, *In Memory*, 19.

21. *Foote's Health Monthly* 1.7 (10–1876): 3–4.

22. Brodie, *Contraception and Abortion*, 238, asserts that the engraved portrait of Foote in the frontispiece of *Medical Common Sense* (1858) shows "an eccentric with unkempt hair, goatee, and unbuttoned coat; the 1864 edition showed a respectable gentleman with white shirt and collar, tie, vest, and carefully buttoned jacket. The goatee, with its reminders of Foote's German background and youthful reformism, was now gone, replaced by a well-trimmed mustache." I would argue that the careless look and facial hair were part of a fashionable bourgeois "look" for young men, signifying a generational identification with European romanticism and radicalism rather than eccentricity or German ethnicity (according to the *Biographical History of Westchester County*, 1:112, the "Foote family is of English origin"). His later portraits do project a stolid patriarchal respectability, as befitting a middle-aged man, but in many ways Foote's radicalism deepened as he grew older.

23. *Divorce: A Review of the Subject from a Scientific Standpoint. . . .* (New York, 1887), backpaper advertisement; *Foote's Health Monthly* 3.4 (4–1878): 6 [house ad]; *Sammy Tubbs*, 1:iii. The fifth volume, bearing an 1874 copyright, was published in early 1875.

24. House ad published in every issue of *Foote's Health Monthly* 1 (1876).

25. *New York Times*, 4-14-1876: 4.

26. The *New York Independent* reviewer, 2-12-1874: 10, found this admission puzzling. On what grounds did Foote object to fiction? Lack of utility? Vulgarity? Morally damaging effects? Foote clearly knew something of juvenile fiction: *Sammy Tubbs* reworks the formula of Jacob Abbott's "Rollo" books, which braided its hero's adventures with lessons in science, morality, history, etc.

27. T. S. Lambert, *Human Anatomy, Physiology and Hygiene* (Hartford, 1854), 2. Lambert, one of Foote's favorite authors, is often cited in *Sammy Tubbs*.

28. *Sammy Tubbs*, 3:78, 4:198.

29. Wakeman, *In Memory*, 54–55: "the Doctor is a member of the Federation of Freethought, the Secular Union, the Manhattan Liberal Club, the Institute of Heredity, the National Defense Association, the New York Public Health and Con-

stitutional Liberty League, the American Psychical Society." Foote belonged to the National Liberal League; in 1880 he traveled to England as a delegate to the International Liberal Convention; *Foote's Health Monthly* 5.9 (1880): 1.

30. Wakeman, *In Memory*, 11. This move effects a kind of gradient universalism: "Mr. Huxley tells us that 'there is one kind of matter common to all living beings, and that their endless diversities are bound together by a physical as well as by an ideal unity.'" (*Sammy Tubbs*, 5:81)

31. Foote concedes that the analogy is not "scientifically correct": "all the higher forms of animal life below man have a Cerebrum, Cerebellum, and Medulla Oblongata" (*Sammy Tubbs*, 4:65).

32. Foote explicitly theorizes the problem of the "atomic" individual in society: "Instead of revolving in their own orbits, and developing themselves individually in accordance with the peculiar constitution of their own mental and physical machinery, [most people] waste their energies in trying to force others to revolve in precisely the same circuit . . . " (*Sammy Tubbs*, 4: 219–20).

33. The publication of *Sammy Tubbs* coincided with the publication of the McLoughlin brothers' popular series of intensely colored—and intensely racist—children's books, such as *Simple Addition by a Little Nigger* (New York, 1874–75?); *Nine Niggers More* (New York, 1874?); *Simple Addition and Nursery Jingles* (New York, 1875?); L. Valentine, *The Funny Little Darkies* (New York, 1875?).

34. See *Sammy Tubbs*, 1:23, 3:37, 4:45, 4:75–76, 4:84–85.

35. Eric Lott, *Love and Theft: Blackface Minstrelsy and the American Working Class* (New York, 1993), 64, 138–53, and *passim.* See also Alexander Saxton, *The Rise and Fall of the White Republic: Class Politics and Mass Culture in Nineteenth-Century America* (New York, 1990), ch. 7, esp. 170; and David R. Roediger, *The Wages of Whiteness: Race and the Making of the American Working Class* (New York, 1991), 115–31.

36. Lott, *Love and Theft*, 64.

37. Robert C. Toll, *Blacking Up: The Minstrel Show in 19th-Century America* (New York, 1974), 70–71, quoting *Negro Forget Me Not Songster* (Philadelphia, 1840s?), 109–11; *Charley White's Ethiopian Joke Book* (New York, 1855), 12, 34, 36–37, 54–55; E. F. Dixey, *Dixey's Essence of Burnt Cork* (Philadelphia, 1859), 36–37.

38. Foote was not alone in attempting to domesticate minstrelsy. In the post-bellum era the meaning of minstrel show performance was diversifying. While a rough version of minstrelsy continued throughout the century, a glitzier, more sentimental, domesticated version, aimed at a broader, more middle-class and sexually mixed audience, flourished in the period after the Civil War. Cf. Alexander Saxton, *Rise and Fall*, 165, who argues for no "basic change in minstrelsy," only the "gradual success of the Republican coalition in capturing segments of the Democracy" that made up the minstrel show's audience.

39. Foote does not acknowledge that anatomy had its own carnivalesque; see chap. 3 above.

40. *Sammy Tubbs*, 4:45, 84–85.

41. "Light and Shade: In the Jaws of Death," *New York World*, 2-24-1874: 7. Variations on this scenario show up all over the cultural landscape, most famously in Hollywood films of the 1930s and 1940s, and even in Gertrude Stein, *Three Lives* (1913; New York, 1990), 23: "She [a German maid] loved to make sport with the

skeletons the doctor had, to make them move and make strange noises till the negro boy shook in his shoes and his eyes rolled white in his agony of fear."

42. Cf. Lott, *Love and Theft*, 148, which discusses the ways in which blackness's contaminating effect was transvalued into a realm of freedom and excess in the minstrel show.

43. For the demographics of medical school cadavers, see David C. Humphrey, "Dissection and Discrimination: The Social Origins of Cadavers in America, 1760–1915," *Bulletin of the New York Academy of Medicine* 49 (1973): 819–27. Cf. the nearly contemporary account of anatomical dissection in Mark Twain and Charles Dudley Warner, *The Gilded Age: A Tale of To-Day* (New York, 1873; rpt. New York, 1915), ch. 15, esp. 1: 153 (discussed above in chap. 3).

44. Foote here is recirculating the notion that the racial characteristics of black people (childishness, plasticity) make them good material for the self-making projects of the middle-class, an idea that had currency in some antebellum antislavery circles. Black tractability is a reproach and a spur to the less tractable Irish and recalcitrant children. See Lott, *Love and Theft*, 32; George Fredrickson, *The Black Image in the White Mind: The Debate on Afro-American Character and Destiny, 1817–14* (New York, 1971), 50, 101.

45. Lott, *Love and Theft*, 118.

46. Foote believed that only use of greco–latinate terms for body parts could legitimize public discussion of the body, especially the sexual body. With less enthusiasm, a decade later he supported the right of "free lovers" to print non-latinate profane words like "cock" and "fuck." For the politics of sexual nomenclature, see Jesse F. Battan, "'The Word Made Flesh': Language, Authority, and Sexual Desire in Late 19th-Century America," *Journal of the History of Sexuality* 3 (1992): 223–44.

47. *Sammy Tubbs*, 1:39–43, 53–55.

48. *Sammy Tubbs*, 1:42–43, 4:22.

49. For nineteenth-century conceptions of body as machine, see Anson Rabinbach, *The Human Motor: Energy, Fatigue, and the Origins of Modernity* (New York, 1990) and Mark Seltzer, *Bodies and Machines* (New York, 1992).

50. Foote respects the cultural demand that the cadaver serve as a sacralized object in a ritual honoring the life and spirit of the departed, but holds that this can be reconciled with a utilitarian ethos. The discussion emerges when Sammy decides to dissect the bodies of a pet dog and Sponsie 1 to demonstrate the anatomy of the nervous system for a lecture. Dr. Hubbs: "having the bodies of your dead pets before you will constantly remind you of your bereavement. . . . " Sammy replies: "I can . . . make good use of their brains and nerves before my class . . . and then . . . bury their remains just as decently as if they had not served a useful purpose" (4:222–23).

51. Foote's ideas on heredity were influenced by R. T. Trall, *Sexual Physiology: A Scientific and Popular Exposition of the Fundamental Problems in Sociology* (New York, 1866) and Haeckel's synthesis of Darwin and Lamarck, but also conserved an older strain of obstetrical lore: pregnancy as a perilous time of hyperimpressionability for the fetus; see *Sammy Tubbs*, 5:211–12.

52. *Foote's Health Monthly* 1.1 (1876): 1.

53. Brodie, *Contraception and Abortion*, 241–42, argues that Foote "recognized

the new and growing importance of women as customers" and "emphasized in publications . . . the ease with which women . . . could obtain his [mail order] products and the secrecy with which they could use them."

54. *Foote's Health Monthly* 1 (1876); the ad appeared before the publication of book 5.

55. *New York Independent*, 11-26-1874: 9; the *Independent* was edited by Theodore Tilton.

56. Through 1874, the *New York Times* took no notice of Foote's heterodox medical politics; 2-21-1874: 9 and 12-3-1874: 3. In 1876, however, the *Times* did take notice; "A Blow to Quack Doctors," *New York Times*, 3-29-1876: 8, and Foote's reply, *New York Times*, 4-14-1876: 4. In *Foote's Health Monthly* 1.1 (1876): 2, Foote complained that the *Times* refused to "teach its readers anything of those organs which the Creator assigned to the important function of reproduction, or, if it thinks this information should be conveyed through medical works . . . worded as to reach the popular mind[,] . . . allow its advertising columns to be used in calling attention to such publications." The fifth volume received a brief favorable notice in *Medical Eclectic* 2.2 (3-15-1875): 77–78.

57. See Battan, "Word Made Flesh"; Sears, *Sex Radicals*. Other events that worked to break up the alliance were the publication of J. W. Draper, *The History of the Conflict Between Science and Religion* (New York, 1875); the 1875 Beecher-Tilton adultery trial (which served to discredit liberal evangelicalism); and the championing of materialism by John Tyndall and other prominent European physiologists and evolutionists.

58. *Foote's Health Monthly* 1.9 (1876): 6.

59. Ibid., 10.12 (1885): 11; these figures probably lump together sales of individual volumes with four- and five-volume sets. Portions of the first book were reprinted in *Foote's Health Monthly* 1 (1876); the fifth book was later released under the title *Sexual Physiology for the Young* (New York, 1882). For Foote's complaint that sales of *Sammy Tubbs* did not equal the "250,000 copies which . . . Medical Common Sense enjoyed," see *Foote's Health Monthly* 5.12 (1880): 8. The series was sold via mail and through a network of agents. *Moore's Rural New-Yorker* (Rochester), 3-21-1874: 200; 3-28-1874: 216; 4-4-1874: 232, has an ad on the back page: "New Book. Nothing Like it in Literature. Agents wanted. . . . Select your territory. . . ."

60. Comstock began taking aim at Foote well before the 1875 publication of *Sammy Tubbs*, vol. 5. In *Frauds Exposed, or How the People are Deceived and Robbed, and Youth Corrupted* (New York, 1880), 426, Comstock claimed that "the first thing accomplished after the signing of the [federal Comstock Act] in 1873 by President Grant was to oblige . . . Mr. E. B. Foote . . . to suppress several thousands of circulars, advertisements, and books that he was sending through the mail. . . . "

61. Thanks to Gina M. Camodeca for raising the issue of anthropomorphized female genitalia (email message, 12-4-1995).

62. Such issues were debated in advance of Foote's entry into the field. T. S. Lambert, *Human Anatomy, Physiology and Hygiene*, omitted any discussions or illustrations of sexual organs in his 1854 secondary school textbook on "physiological anatomy," and argued defensively that "It is not . . . desirable that the young scholar should study the dry details of Anatomy or the great philosophical truths

of Physiology, or learned hypotheses and extended experiments. The general student needs only the general principles" (27).

63. *Sammy Tubbs*, 5:96–97. The erect penis and singing vagina (drawn by H. L. Stephens) are included in an edition that bears an 1874 imprint (owned by Florida State University). In other editions bearing an 1874 imprint (owned by Purdue University and the American Antiquarian Society), and in some subsequent editions, they are replaced by pictures of yeast cells, "common moulds," and the "conjugation" of a simple animal (taken from a contemporary textbook), and a small revision of the written text (which is put in unexplained brackets). Volume 5 was not published until 1875; both Florida State and Purdue have a volume 4 with an 1876 imprint, but textually identical to the 1874 edition. An 1876 five-in-one edition (owned by Johns Hopkins University) has the anthropomorphic vagina and erect penis on 5:96 and 97, but not the anatomical diagrams of the male and female reproductive organs. *Sexual Physiology for the Young* (New York, 1882), a separately released edition of the fifth volume, has the anatomical diagrams but not the anthropomorphic vagina. (Thanks to Charles Rosenberg for making available to me his copy.) An 1887 five-in-one edition (owned by the University of Rochester) lacks the anthropomorphic vagina and erect penis on 5:96–97 and the anatomically explicit diagrams on 5:180½ and 180¾.

64. *Sammy Tubbs*, 5:95. Italicized text indicates material in the 1874 Florida State and 1876 Johns Hopkins "erect penis" copies but omitted from the 1874 Purdue, AAS, and 1887 University of Rochester copies.

65. Identical or similar illustrations appear in William Alcott, F. C. Hollick, Mary Gove, Catherine Beecher, Calvin Cutter, T. S. Lambert, and other popular and pedagogical anatomies.

66. But no popular work was as explicit, transgressive, wide ranging, or entertaining as *Sammy Tubbs*; none was aimed at as young or as wide a readership. Burt Green Wilder's *What Young People Should Know: The Reproductive Function in Man and the Lower Animals* (Boston, 1875) is as explicit as *Sammy Tubbs*, but highly technical and detailed. Wilder's "young people" were male college students. In the late 1870s Wilder, a professor at Cornell, taught a controversial but popular course for seniors on "Physiology and Hygiene," also known as the "lecture on certain duties of men before and after marriage." See Leach, *True Love*, 47–51.

67. Sarah Hackett Stevenson, *The Physiology of Woman* (Chicago, 1881), 173.

68. Wakeman, *In Memory*, 10–11.

69. Comstock was Foote's principal antagonist, but there were others. Caroline Winslow and Lucinda Chandler, advocates of sexual purity, agreed with much of Foote's agenda, but parted company over his contention that "Sexual Continence is not Conducive to Health"; see *Foote's Replies to the Alphites. . . .* (New York, 1889); Leach, *True Love*, 94–98. Stevenson, *Physiology of Woman*, 47, warned that "much mischief has been bred by a pseudo-scientific literature under the name of Biology, Psychology, Phrenology, and even Physiology, for there is no domain these prolific writers will not dare to enter. . . . " Wilder, *What Young People Should Know*, 135–40, cautioned against popular books on sexual topics and "advertising quacks" who specialized in sexual problems.

70. Foote, of course, made a prior claim for direct knowledge of the body, as a dissector, but this claim was more citational than real: he was no anatomist, did no

original research, and probably had very limited training in dissection. His claims for epistemological privilege in assessing canonical medical texts rested on his (self-avowed) vocation as a "gifted healer" and as the possessor of a masculinist, transcendently self-affirmative will.

71. "Every man his own physician," a slogan of the Thomsonians, goes back at least as far as John Theobald's *Every Man his Own Physician* (London, 1754); Charles Rosenberg, *Explaining Epidemics* (Cambridge, 1992), 35.

72. See *Report of the American Humane Association on Vivisection and Dissection in Schools* (Chicago, 1895).

73. Foote flirted with a variety of positions on vaccination before finally endorsing the noncompulsory use of bovine virus (with the caveat that impure and incompetently administered vaccine was dangerous and that the matter bore further study); *Foote's Health Monthly* 2.3 (1877): 11–12; 5.3 (1880): 10; 7.3 (1882): 4. He defended vivisection, with varying degrees of fervor; *Foote's Health Monthly* 1.7 (1876): 2 and 6.12 (1881): 10. By 1894 he likely agreed with his son, who labeled himself "an anti-vaccinationist, but a believer in the utility of vivisection, *limited*"; Putnam, *Four Hundred Years*, 732. The limitation on vivisection still put the Footes at some distance from the medical establishment—and from the anatomical self-making of *Sammy Tubbs*.

74. See J. B. Blake, "The Development of American Anatomy Acts," *Journal of Medical Education* (1955) 30: 431–39; A. M. Lassek, *Human Dissection: Its Drama and Struggle* (Springfield, IL, 1958); and Ruth Richardson, *Death, Dissection and the Destitute* (London, 1987). Foote condemned opposition to dissection (which he attributed to "religious prejudices" and "superstition") and supported anatomy acts; *Sammy Tubbs*, 1:39–43. In 1878—the peak year for anatomy scandals, which were widely publicized in the popular press—a cresting wave of popular revulsion against body snatching caused Foote to soft-pedal his advocacy of dissection. Foote's unconvincing solution was to advocate the passage of laws providing medical schools with the bodies of "unfortunates . . . who die in the wards of hospitals friendless and alone," while replacing cadavers with anatomical "manikins" for "all students except those who wish to become accomplished surgeons"; these anatomical models could also be "supplemented with the bodies of the lower orders of animal life" (a solution opposed, of course, by antivivisectionists). Foote proposed that dissections of the human body could be limited to "a few surgical colleges," but held fast to the idea that "knowledge of the human body should become more general rather than circumscribed" and that "the welfare of the living" made it necessary "that human bodies should be dissected"; *Foote's Health Monthly* 3.11 (1878): 5–6.

CHAPTER NINE: "ANATOMY OUT OF GEAR"

1. *New York Tribune*, 1-10-1888. In this chapter, omission of page numbers for newspaper items indicates that the article is in the District Attorney's scrapbook, Municipal Archives, New York City.

2. *New York Herald*, 1-10-1888.

3. Ibid.; *New York Times*, 1-10-1888: 8; *New York World*, 1-10-1888; *New York Herald*,

1-10-1888; *New York Sun,* 1-10-1888; *New York Morning Journal,* 1-10-1888: 2; *New York Tribune,* 1-10-1888; *New York Star,* 1-10-1888: 2.

4. See for example, F. J. Cole, *History of the Anatomical Museum* (London, 1914); Stewart H. Holbrook, *The Golden Age of Quackery* (New York, 1959).

5. George C. D. Odell, *Annals of the New York Stage* (New York, 1931), 5: 66, 228, 305, 400, 585, 6: 80–81, 7: 95, 527, 9: 88, 478, 10: 95, 11: 586, 15: 771; Richard D. Altick, *The Shows of London* (Cambridge, MA, 1978), 1, 27–28, 54–56, 260–61, 338–42; Neil Harris, *Humbug; the Art of P. T. Barnum* (Boston, 1973); Brooks McNamara, *Step Right Up* (rev. ed., Jackson, MS, 1995), 37–41. Writing in the 1930s, Odell dismissed anatomy museums as a particularly vulgar type of plebeian entertainment. His bemused disdain was a typical bourgeois response (another being unbemused disdain): "I hate to sink to the level of Dr. Kahn's Museum of Anatomy. . . . " [15: 771].

6. See, for example, Joel J. Orosz, *Curators and Culture: The Museum Movement in America, 1740–1870* (Tuscaloosa, 1990); Sally Kohlstedt, "Curiosities and Cabinets: Natural History Museums and Education on the Antebellum Campus," *Isis* 79 (1988): 405–26; David R. Brigham, *Public Culture in the Early Republic: Peale's Museum and its Audience* (Washington, 1995).

7. Paula Findlen, *Possessing Nature: Museums, Collecting and Scientific Culture in Early Modern Italy* (Berkeley, 1994); Lorraine Daston and Katharine Park, *Wonders and the Order of Nature, 1150–1750* (New York, 1998).

8. According to Lorraine Daston, rev., "The Factual Sensibility," *Isis* 79 (1988): 452–67, "fact" derives from the French word *faire* and in seventeenth-century Europe retained that connotation, something more active than the present meaning: a deed, a proving, or even a crime.

9. Mark Dery, "Anatomy Lesson: The Visceral Pleasures of Medical Museums," in Sara Diamond and Sylvere Lotringer, ed. *Flesh Eating Technologies* (New York, 1999); thanks to Mark Dery for sharing a draft of his article with me.

10. *Catalogue of the Surgical and Pathological Museum of Valentine Mott . . . and . . . Alexander B. Mott. . . .* (New York, 1858), 45. The Mott collection had a variety of bones from Waterloo, 16, 74; a cast of the skull and head of Gibbs the pirate, 49, 64; and the skulls of "the celebrated Davy Crockett, from an undoubted source," 74, and "Bob, the celebrated Georgia bandit," 67. The catalogue provides an account of Bob's capture.

11. John V. Pickstone, "Museological Science? The Place of the Analytical/Comparative in 19th-Century Science, Technology and Medicine," *History of Science* 32.2 (1994): 111–38.

12. See, for example, "Letter from Albany," *The National Era,* 6-10-1847: 3, a report of a group tour of the anatomical museum of the Albany Medical Institute.

13. Altick, *Shows of London,* 54–55.

14. *A Descriptive Catalogue . . . of Rackstrow's Museum. . . .* (London, 1794), 17–18 [NYHS]; Altick, *Shows of London,* 55–56.

15. *Dunlap's Pennsylvania Packet* [Philadelphia], 10-10-1774, 11-28-1774, 12-3-1774, 1-8-1778; Orosz, *Curators and Culture,* 21–22.

16. *Royal Gazette* (New York), 3-17-1781. Yeldall's lecture and exhibition may have been connected to some kind of traveling medicine show. A decade earlier, he toured the colonies with a troupe, including a clown named Merry Andrew,

selling "Public Medicines," *Pennsylvania Journal,* 11-21-1771; William Helfand, "Advertising Health to the People," *"Every Man his own Doctor": Popular Medicine in Early America,* exhibition catalogue, Library Company of Philadelphia (Philadelphia, 1998), 26.

17. *Diary of William Bentley, D.D., pastor of the East Church, Salem, Massachusetts* (Gloucester, MA, 1962), 4:441 (3-10-1817). Thanks to Brett Mizelle, for alerting me to this passage, and Thomas Horrocks, Countway Library, for help with research on H. Williams. See also *To the Patrons of the Arts: Messrs. Stowell and Bradley Respectfully Inform the Ladies and Gentlemen of Salem and its Vicinity, that They Have Opened for a Short Time an Elegant Museum* (Salem, 1817) [AAS].

18. *New York Medical Inquirer* 1.5 (1830): 237–38.

19. *Boston Medical and Surgical Journal,* 11-4-1846: 282–83.

20. Altick, *Shows of London,* 54–56, 338–42.

21. *New York Times,* 1-10-1888: 8.

22. *Guide to the European Anatomical, Pathological and Ethnological Museum of Professor Charles Kreutzberg* (Philadelphia, 1876?) [Atwater Kent Museum, Philadelphia]. The "moral purpose" formula is recycled in *Neurasthenia, or Nervous Exhaustion, Its Nature, Cause and Cure,* a 25¢ pamphlet of lectures given at Dr. Baskette's Gallery of Anatomy, Chicago (late 19th century?) [Collection of William H. Helfand].

23. *Catalogue of the Grand Anatomical Museum, or National Academy of Natural, Anatomical and Pathological Science* (New York, 1854) [FC].

24. Quote is from *Catalogue of the New York Anatomical Gallery and Academy of Natural, Medical, and Moral Sciences* (New York, 1847); other catalogues surveyed include those already cited in this chapter, plus *Catalogue of the Grand Anatomical Museum* (New York, 1854); *Catalogue of the New-York Museum of Anatomy* (New York, 1863) [NLM]; *A Visit to the New York Museum of Anatomy* (New York, 1867?) [NYHS]; *Dr. Hallock & Co.'s Museum of Anatomy and Medical Institute* (Boston, ca. 1870) [FC]; *Hand Book and Descriptive Catalogue of Dr. Kahn's Museum of Anatomy and Natural Science* (New York, n.d., [ca. 1869–88]) [collection of William H. Helfand]; *Catalogue of the New-York Museum of Anatomy* (New York, 1870); *Catalogue: Dr. Baskette's Gallery of Anatomy* (Chicago, ca. 1870) [collection of William H. Helfand].

25. *Guide to the European Anatomical Museum* (Philadelphia, 1876), 2.

26. *A Visit to the New York Museum of Anatomy* (New York, 1867?), 3.

27. *Catalogue of the Grand Anatomical Museum* (New York, 1854), 5, 7–8.

28. Ibid.

29. Ibid.

30. "The Sea-Serpent Factory," *New York World,* 11-6-1887: 1.

31. Edward Kahn owned an anatomy museum in London in the 1850s; Louis J. Kahn, who established his own museum in New York in the late 1860s, claimed a family connection. Henry J. Jordan established a museum in New York in the mid-1860s and perhaps earlier; his 1863 collection seems to be British in origin (e.g., it has displays on British rather than American criminals). Phillip Jordan and Louis J. Jordan (probably an alias for Louis J. Kahn) also operated museums in New York in the 1870s and 1880s. The name of Henry J. Jordan later pops up in connection with a Philadelphia museum. Robert Jourdain operated a museum in Boston. The precise connections between the Jordans is not presently known.

32. Charles Gibbs and Thomas Wansley, pirates based in Havana, were caught by the U.S. Navy and tried in New York in 1831. Gibbs confessed to the hijacking of eight ships and the murder of their crews, nearly 400 people. He and Wansley were sentenced to be hanged and then given to the College of Physicians and Surgeons for dissection; *Mutiny and Murder; Confession of Charles Gibbs* (Providence, 1831), 24 [NYHS]. The "fac simile" of Gibbs's penis may have been copied from an object in the museum of the College of Physicians and Surgeons of New York.

33. New York City, District Attorney Indictment Papers, Court of General Sessions; People vs. Horace P. Tolles and Wooster Beach, 11-22-1850 [NYMA].

34. Circus and tableaux vivant performers wore flesh-colored tights, but over the course of the century the stricture on uncovered skin relaxed a bit. Robert C. Toll, *Blacking Up: The Minstrel Show in 19th-Century America* (New York, 1974), 136–37; Robert Allen, *Horrible Prettiness: Burlesque and American Culture* (Chapel Hill, 1993); Peter G. Buckley, "The Culture of 'Leg-Work': The Transformation of Burlesque after the Civil War," in James Gilbert et al., eds., *The Mythmaking Frame of Mind: Social Imagination and American Culture* (Belmont, CA, 1993).

35. New York City, District Attorney Indictment Papers, Court of General Sessions; People v. Horace P. Tolles and Wooster Beach, 11-22-1850 [NYMA]; F. C. Hollick, *The Origin of Life.* . . . (New York, 1878), x; Hollick's emphasis. The medical elite did not universally endorse Beach's museum. *Boston Medical and Surgical Journal,* 11-4-1846: 282–83, complained that his "midwifery department, . . . to which he invites the public, old and young indiscriminately, for a few shillings and the ladies especially" contained "mysteries" that were "not fit objects for young people of either sex to look upon, nor should females be permitted to see such sights. . . . Nor should such any anatomical exhibitions be countenanced by the public, unless . . . assurance is given that no indelicate or improper features deform the collection, nor unless the respectable character of the exhibiter afford a guarantee to this effect." Beach may not have been up to the journal's standard, but he had taught as professor of clinical medicine at the Eclectic Medical College of Cincinnati.

36. W[ooster] Beach, *A Treatise on Anatomy, Physiology, and Health,* . . . *for students, schools, and popular use* (New York, 1847) [AAS], was offered for sale at the museum, with colored plates for $3, uncolored plates for $2.50, and without plates for $2. *Treatise,* 128–29, explains how readers could make anatomical preparations at home, using directions given in F. C. Hollick's *American Class-book.* For the museum's phrenological office, see B. J. Gray, *Catalogue of the New York Anatomical Gallery* (1847).

37. A. H. Saxon, *P. T. Barnum: The Legend and the Man* (New York, 1989), 80, 234; *New York Sun,* 2-26-1836: 2; *New York Herald,* 2-27-1836: 1, 3-1-1836: 2, 3-2-1836: 1; Benjamin Reiss, "P. T. Barnum, Joice Heth and Antebellum Spectacles of Race," *American Quarterly* 51 (1999): 78–107.

38. See Richard Butsch, "Bowery B'hoys and Matinee Ladies: The Re-Gendering of Nineteenth-Century American Theater Audiences," *American Quarterly* 46 (1994): 374–405.

39. *Guide to the European Anatomical Museum* (Philadelphia, 1876), 2.

40. *New York Star,* 1-10-1888: 2.

41. In 1869, Henry J. Jordan experimented with a small Ladies' New York Museum of Anatomy at 600 Broadway, but it flopped. After a few months he trans-

ferred the collection to his New York Museum of Anatomy; Odell, *Annals of the New York Stage*, 8: 516, 650.

42. Felix Riesenberg, *East Side West Side* (New York, 1927), 143–45, 198–99.

43. H. W. Felter, "Pathfinders," *National Eclectic Medical Quarterly* 1.2 (12–1909): 94; *Catalogue of the Grand Anatomical Museum* (New York, 1854).

44. David R. Brigham, *Public Culture in the Early Republic: Peale's Museum and its Audience* (Washington, 1995).

45. Orosz, *Curators and Culture*, 221.

46. Bluford Adams, *E Pluribus Barnum: the Great Showman and the Making of U.S. Popular Culture* (Minneapolis, 1997); Harris, *Humbug*; Charlotte M. Porter, "The Natural History Museum," in Michael S. Shapiro, ed., with Louise Ward Kemp, *The Museum: A Reference Guide* (New York, 1990), 8.

47. See for example, *Dr. Hallock & Co.'s Museum of Anatomy and Medical Institute* (Boston, ca. 1870?); Robert J. Jourdain, *Catalogue of the Parisian Gallery of Anatomy and Medical Science* (Boston, 1869) [FC].

48. See Brooks McNamara, *Step Right Up* (New York, 1976), esp. 39–44.

49. In 1887, Comstock had campaigned against dealers of fine-art prints and stirred up considerable public resistance to his efforts to censor a cultural domain that made plausible claims to respectability. In this context, the popular anatomical museums probably seemed a safe and inviting target to Comstock, like the contraceptives and sexually explicit printed materials that made him his name. Thanks to Elizabeth Hovey for sharing her research on Comstock.

50. *New York Herald*, 1-10-1888.

51. *Visit to the New York Museum of Anatomy* (New York, 1867?), 3.

52. *Catalogue of the Grand Anatomical Museum* (New York, 1854), 4.

53. *New York Tribune*, 1-10-1888.

54. *Guide to the European Anatomical Museum* (Philadelphia, 1876), 45–46.

55. *New York Morning Journal*, 1-10-1888: 2.

56. *New York Sun*, 1-10-1888.

57. *New York Morning Journal*, 1-10-1888: 2.

58. *New York Star*, 1-22-1888.

59. "Reminiscences of a Prosector and Appreciation of Leidy's Work as an Anatomist," in *The Joseph Leidy Commemorative Meeting, held in Philadelphia, December 6, 1923* (n.p., n.d.), 62–65. Thanks to Gretchen Worden for bringing this memoir to my attention.

60. *New York World*, 1-10-1888; see also *New York Sun*, 1-10-1888; *New York Herald*, 1-10-1888.

61. *New York World*, 1-10-1888.

62. L. J. Kahn, *Value of the Microscope: Examinations of the Urine and Chronic Diseases* (New York, 1876).

63. *New York Sun*, 1-10-1888.

64. *New York Times*, 1-12-1888: 5; *Medico-Legal Journal*, 3–1888: 486–87; thanks to Maureen Beyer, Historical Library, Yale Medical College, for this reference. George M. Beard, coiner of the term *neurasthenia*, was a member of the Society until his death in 1885. The doctors of the Society and the popular anatomical museums had shared interests. Both cautioned against "nervous debility," "nervous exhaustion," and the medical dangers of masturbation and promiscuity. Wil-

liam A. Hammond, for example, wrote *On Certain Conditions of Nervous Derangement* . . . (New York, 1881); and *Sexual Impotence in the Male and Female* (Detroit, 1887). Anatomical museum lecturers enthusiastically adopted Beard's "neurasthenia" diagnosis and the sexual etiology of neurasthenia.

65. *New York Star*, 1-10-1888: 2.

66. *New York Tribune*, 1-20-1888.

67. Anthony Comstock, notes, "Persons arrested under the Auspices of the New York Society for the Suppression of Vice," vol. 2, 1888, Manuscript Division, Library of Congress: "Had wax figures of females life size, some pregnant & some otherwise & 37 cases of filthy penises. These cases were disposed of before Judge Gildersleeve (it would be hard by justi. to say tried). He allowed the defense greatest latitude, and after they had prepared, altered and fixed up their museum, Gildersleeve allowed the jury to go up & see how they had afixed it up. He also sent them to hdq'rs Police, to see matters seized, and also allowed persons to testify about their exhibits, without ever going there to see them, or without knowing what the things actually seized were, but they testified in a general way upon days and dates other than the day of arrest. Larry Jerome's son was the Asst. Dist. Atty. in charge of case & the stenographers note will bear out the statement that the case was very poorly tried. G. in his charge to Jury ignored the words "filthy" and "disgusting" in statute, the record in muller case, while he pretended to charge them in the words of the Ct. of Apps. in that case." I want to thank Elizabeth Hovey for her generosity in sharing her research on Anthony Comstock with me.

68. *Descriptive Catalogue of Dr. Kahn's Museum of Anatomy and Medical Science* ["price 5 cents"] (New York, n.d., [ca. 1905]) [collection of William H. Helfand] lists Kahn's address as 312 Bowery ("Above Houston Street"). In addition to Kahn's, there existed in the early twentieth century the David DiBol College of Anatomy and Gallery of Science and perhaps others on the Bowery.

69. Police Court, 3d Dist., New York County, 10-12-1887 to 2-1-1888 (roll #30); Magistrate's Court Docket Book, 3d Dist. [New York City Municipal Archives]. Nativity of those arrested: Italy 7; Germany 6; Austria 2; Hungary 1; United States 1.

70. *New York Tribune*, 1-10-1888.

71. *New York Herald*, 1-10-1888.

72. See, for example, Brigham, *Public Culture in the Early Republic*.

CONCLUSION

1. Benjamin Rush, "An Inquiry into the Cause of Animal Life, in three lectures, delivered in the University of Pennsylvania" in Rush, *Medical Inquiries and Observations* (2d ed., Philadelphia, 1805), 2: 372–73 [CPP].

2. In turn, J. W. Draper, the mid-nineteenth-century chemist-physiologist, found eighteenth-century anatomy "static," "a dry, though accurate, enumeration of parts and functions," compared to the "dynamic" nineteenth-century Parisian school; obituary, *Medical Register of New York, New Jersey and Connecticut* 20 (1882): 227.

3. D. H. Agnew, *Lecture Introductory to the One Hundred and Fifth Course of Instruc-*

tion in the Medical Department of the University of Pennsylvania, delivered Monday, October 10, 1870 (Philadelphia, 1870), 25. Agnew attributed the indifference not to the shift to clinical or laboratory medicine, but rather to "illustrated works on anatomy, colossal models and diagrams" that gave students an alternative to dissection, "which is repugnant to many."

4. E. W. Holmes, "The Dissecting Room," *Transactions of the Pan-American Medical Congress* 2 (1893): 1153.

5. *Cincinnati Commercial*, 5-3-1878, qtd. in Harry J. Sievers, *The Harrison Horror* (Fort Wayne, IN, 1956), 10.

6. Linden F. Edwards, "The Famous Harrison Case and Its Repercussions," *Bulletin of the History of Medicine* 31 (1957): 162–71; "The Ohio Anatomy Law of 1881," *Ohio State Medical Journal* 46 (1950): 1190–92 and 47 (1951): 49–53, 143–46; Sievers, *Harrison Horror.*

7. Edwards, "Ohio Anatomy Law of 1881," 49–52, 143–46; "Famous Harrison Case," 168–69.

8. Benjamin Butler, *Address of his Excellency Benjamin F. Butler, to the Two Branches of the Legislature of Massachusetts, January 4, 1883* (Boston, 1883); *Argument before the Tewksbury Investigation Committee. . . .* (n.p., 1883); *Autobiography and Personal Reminiscences of Major-General Benjamin F. Butler. . . .* (Boston, 1892), 969, 975–76 [MHS]; Massachusetts House of Representatives, Doc. 300, *Report of Hearings Before the Joint Standing Committee on Public Charitable Institutions: under the Order for Said Committee to Investigate the Mismanagement, Control and Condition of the Public Charitable Institutions, and the Special Charges of the Mismanagement of the State Almshouse at Tewksbury* (Boston, 1883), 2 vols. [NLM]. The Massachusetts Historical Society has an envelope, embossed with the words "House of Representatives, Boston" and marked "Piece of Tanned human skin from Tewksbury hearing R Walcott Esq."

9. Suzanne M. Shultz, *Body Snatching: The Robbing of Graves for the Education of Physicians in Early Nineteenth Century America* (Jefferson, NC, 1992), 72–77; *Cincinnati Evening Post*, 2-23-1884: 1.

10. See, for example, H. Lenox Hodge, *Anatomical Rooms: Plan for their Construction, Ventilation, and Hygienic Management* (Richmond, 1875; rpt. *Virginia Medical Monthly*, 10–1875); Charles L. Bardeen, *Anatomy in America* (Madison, 1905), 138–41, 153–54.

11. Robert D. Lyons, *A Handbook of Hospital Practice. . . .* (New York, 1860), 119.

12. Arthur E. Hertzler, *The Horse and Buggy Doctor* (New York, 1938), 43.

13. U.S. Department of Commerce, *Historical Statistics of the United States* (Washington, 1975), 1: 163–65 (Series D 705–738). The approximate figures given are for the antebellum and Civil-War era; in the postbellum era, wages rose by approximately 50%.

14. H. A. Kelly, "The Barred Road to Anatomy," *Johns Hopkins Hospital Bulletin* 208 (7–1908): 196–201.

15. *[Indianapolis] Recorder*, 3-15-1902: 1; qtd. from the *Christian Index.*

16. Stanley Buder, *Pullman: An Experiment in Industrial Order and Community Planning, 1880–1930* (New York, 1967), 209–10.

17. There was a long medical tradition of private autopsies on the bodies of practitioners, often performed by friendly colleagues.

18. Philip Van Ingen, *The New York Academy of Medicine: Its First Hundred Years* (New York, 1949), 336.

19. Jarvis Means Morse, *A Neglected Period in Connecticut's History, 1818–1850* (New Haven, 1933), 294, citing Connecticut State Records, 1834, 169–70; *Connecticut Courant*, 5-5-1834; 6-9-1834.

20. The disciplinary boundary between medicine and the social sciences was not sharply defined; e.g., surgeon Valentine Mott addressed the ASSA on the subject of rabies.

21. Wines to Dall, 9-22-1868 [Dall papers, MHS], qtd. in Leach, *True Love and Perfect Union*, 324; see also 341.

22. *What Social Classes Owe to Each Other* (Caldwell, ID, 1995), 101. Sumner's answer to the title question: absolutely nothing.

23. Cf. Dorothy Ross, *The Origins of American Social Science* (Cambridge, 1991), which neglects anatomy as a discursive source of professionalism.

24. D. M. Bennett, *The World's Sages, Thinkers, and Reformers* (New York, 1876), 970.

25. Emerson, "Historic Notes of Life and Letters in New England" [1880], *Lectures and Biographical Sketches* (Boston, 1904), 329. This quote came to my attention via a query advanced by Russ Castronovo (University of Miami, Florida) on H-AMSTDY, 3-5-1997; the citation was identified by Jeffrey Steele, University of Wisconsin, Madison.

26. Joseph Leidy, *Introductory Lecture to the Course on Anatomy, Delivered in the University of Pennsylvania, October 11th, 1859* (Philadelphia, 1859), 3 [CPP].

27. C. M. Ellis, Baltimore County, to Joseph Leidy, Philadelphia, 3–1861 [CPP].

28. *New York Times*, 9-3-1993: 16; Jordan Bonfante, "The Anatomy of Death," *Time Magazine*, 12-15-1997.

BIBLIOGRAPHY

AAS = American Antiquarian Society, Worcester, MA
CPP = Library of the College of Physicians, Philadelphia
FC = Francis Countway Library of Medicine, Harvard University
HS = Health Sciences Library, Special Collections, Columbia University
MHS = Massachusetts Historical Society, Boston
NLM = National Library of Medicine
NYAM = New York Academy of Medicine
NYHS = New-York Historical Society
NYMA = Municipal Archives, New York City
NYPL = New York Public Library, Rare Book and Manuscript Collection
NYU = Ehrmann Medical Library, New York University

MANUSCRIPTS

Zabdiel Boylston Adams, "Interesting reminiscences of a long professional life," typescript, 3-6-1894 [FC].

C. C. Carlos Barne?, to J. C. Warren, 8-22-1830 [J. C. Warren Papers, MHS].

Rev Mr Milton P[almer] Braman, Danvers, MA?, to J. C. Warren, 10-13-1830 [J.C. Warren Papers, MHS].

College of Physician & Surgeons, New York, Minutes, 1814 [HS].

Anthony Comstock, notes, New York Society for the Suppression of Vice, "Persons arrested under the Auspices of the New York Society for the Suppression of Vice," Vol. 2, 1888 [Manuscript Division, Library of Congress].

Samuel Craddock, Jr., Geneva, NY, to D. E. Craddock, Weedsport, NY, 10-25-1847, Williams and Craddock Family Papers, Cornell University, Dept. of Manuscripts and University Archives.

Samuel A. Edgerly, New York City, diary, 1859–1860 [NYPL].

C. M. Ellis, Baltimore County, to Joseph Leidy, Philadelphia, 3–1861 [CPP].

William Eustis, Boston, to John Warren, Salem, 11-17-1773 [J. C. Warren Papers, MHS].

John D. Fisher, Hayward Plain, to J.C. Warren, 9-30-1829 [J. C. Warren Papers, MHS].

Nathaniel Freeman to Robert Andrews, Hanover, NH, 7-7-1832 [FC].

J[ohn D.] Godman, New York City, to J. C. Warren, 6-7-1828 [J. C. Warren Papers, MHS].

——— to J. C. Warren, Saratoga Springs, NY, 6-?-1828 [J. C. Warren Papers, MHS].

——— to J. C. Warren, Boston, 9-29-1828 [J. C. Warren Papers, MHS].

——— to J. C. Warren, 1-1-1829 [J. C. Warren Papers, MHS].

Edward Everett Hale to H. P. Bowditch, Roxbury, MA, 1-3-1896 [FC].

James Henderson, New York, to J. C. Warren, 12-23-1828 [J. C. Warren Papers, MHS].

Oliver Wendell Holmes (Boston) to W. W. Keen (Philadelphia), 1-15-1875 [NYAM].

W.E. Horner, Philadelphia, to J. C. Warren, Boston, 11-30-1824 [J. C. Warren Papers, MHS].

Alex[ander] E. Hosack, New York, to J. C. Warren, 1-20-1844 [J. C. Warren Papers, MHS].

John T. Kirkland, Cambridge, to John C. Warren, Boston, 3-28-1814 [J. C. Warren Papers, MHS].

Samuel H. Parkman, Boston, to J. C. Warren, New York, 10-1-1843, 12-12-[1848?] [J. C. Warren Papers, MHS].

Police Court, 3d Dist., New York County, 10-12-1887 to 2-1-1888 (roll #30); Magistrate's Court Docket Book, 3d Dist. [New York City Municipal Archives].

John Revere, New York, to J. C. Warren, 11-6-1827, 12-14-1827, 3-6-1828 [J. C. Warren Papers, MHS].

Jerome Van Crowninshield Smith, Boston, to J. C. Warren, 1-31-1825, 5-16-1825 [J. C. Warren Papers, MHS].

University of Pennsylvania Medical Department, Department of Anatomy, Accounts of the Anatomical Chair, 10-1-1839 to 6-6-1853 (in the handwriting of W. E. Horner up to 2-1-1853 and unidentified hand to 6-6-1853) [CPP].

John Warren and Aaron Dexter, "Memorial & Petition for the Removal of Med. Lect. to Boston," 2-20-1810 [J. C. Warren Papers, MHS].

J. C. Warren journals, 1838–1846 [J. C. Warren Papers, MHS].

——— to Delavan?, 6-25-1842 [J. C. Warren Papers, MHS].

——— to J.M. Warren, 7-14-1842 [J. C. Warren Papers, MHS].

Cyrus Weeks, New York, to J. C. Warren, 1-24-1837, 10-5-1848 [J. C. Warren Papers, MHS].

——— [C.W.], New York, to J. C. Warren, Boston, 10-15-1843 [J. C. Warren Papers, MHS].

N. P. Wiley to I. B. Van Schaick, New York, 1-14-1820? [NYAM].

Jeffries Wyman, Richmond, VA, to Elizabeth A. Wyman, Boston, 1-31-1846 [FC].

Primary Works

D. H. Agnew, *Lecture Introductory to the One Hundred and Fifth Course of Instruction in the Medical Department of the University of Pennsylvania, delivered Monday, October 10, 1870* (Philadelphia, 1870) [CPP].

William A. Alcott, *The House I Live In . . . Pt. 1: the Human Frame* (Boston, 1834).

———, *The House I Live In . . .* (2d ed., Boston, 1836).

———, "The Science of Human Life," *The Moral Reformer and Teacher of the Human Condition* 2.1 (Boston, 1–1836): 5–8.

———, *The House I Live In . . . (Lu Kuiy' Khan' dha 'aim' e 'a Kron' ca)*, trans. Stella Kneeland Bennett (1st Burm. ed., Tavoy-Rangoon, Burma, 1843; 3d Burm. ed., Rangoon, 1875; 4th Burm. ed., Rangoon, 1884).

———, *The Laws of Health; or the Sequel to "The House I Live In"* (Boston, 1857).

———, *Forty Years in the Wilderness of Pills and Powders; or, the Cogitations and Confessions of an Aged Physician* (Boston, 1859).

American Humane Association, *Report of the American Humane Association on Vivisection and Dissection in Schools* (Chicago, 1895).

[Anonymous], *Barnyard Rhymes; showing what opinions the turkey, the cock, the goose, and the duck entertain of allopathia, homeopathia, electro-galvanism and the animalcule doctrines* (New York, 1838) [NLM].

[Anonymous], *From a Dying Libertine to His Friend, Together with the Dying Words of a young Man* (n.p. [ca. 1790–1810]) [AAS].

[Anonymous], *The Gypsy Dream Book and Fortune Teller, with Napoleon's Oraculum* (New York: M.J. Ivers & Co., n.d. [ca. 1850]).

[Anonymous], "Influence of death," *The American Museum, or, Universal Magazine* 8 (1790): 227–29.

[Anonymous], *Life of the Notorious Kidnapper, George F. Alberti, by a member of the Philadelphia Bar (Authorized Edition)* (Philadelphia, 1851) [NYHS].

[Anonymous; "by the author of Cobweb Papers"], "Pen, Press, and Pencil," *Potter's American Monthly* 12 (1878): 350–51.

[Anonymous], rev. of Amariah Brigham, *Remarks on the Influence of Mental Cultivation and Mental Excitement upon Health* (2d ed., Boston, 1833), in *Annals of Phrenology* 2 (1835): 488, rpt. from *Edinburgh Phrenological Journal* 45 (1833?).

[Anonymous; "by the author of 'The Pastoral Life and Manufactures of the Ancients"], *The Wonders of Nature and Art; or, Truth Stranger than Fiction; Adapted to Interest and Instruct, to Enliven the Social and Beguile the Solitary* (New York, 1847).

Association for the Benefit of Colored Orphans, *Annual Reports* (New York, 1837–50).

Association of American Anatomists, "Extract from Proceedings of Eighth Session held at Philadelphia, Pa., Dec. 27 and 28, 1895," *Science*, n.s. 3.55 (1-17-1896) [HS].

Azel Backus, *An Inaugural Discourse, delivered in the Village of Clinton, December 3, 1812 by the Rev. Azel Backus, D.D., on the day of his Induction into the office of the President of Hamilton College* (Utica, 1812).

[George Bancroft, rev.], "*Address to the Community, on the Necessity of Legalizing the Study of Anatomy* . . . , 1829," *North American Review* 70 (1–1831): 64–73.

W[ooster] Beach, *The American Practice of Medicine.* . . . (New York, 1836; many editions thereafter).

———, *A Treatise on Anatomy, Physiology, and Health, designed for students, schools, and popular use* (New York: Published by the author, at the Anatomical Museum, corner of Bowery and Division St., 1847) [AAS].

———, *The Improved System of Midwifery.* . . . (New York, 1847).

Thomas Beddoes, *Hygëia: or Essays Moral and Medical, on the Causes Affecting the Personal State of our Middling and Affluent Classes* (London, 1802–3).

Gunning S. Bedford, *A General Introductory Lecture to a Course of Lectures on Popular Anatomy and Physiology, delivered at the Hall of the Stuyvesant Institute, Wednesday, Nov. 26* ([New York,] 1840).

Catharine Beecher, *A Treatise on Domestic Economy, for the use of Young Ladies at Home* (1st ed., Boston, 1841; rev. 2d ed., Boston, 1843; 3d ed., New York, 1856).

———, *Physiology and Calisthenics, for Schools and Families* (New York, 1871; copyright 1856).

————, and H.B. Stowe, *American Woman's Home, or Principles of Domestic Science: Being a guide to the formation and maintenance of economical, healthful, beautiful and Christian homes* [New York, 1869] (Hartford, CT: Stowe-Day Foundation, 1975).

Ezekiel Porter Belden, *New-York: Past, Present and Future* (New York, 1849).

D. M. Bennett, *The World's Sages, Thinkers, and Reformers* (New York, 1876).

Diary of William Bentley, D.D., pastor of the East Church, Salem, Massachusetts (Gloucester, MA: Peter Smith, 1962), 4 vols.

Jacob Bigelow, *Remarks on the Dangers and Duties of Sepulture: or, Security for the Living, with Respect and Repose for the Dead* (Boston, 1823).

The Biographical History of Westchester County (Chicago, 1899).

Isabella Lucy Bird, *The Englishwoman in America* [1856] (Madison, WI: University of Wisconsin Press, 1966).

Elizabeth Blackwell, *Counsel to Parents on the Moral Education of Their Children* (New York, 1883).

————, *Pioneer Work in Opening the Medical Profession to Women* [London, 1895] (New York: Schocken, 1977).

Andrew Boardman, *An Essay on the Means of Improving Medical Education and Elevating Medical Character* (Philadelphia, 1840) ["from the Eclectic Journal of Medicine, for April, 1840"].

Robert Boyle, *Disquisition About the Final Causes of Natural Things* (London, 1688).

Joseph Brevitt, *The History of Anatomy from Hippocrates who lived 400 years before Christ, together with the discoveries and improvements of succeeding Anatomists in the regular succession of time in which they lived to the present time* (Baltimore, 1794).

Henry Arthur Bright, *Happy Country This America: The Travel Diary of Henry Arthur Bright* [1852], ed. Anne Henry Ehrenpreis (Columbus, OH: Ohio University Press, 1978).

H. Brooke, compil., *Tragedies on the Land . . .* (Philadelphia, 1847).

John Brooks, *A Discourse Delivered Before the Humane Society of the Commonwealth of Massachusetts, 9th June, 1795* (Boston, 1795).

J. Ross Browne, *Confessions of a Quack, or the Autobiography of a Modern Æsculapian* (Louisville, 1841).

James Silk Buckingham, *America, Historical, Statistic and Descriptive* (London, 1841), 2 vols.

William Burke, *A Popular Compendium of Anatomy; Or A concise and clear description of the human body and physiology, or natural history, the various actions and funcitons of its different organs, and Containing also an article on suspended animation, with the proper means to be used for drowned persons* (London, 1805).

Charles Caldwell, *Thoughts on the Impolicy of Multiplying Schools of Medicine* (Lexington, 1834).

Joseph Carson, *A History of the Medical Department of the University of Pennsylvania, from its Foundation in 1765, with Sketches of the Lives of Deceased Professors* (Philadelphia, 1869).

Catalogue. Dr. Baskette's Gallery of Anatomy (Chicago, n.d. [ca. 1875]) [collection of William Helfand].

Catalogue of the Grand Anatomical Museum, or National Academy of Natural, Anatomical and Pathological Science (New York, 1854).

Catalogue of the New York Anatomical Gallery, and Academy of Natural, Medical and Moral Science (New York, 1847; 1850).

Catalogue of the Parisian Gallery of Anatomy and Medical Science (Boston, 1869) [FC].

D. W. Cathell, *The Physician Himself and What He Should Add to the Strictly Scientific* (Baltimore, 1882).

———, *The Physician Himself and What He Should Add to His Scientific Acquirements in Order to Secure Success* (4th ed., Baltimore, 1885).

[Walter Channing?], *Remarks on the Employment of Females as Practitioners in Midwifery* (Boston, 1820).

Heber Chase, *The Medical Student's Guide; Being a Compendious View of the Collegiate and Clinical Medical Schools, the Courses of Private Lectures, the Hospitals and the Almshouses, and Other Institutions Which Contribute Directly or Indirectly to the Great Medical School of Philadelphia* (Philadelphia, 1842) [CPP].

S. W. Clark, *From the Ridiculous to the Sublime* (Chicago, 1875).

Cleave's Biographical Cyclopædia of Homœopathic Physicians and Surgeons (Philadelphia, 1873).

V[air] Clirehugh, *A Treatise on the Anatomy and Physiology of the Skin and Hair, as Applied to the Causes, Treatment and Prevention of Baldness and Grey Hair; the Removal of Scurf, Dandriff . . .* (New York, n.d., [ca. 1838–42]) [AAS].

John Gorham Coffin, *A Discourse on Medical Education and on the Medical Profession* (Boston, 1822).

Andrew Combe, *Principles of Physiology Applied to the Preservation of Health and to the Improvement of Physical and Mental Education* (New York, 1836).

George Combe, *The Constitution of Man Considered in Relation to External Objects* (Edinburgh, 1828).

Anthony Comstock, *Frauds Exposed, or How the People are Deceived and Robbed, and Youth Corrupted* (New York, 1880).

Joseph Comstock, "On the Study of Living Anatomy," *Boston Medical and Surgical Journal* 49 (1-18-1854): 500–2.

F. A. Conkling, *Remarks of Mr. F. A. Conkling on the Bill for the Promotion of Medical Science, in Assembly, February 28, 1854* (Albany, NY, 1854).

C. B. Coventry, *Address to the Graduates of the Medical Institution of Geneva College, delivered January 25th, 1842* (Utica, 1842).

Robert Crowell, *Interment of the Dead, a Dictate of Natural Affection . . .* (Andover, MA, 1818) [NYHS]

John McNabb Currier, *Song of the Hubbardton Raid* (Castleton, VT, 1880).

[J.] Calvin Cutter, *The Physiological Family Physician, designed for Families and Individuals* (West Brookfield, MA, 1845).

——— *First Book on Anatomy and Physiology* (Boston, 1847).

———, *Anatomy and Physiology: Designed for Academies and Families* (Boston, 1847; 4th stereotype ed., Boston 1847; 15th ed., Boston 1848).

———, *A Treatise on Anatomy, Physiology and Hygiene: Designed for Colleges, Academies, and Families* (Boston, 1850) [CPP].

———, *Anatomy, Physiology, and Hygiene (in Sgau Karen)*, trans. and adapt. Mrs. J.G. Binney, from the rev. ed. (Rangoon, 1872).

Andrew Jackson Davis, *The Principles of Nature, Her Divine Revelations, and a Voice to Mankind* (35th ed. Boston, 1847).

——, *The Great Harmonia; Being a Philosophical Revelation of the Natural, Spiritual, and Celestial Universe* (Boston, 1850).

——, *The Harbinger of Health; Containing Medical Prescriptions for the Human Body and Mind* (New York, 1861; 19th ed., Rochester, NY, 1909).

——, *Events in the Life of a Seer: Being Memoranda of Authentic Facts in Magnetism, Clairvoyance, Spiritualism by Andrew Jackson Davis* (6th ed., Boston, 1868).

George E. de Schweinitz, "Reminiscences of a Prosector and Appreciation of Leidy's Work as an Anatomist," in *The Joseph Leidy Commemorative Meeting, held in Philadelphia, December 6, 1923* (n.p., n.d.).

Chester Dewey, *Introductory Lecture Delivered to the Medical Class of the Berkshire Medical Institution; August 5, 1847* (Pittsfield, MA, 1847).

Samuel Dickson, *The Principles of the Chrono-Thermal System, with an introduction and notes by William Turner* [1839] (13th ed., New York, 1850) [HS].

[Edward H. Dixon], "Scenes in a Medical Student's Life—Resurrectionizing," *The Scalpel* 7 (1855): 93–100.

——, "An M.D., or a Modern Doctor of Medicine; Pursuit of Practice under Difficulties," *The Scalpel* 10.3 (10–1858): 407–8.

Frederick Douglass, *Narrative of the Life of Frederick Douglass, An American Slave, Written by Himself* [1845], ed. Houston A. Baker (New York: Viking Penguin, 1986).

Daniel Drake, *An Introductory Lecture, On the Means of Promoting the Intellectual Improvement of the Students and Physicians of the Valley of the Mississippi, Delivered in the Medical Institute of Louisville, November 4th, 1844* (Louisville, 1844).

Francis S. Drake, *Dictionary of American Biography. . . .* (Boston, 1872).

John W. Draper, *University of New-York Medical Department: a Valedictory Lecture, Delivered by Professor Draper* (New York, 1842) [CPP].

——, *Petition of the Medical Faculty of the University of the City of New-York to the . . . Senate and Assembly of the State of New-York. . . .* (New York, 1853).

——, "An Appeal to the State of New York to Legalise the Dissection of the Dead, Being an Introductory Lecture, Delivered at the Opening of the Session of the Medical Department of the University of New York," *Nelson's American Lancet* 8 (Winter 1853–54): 105–12; 133–41.

——, *Human Physiology, Statistical and Dynamical; The Conditions and Course of the Life of Man* (New York, 1856; 2d ed., New York, 1858) [CPP].

——, *History of the Conflict Between Religion and Science* (New York, 1876).

Henry William Ducachet, *Tribute to the Memory of Jacob Dyckman, M.D., Late Health Commissioner of the City of New-York, &c., Being a Discourse Pronounced by His Friend, Henry William Ducachet, M.D., on Monday, January 6th, 1823. . . .* (New York, 1823) [HS].

Robley Dunglison, *The Medical Student; or, Aids to the Study of Medicine. . . .* (Philadelphia, 1837).

——, *An Introductory Lecture to the Course of Institutes of Medicine, &c. Delivered in Jefferson Medical College, November 1, 1841* (Philadelphia, 1841).

Henry Dunnel, "Annual Report of the Interments in the City and County of New York, showing their Age, Sex, Colour and Places of Nativity, for the year 1837," *American Journal of the Medical Sciences* 13 (1838): 242.

H. Milne Edwards, *Outlines of Anatomy and Physiology*, trans. J.F.W. Lane (Boston, 1841).

George Eliot, *Middlemarch* (London, 1871–72; rpt. London: Dent, 1959).

Samuel Hayes Elliot, *New England's Chattels: or, Life in the Northern Poor-house* (New York, 1858).

Ralph Waldo Emerson, "Historic Notes of Life and Letters in New England" [1880], *Lectures and Biographical Sketches* (Boston: Houghton Mifflin, 1904).

Paul F. Eve, "Introductory Lecture delivered in the Medical College of Georgia, November 5th, 1849," in W.H. Goodrich, *The History of the Medical Department of the University of Georgia* (Augusta, GA: University of Georgia Press, [1928]).

Marianne Finch, *An Englishwoman's Experience in America* (London, 1853; rpt. New York: Negro Universities Press, 1969).

Austin Flint, Sr., *The Reciprocal Duties and Obligations of the Medical Profession and the Public: A Public Introductory Lecture Delivered at Rush Medical College. . . .* (Chicago, 1844).

———, "The First Century of the Republic: Medical and Sanitary Progress," *Harper's New Monthly Magazine* 53 (6–1876): 70–84.

Edward Bliss Foote, *Medical Common Sense* (New York, 1859–60; rpt. 1864).

———, *Plain Home Talk* (New York, 1870).

———, *Sammy Tubbs, the Boy Doctor, and "Sponsie," the Troublesome Monkey* (New York, 1874–75), 5 vols.

———, *Divorce: A Review of the Subject from a Scientific Standpoint, in answer to Msgr. Capel, the Rev. Dr. Dix, the New-England Divorce Reform League and others who desire more stringent Divorce Laws* (New York, 1887).

———, *Dr. Foote's Replies to the Alphites, giving some cogent reasons for believing that Sexual Continence is not Conducive to Health* (New York, 1889) [FC].

Edward Bond Foote, *The Radical Remedy in Social Sciences; or Borning Better Babies through Regulating Reproduction by Controlling Contraception* (New York, 1886).

Orson Fowler, *Love and Parentage* (New York, 1851).

Samuel W[ard] Francis, *Memoir of the Life and Character of Prof. Valentine Mott. . . .* (New York, 1865.

———, *Biographical Sketches of Distinguished Living New York Physicians* (New York, 1867).

J. O. G., "Religio Medicorum," letter to *Boston Medical and Surgical Journal* (7-19-1854): 501–4.

Galen, *On Anatomical Procedures*, trans. Charles Singer (Oxford: Oxford University Press, 1956).

Marlin Gardner and Benjamin H. Aylworth, *The Domestic Physician and Family Assistant* (Cooperstown, NY, 1836).

[Charles Gibbs], *Mutiny and Murder; Confession of Charles Gibbs, a Native of Rhode Island, who, with Thomas J. Wansley, was doomed to be hung in New York on the 22nd of April last, for the murder of the Captain and Mate of the Brig Vineyard, on her passage from New-Orleans to Philadelphia, in November 1830. GIBBS confesses that within a few years he has participated in the murder of nearly 400 human beings!* (Providence, 1831), 24 [NYHS].

John Davidson Godman, *Contributions to Physiological and Pathological Anatomy; con-*

taining the Observations made at the Philadelphia Anatomical rooms during the session of 1824–25 (Philadelphia, 1825).

———, *Anatomy Taught by Analysis: A Lecture Introductory to the Course, Delivered in the Philadelphia Anatomical Rooms, Fifth Session, 1825–6* (Philadelphia, 1826).

———, *Introductory Lecture to the Course of Anatomy and Physiology, in Rutgers Medical College, New-York, Delivered, November 11, 1826* (New York, 1826).

———, *Introductory Lecture to the Course of Anatomy and Physiology, in Rutgers Medical College, New-York, Delivered on Friday, November 2, 1827* (New York, 1827).

S. G. Goodrich, *Peter Parley's Farewell* (Boston, 1839) [AAS].

Mary Gove, "Lectures to Ladies on Anatomy and Physiology," *Graham's Journal* 2.21 (1838): 325–30; 2.22 (10-28-1838): 338–42.

Sylvester Graham, *A Lecture on Epidemic Diseases Generally, and Particularly the Spasmodic Cholera . . . With an Appendix, Containing Several Testimonials, and a Review of Beaumont's Experiments on the Gastric Juice* (rev. ed., Boston, 1838).

Great Britain, Parliament, House of Commons, *Report from the Select Committee on Anatomy* [Session 29 January to 28 July 1828, v. 7].

Angelina Grimké, *Appeal to the Christian Women of the South* (New York, 1836).

Samuel Hahnemann, *Organon of Homœopathic Medicine* [1810] (1st Amer. ed. from Brit. trans. of 4th German ed., Allentown, PA, 1836).

———, *Organon of Homœopathic Medicine* (3d Amer. ed., New York, 1849).

———, *The Chronic Diseases, Their Peculiar Nature and Their Homœopathic Cure* [1828; 2d enlarged German ed., 1835], ed. Louis H. Tafel, (Philadelphia, 1904).

———, *Lesser Writings of Samuel Hahnemann*, coll. and trans. R.E. Dudgeon (New York, 1852).

F. Hallock, *Dr. Hallock & Co.'s Museum of Anatomy and Medical Institute* (Boston [ca. 1870?]) [FC].

F[rank] H. Hamilton, *Introductory Address, and Catalogue of Students attending the Annual Course of Lectures on Anatomy and Surgery* (Auburn, NY, 1837).

———, *Address to the Graduates in Medicine at the University of Buffalo, April 27, 1853* (Buffalo, 1853).

William A. Hammond, *Cerebral Hyperaemia the Result of Mental Strain or Emotional Disturbance* (New York, 1878).

———, *On Certain Conditions of Nervous Derangement, Somnambulism* (New York, 1881).

———, *Sexual Impotence in the Male and Female* (Detroit, 1887).

Edward M. Hartwell, *The Study of Human Anatomy, Historically and Legally Considered: A Paper Read at the Meeting of the American Social Science Association, September 9, 1880* (Boston, 1881), rpt. from *Journal of Social Science.*

Charles Haswell, *Reminiscences of New York by an Octogenarian (1816 to 1860)* (New York, 1896).

Hermann von Helmholtz, "On the Relation of Natural Science to General Science, Academical Discourse Delivered at Heidelberg, November 22, 1862," trans. H.W. Eve, in *Popular Lectures on Scientific Subjects* (London, 1873).

W. T. Helmuth, *Surgery and its Adaptation into Homeopathic Practice* (Philadelphia, 1855).

Thomas Hersey, *The Midwife's Practical Directory; or, the Woman's Confidential Friend* (2d ed., Columbus, OH, 1838).

Edward Hitchcock and Edward Hitchcock, Jr., *Elementary Anatomy and Physiology, for Colleges, Academies, and other schools* (rev. ed., New York, 1860).

H. Lenox Hodge, *Anatomical Rooms: Plan for their Construction, Ventilation, and Hygienic Management* (Richmond, 1875); rpt. from *Virginia Medical Monthly* (10–1875).

William H. Holcombe, *How I Became a Homoeopath* (Philadelphia, 1866) [AAS].

F. C. Hollick, *An Inquiry into the Rights, Duties, and Destinies, of the Different Varieties of the Human Race, with a view to a proper consideration of the subjects of slavery, abolition, amalgamation, and aboriginal rights* (New York, 1843).

—————, *The Origin of Life: A Popular Treatise on the Philosophy and Physiology of Reproduction, in Plants and Animals, including The Details of Human Generation, with a full description of the Male and Female Organs* (10th stereotype ed.; original ed., New York, 1845).

—————, *Neuropathy; or the true principles of the art of healing the sick* (Philadelphia, 1847) [AAS].

—————, *Practical Facts in the Medical Application of Galvanism and Electro-Magnetism* (New York, 1848) [AAS].

—————, *Outlines of Anatomy and Physiology for Popular Use* (Philadelphia, 1847) [AAS].

—————, *The Marriage Guide, or Natural History of Generation; a Private Instructor for Married Persons and Those About to Marry, both Male and Female; in every thing concerning the physiology and relations of the sexual system and the production or prevention of off spring—including all the new discoveries, never before given in the English language* (New York, 1850; facs. rpt. New York: Arno Press, 1974).

—————, *A Popular Treatise on Venereal Diseases, in All Their Forms* (New York, 1852) [AAS].

—————, *The American Class-Book of Anatomy and Physiology and their application to the preservation of health* (New York, 1853) [AAS].

————— *The Male Generative Organs in Health and Disease, from Infancy to Old Age. . . .* (New York, 1853).

Edmund W. Holmes, "The Dissecting Room," *Transactions of the Pan-American Medical Congress* 2 (1893): 1152–54.

Oliver Wendell Holmes, Sr., *Elsie Venner* (Boston, 1861).

—————, *Medical Essays, 1842–1882* (Cambridge, MA, 1891).

George Jacob Holyoake, *Sixty Years of an Agitator's Life* (London, 1892), 2 vols.

Worthington Hooker, *Physicians and Patients* (New York, 1849).

—————, *Lessons From the History of Medical Delusions* (New York, 1850).

Francis Hopkinson, *An Oration, Which Might Have Been Delivered to the Students in Anatomy of the Late Rupture Between the Two Schools in this City* (Philadelphia, 1789) [AAS].

The Confession of Adam Horn (Baltimore, 1843) [Historical Society of Pennsylvania].

Harriot K. Hunt, *Glances and Glimpses; or Fifty Years Social, including Twenty Years Professional Life* (Boston, 1856).

William Hunter [1718–83], *Two Introductory Lectures. . . . to his Last Course of Anatomical Lectures . . .* (London, 1784) [CPP].

J[edediah] Vincent Huntington, *Rosemary, or Life and Death* (New York, 1860).

Thomas Jefferson, *The Writings of Thomas Jefferson*, ed. H.A. Washington (Washington, DC: U.S. Congress, 1853–54).

———, *The Writings of Thomas Jefferson*, ed. Paul Leicester Ford (New York: Putnam & Sons, 1892–99).

B. F. Joslin, *Principles of Homœopathy* (New York, 1850).

[L. J.] Kahn, *Hand Book and Descriptive Catalogue of Dr. Kahn's Museum of Anatomy and Natural Science* (New York, n.d. [ca. 1869–88]) [collection of William Helfand].

———, *Value of the Microscope: Examinations of the Urine and Chronic Diseases* (New York, 1876) [NLM].

——— and [L.J.?] Jordan, *Nervous Exhaustion: A Series of Lectures on the Diseases of the Genito-Urinary Organs* (New York, 1897) [HS].

———, *Descriptive Catalogue of Dr. Kahn's Museum of Anatomy and Medical Science* (New York: Isaac Goldmann Co., Printers, n.d. [ca. 1900–5]) [collection of William Helfand].

Elizabeth Keckley, *Behind the Scenes, or, Thirty Years a Slave, and Four Years in the White House* (New York, 1868).

W. W. Keen, *A Sketch of the Early History of Practical Anatomy: The Introductory Address to the Course of Lectures on Anatomy at the Philadelphia School of Anatomy, Tuesday, October 11, 1870* (Philadelphia, 1870).

———, *A Sketch of the Early History of Practical Anatomy: The Introductory Address to the Course of Lectures on Anatomy at the Philadelphia School of Anatomy, Tuesday, October 6, 1874* (Philadelphia, 1874).

———, *History of the Philadelphia School of Anatomy* (Philadelphia, 1875).

Dan King, *Quackery Unmasked: or a Consideration of the Most Prominent Empirical Schemes of the Present Time* (Boston, 1858) [AAS].

Charles Kreutzberg, *Guide to the European, Anatomical, Pathological and Ethnological Museum of Professor Charles Kreutzberg* (Philadelphia, 1876) [Atwater Kent Museum, Philadelphia.]

T[homas] S[cott] Lambert, *Pictorial Anatomy* (Portland, ME, 1851).

———, *Hygienic Physiology* (Portland, ME and New York, 1852).

———, *Human Anatomy, Physiology and Hygiene* (Hartford, CT, 1854) [CPP].

Charles Lawrence, *History of the Philadelphia Almshouse and Hospitals from the Beginning of the Eighteenth to the Ending of the Nineteenth Century. . . .* (Philadelphia, 1905).

William Lawrence, *Lectures on the Physiology, Zoology and the Natural History of Man, delivered at the Royal College of Surgeons* (Salem, MA, 1828).

Andrew J. Leavitt, *The Body Snatchers: A Negro Sketch in Two Scenes* (New York, 1879).

Joseph Leidy, *Lecture Introductory to the Course on Anatomy in the University of Pennsylvania for the Session 1858–59* (Philadelphia, 1859).

———, *Introductory Lecture to the Course on Anatomy, Delivered in the University of Pennsylvania, October 11th, 1859* (Philadelphia, 1859) [CPP].

A. Le Pileur, *Wonders of the Human Body* (New York, 1870) [CPP].

George Lippard, *The Quaker City, or the Monks of Monk Hall* (1845; rpt. Philadelphia: Leary, Stuart, n.d. [ca. 1876]).

———, *The Quaker City*, ed. and intro. David S. Reynolds (Amherst: University of Massachusetts Press, 1995).

——, *The Nazarene; or, the Last of the Washingtons, a Revelation of Philadelphia, New York, and Washington, in the Year 1844* (Philadelphia, 1846).

——, *The Monk of Wissahikon* (Wissahikon, PA, 1848).

——, *The Empire City; or, New York By Night and Day, Its Aristocracy and Its Dollars* [1850] (Philadelphia, 1864).

——, *New York: Its Upper Ten and Lower Million* (Cincinnati, 1853).

Robert D. Lyons, *A Handbook of Hospital Practice*. . . . (New York, 1860).

James M'Clintock, *Introductory Lecture to the Course on Anatomy and Physiology, in the Vermont Academy of Medicine, delivered April 7, 1841* (Castleton, VT, 1841).

W. J. McKnight, *Brookville's Pioneer Resurrection, or "Who Skinned the Nigger"* (n.p., n.d.), rpt. from *Jeffersonian Democrat* (1–1897).

——, *The Pioneer Doctor: "Who Skinned the Nigger" or the Origin and Enactment of Pennsylvania's State Anatomical Law* (n.p., n.d.), rpt. from *Brookville Republican* (3-1-1915).

McLoughlin Brothers, *Simple Addition by a Little Nigger* (New York, 1874–75?) [AAS].

——, *Nine Niggers More* (New York, 1874?) [AAS].

——, *Simple Addition and Nursery Jingles* (New York, 1875?) [AAS].

[Nathaniel S. Magoon], *Thomson's Almanac for the Year 1844* (Boston, n.d. [1843]).

Harriet Martineau, *Retrospect of Western Travel* (London, 1838; rpt. New York: Haskell House, 1969), 3 vols.

Andrew Marvell, "A Dialogue Between the Soul and Body" (1681), in M.E. Abrams et al. (ed.), *The Norton Anthology of English Literature* (New York: Norton, 1968), 1:985–86.

Massachusetts General Court, House of Representatives, Select Committee (HR doc. #4), *Report of the Select Committee of the House of Representatives on so much of the Governor's Speech, at the June Session, 1830, as related to Legalizing the Study of Anatomy* (Boston, 1831).

——, (HR doc. #300), *Report of Hearings Before the Joint Standing Committee on Public Charitable Institutions: under the Order for Said Committee to Investigate the Mismanagement, Control and Condition of the Public Charitable Institutions, and the Special Charges of the Mismanagement of the State Almshouse at Tewksbury* (Boston, 1883), 2 vols. [NLM].

Massachusetts Medical Society, *Proceedings of the Counsellors* [J. C. Warren, John Dixwell, George Hayward] (Boston, 1826) [MHS].

——, *Address to the Community, on the Necessity of Legalizing the Study of Anatomy* (Boston, 1829).

Cotton Mather, *Addresses to Old Men* (Boston, 1690).

Medical Society of Maine, *Address to the Community on the Necessity of Legalizing the Study of Anatomy* (Brunswick, ME, 1832) [MHS].

John Morgan, *A Discourse upon the institution of Medical Schools in America; Delivered at a Public Anniversary Commencement, held in the College of Philadelphia May 30 and 31, 1765. With a Preface Containing, amongst other things, the Author's Apology For attempting to introduce the regular mode of practising Physic in Philadelphia* (Philadelphia, 1765).

Valentine Mott, *Reminiscences of Medical Teaching and Teachers in New York: An Address Introductory to a Course of Lectures at the College of Physicians and Surgeons, New York, Session of 1850–51* (New York, 1850).

————, *Catalogue of the Surgical and Pathological Museum of Valentine Mott, M.D., . . . and of his son Alexander B. Mott. . . .* (New York, 1858) [CPP].

————, *Address of Valentine Mott, M.D., LL.D., Emeritus Professor of Surgery, Etc., Etc., Before the Graduates of 1860 of the University Medical College of New York* (New York, 1860).

Fr. Moulton, *The Compleat Bone-Setter, . . . the Method of Curing Broken Bones and Strains and Dislocated Joynts, together with Ruptures, commonly called Broken Bel-lyes. . . . Written originally by frier Moulton. . . . Revised, Englished, and Enlarged by R[obert] Turner* (2d ed., n.p., 1665).

George Henry Napheys, *The Transmission of Life: Counsels on the Nature and Hygiene of the Masculine Functions* (New York, 1872).

National Cyclopædia of American Biography (New York, 1893).

New York City, Board of Aldermen, *Report on Deaths in the City of New-York,* #63, 2-10-1845: 826 [NYMA].

————, Board of Aldermen, *Documents of the Board of Aldermen of the City of New York,* 5–1847 to 5–1848 [NYMA].

————, Board of Assistant Aldermen, *Annual Report of the City Inspector of the Number of Deaths and Interments in the City and County of New York, for the Year 1847,* #21, 3-27-1848: 94 [NYMA].

The New-York Medical Almanac and Repository of Useful Science and Amusement, for the year 1824 (New York, 1824).

New York Museum of Anatomy, *A Visit to the New York Museum of Anatomy* (New York, n.d. [1867?]) [NYHS].

New York State, Assembly, *Report of the minority of the select committee on the petition of John Thompson and others, relative to the Thompsonian practice of physic, etc,* Document 235, 3-28-1828.

New York State, Education Department, *Fifteenth Annual Report* (Albany, 1919).

Elisha North, *Outlines of the Science of Life* (New York, 1829).

Robert Dale Owen, *Moral Physiology; or, A Brief and Plain Treatise on the Population Question* (New York, 1831).

P&S Faculty, *Response to the Report of the Regents* [2-18-1826] (New York, 1826): 150–51 [HS].

William Paley, *Natural Theology; or Evidence of the Existence and Attributes of the Deity, Collected from the Appearance of Nature* (London, 1802).

Usher Parsons, *The Importance of the Sciences of Anatomy and Physiology as a Branch of General Education; being an Introduction to a Course of Lectures to the upper classes of Brown University* (Cambridge, 1826) [MHS].

Granville Sharp Pattison, *Syllabus of a Popular Course of Lectures on General Anatomy and Physiology, as Illustrative of the Natural History of Man* (Philadelphia, 1819).

E. R. Peaslee, *The Moral Character of the Medical Profession: An Address introductory . . . in the New York Medical College, Session of 1852–53* (New York, 1852).

Edgar Allan Poe, "The Magnetizer; or, Ready for Any Body," *Broadway Journal* (9-6-1845): 133–34.

————, "The Philosophy of Composition" (n.p., 1846).

Ann Preston, *Valedictory Address to the Graduating Class of the Female Medical College of Pennsylvania, for the Session of 1857–58* (Philadelphia, 1858) [CPP].

James Cowles Prichard, *Researches in the Physical History of Mankind* (2d ed., London, 1826), 2 vols.

Samuel P. Putnam, *Four Hundred Years of Freethought* (New York, 1894).

Rackstrow's Museum, *A Descriptive Catalogue . . . of Rackstrow's Museum: Consisting of a large and very valuable Collection of most curious Anatomical Figures and Real Preparations; Also Figures Resembling Life; with a Capital Collection of Natural and Artificial Curiosities* (London, 1794) [NYHS].

Alexander Ramsay, *Prospectus of Fifteen Lectures on the Animal and Intellectual Economy of Man: Adapted to the Purposes of the Medical Practitioner, the Speculative Philosopher, the Parent, and the Youth, as the medium of that knowledge of God and ourselves, which seems connected with health, piety, and religion* (New York, 1816).

———, *Announcement and Prospectus of Lectures of Alexander Ramsay* (New York, 1817) [NYAM].

———, *Farewell Discourse* (Montreal, 1818, 1820?) [NYAM].

———, *Address and Anatomical Prospectus* (Concord, 1819).

David Meredith Reese, *Humbugs of New-York: Being a Remonstrance Against Popular Delusion; Whether in Science, Philosophy, or Religion* (New York, 1838).

Report of a Committee of the Regents of the University, Appointed to Visit the College of Physicians and Surgeons in the City of New-York, Made to the Regents, January 12, 1826 (Albany, 1826).

Sumner Rhoades, *Address Introductory to the Course of Instruction in the Anatomical Rooms of Geneva Medical College* (Geneva, NY, 1841).

John B. Roberts, "The Remedy for the Annual Scarcity of Dissecting Material" [unattributed magazine clipping, 1890] [CPP].

——— "Some Defects in Anatomical Teaching in the Medical Schools of the United States," *Transactions of the First Pan-American Medical Congress Held in the City of Washington, D.C., U.S.A., September 5, 6, 7, and 8, A.D. 1893* (Washington, DC, 1895).

John Hovey Robinson, *Marietta or the Two Students: A Tale of the Dissecting Room and Body Snatching* (Boston, 1846).

———, *Silver-Knife, or the Hunter of the Rocky Mountains; A Romance of the Wild West* (Boston, 1850).

William Rowley, *On the Absolute Necessity of Encouraging, instead of Preventing and Embarrassing, the Study of Anatomy; with a Plan to Prevent Violating the Dormitories of the Defunct. Addressed to the Legislature of Great Britain, and sent to every Honourable Member*, in *A Treatise on the Causes and Cure of Swelled Legs . . . to which is added, A Tract on the absolute Necessity of Encouraging the Study of Anatomy, &c to supply the Army, Navy, and Country, with skilful Physicians and Surgeons, &c. Addressed to the Legislature of Great Britain* (London, 1796) [CPP, HS].

David Ruggles, *The "Extinguisher" Extinguished! or David M. Reese, M.D. "Used Up"* (New York, 1834).

W. S. W. Ruschenberger, *Elements of Anatomy and Physiology: Prepared for the Use of Schools and Colleges . . . from the text of Milne Edwards and Achille Comte* (Philadelphia, 1847).

John F. Sanford, *Introductory Lecture, Delivered in the College of Physicians and Surgeons of the Upper Mississippi, Session of 1849–50* (Davenport, MS, 1849).

M. J. Scarlett, *A Valedictory Address . . . Before the Graduating Class of the Female Medical College of Philadelphia, March 16, 1867* (Philadelphia, 1867) [CPP].

Samuel Seabury III, *Moneygripe's Apprentice: The Personal Narrative of Samuel Seabury III*, ed. Robert Bruce Mullin (New Haven: Yale University Press, 1989).

Henry Hall Sherwood, *New or Electric Symptoms of Chronic Diseases, or Chronic Tuber-cula of the Organs and Limbs . . . and Their Natural or Electric Remedies* (Cincinnati, 1836).

————, *Electro-Galvanic Symptoms, and Electro-Magnetic Remedies, in Chronic Diseases of the Class Hypertrophy, or Chronic Enlargements of the Organs and Limbs, including All Forms of Scrofula, with Illustrative Diagrams and Cases* (3d rev. ed., New York, 1837).

————, "Rpt. . . . on the memorial of Henry Hall Sherwood . . . claiming . . . new and important discoveries in magnetism generally and more particularly in the magnetism of the earth and representing that he is the inventor of . . . the geometer, whereby it is practicable and easy, . . . to determine, merely by the dip of the needle, the latitude and longitude of any place . . . ," *U.S. 25th Cong. 2d Sess. Committee of Naval Affairs* (Washington, DC, 1838) [American Philosophical Society, 996].

————, *Motive Power of Organic Life, and Magnetic Phenomena of Terrestrial and Plane-tary Motions, with the Application of the Ever-Active and All-Pervading Agency of Magnetism, to the Nature, Symptoms, and Treatment of Chronic Diseases* (New York, 1841).

————, *The Motive Power of the Human System, with the Symptoms and Treatment of Chronic Disease* (New York, 1841) [many eds., cont. by Wm. Larned, e.g., *Motive Power of the Human System, with the Duodynamic Symptoms and Treatment of Chronic Diseases. Rev. by H.H. Sherwood's Successor, William Larned* (New York, 1850)].

————, *The Astro-Magnetic Almanac for 1843* (New York, n.d. [1842]).

————, *Manual for Magnetizing, with the Rotary and Vibrating Magnetic Machine, in the Duodynamic Treatment of Diseases* (6th ed., New York, 1845) [11 eds. by 1848].

James Marion Sims, *The Story of My Life* (New York, 1884).

Nelson Sizer, *Forty Years in Phrenology* (New York, 1891).

Adam Smith, *Theory of Moral Sentiment* (London, 1759).

Rev. Gibson Smith [and Andrew Jackson Davis], *Lectures on Clairmativeness: or, Human Magnetism, with an Appendix* (New York, 1845).

Jerome Van Crowninshield Smith, *Mind and Matter; or, familiar conversations on the body and soul* (Boston, 1833).

————, *The Class Book of Anatomy, explanatory of the first principles of Human Organization, as the basis of Physical Education, Designed for Schools* (Boston, 1834).

————, *Animal Mechanism: The Eye* (Scientific Tracts, 1.5) (Boston, n.d. [1834?]).

————, *The Class Book of Anatomy, explanatory of the first principles of Human Organization, as the basis of Physical Education, Designed for Schools* (2d ed., Boston, 1836).

Samuel Stanhope Smith, *An Essay on the Causes of the Variety of Complexion and Figure in the Human Species* [New Brunswick, NJ, 1810], rpt. ed. Winthrop Jordan (Cambridge: Belknap Press of Harvard University Press, 1965).

[Thomas Southwood Smith], "Use of the Dead to the Living," *Westminster Review* 2 (1824): 59–97.

————, *On the Importance of the Study of Anatomy, from the Westminster Review, with some additional remarks* (Boston, 1825) [CPP].

————, *Uses of the Dead to the Living: From the Westminster Review; An Appeal to the Public and to the Legislature, on the necessity of affording Dead Bodies to the Schools of Anatomy, by Legislative Enactment* (Albany, NY, 1827).

William Thayer Smith, *Elementary Physiology and Hygiene: The Human Body and Its Health, a Text-book for Schools, Having Special Reference to the Effects of Stimulants and Narcotics on the Human System* (New York, 1884).

Thomas S. Sozinsky, "Grave-robbing and Dissection," *Penn Monthly* 10 (1879): 206–17.

G. D. Spencer, *A Poem on the Hubbardton Raid, read in the Congregationalist Church Hubbardton, May 12, 1880 . . . in reply to poem of J.M. Currier, M.D.* (Rutland, VT, 1880) [NYHS].

Sarah Hackett Stevenson, *The Physiology of Woman* (2d. ed., Chicago, 1881).

Mrs. Stowell, *To the Patrons of the Arts: Messrs. Stowell and Bradley Respectfully Inform the Ladies and Gentlemen of Salem and its Vicinity, that They Have Opened for a Short Time an Elegant Museum* (Salem, 1817) [AAS].

William Graham Sumner, *What Social Classes Owe to Each Other* [1883] (Caldwell, ID: Caxton Printers, 1995).

Waterman Sweet, *An essay on the science of bone setting . . . By Waterman Sweet, natural anatomist and bone setter. In which the author undertakes to prove, that surgery and anatomy are intuitive sciences, and which can be understood, only by those who have a talent for the profession, and are endowed by nature with the sufficient ability to discharge the duties of one of the most complicated sciences known to man* (Providence, RI, 1829).

————, *Views of Anatomy and the Practice of Natural Bonesetting by a mechanical process different from all book knowledge* (Schenectady, 1844) [HS].

The Narrative of Whiting Sweeting, Who was executed at Albany, the 26th of August, 1792 (Albany, 1794) [Brown University Library].

Mrs. Jane Taylor, *Primary Lessons in Physiology: for Children* [copyright, 1839] (rev. ed. New York, 1848) [AAS].

————, *Wouldst Know Thyself, the Outlines of Human Physiology* (New York, n.d. [ca. 1858]) [AAS].

Samuel Thomson, *Address to the People of the United States* (n.p. [Boston?], 1817).

————, *The Secrets of the Noted Empyric Samuel Thompson, Comprehending the Theory of Disease and Mode of Practice* (n.p., 1818).

————, *An Earnest Appeal to the Public, Showing the Misery Caused by the Fashionable Mode of Practice of the Doctors at the Present Day* (n.p., 1824)

————, *Learned Quackery Exposed* (Boston, 1824).

————, *Learned Quackery Exposed; or Theory According to Art, as Exemplified in the Practice of the Fashionable Doctors of the Present Day* (Boston, 1836)

R. B. Todd and W. Bowman, *Physiological Anatomy and Physiology of Man* (Philadelphia, 1850–57).

Zechariah Touchstone [Rev. Thomas Walter], *The Little-Compton Scourge; or, The Anti-Courant* (Boston, 1721).

Roger S. Tracy, *The Essentials of Anatomy, Physiology, and Hygiene: A Text-Book for Schools and Academies* (New York, 1887).

Russell Thacher Trall, *Sexual Physiology: A Scientific and Popular Exposition of the Fundamental Problems in Sociology* (New York, 1866).

Mark Twain and Charles Dudley Warner, *The Gilded Age: A Tale of To-day* (New York, 1873).

University of Iowa, Homeopathic Medical Department, *Announcement of the Homeopathic Medical Department of the State University of Iowa* (Iowa City, 1877).

University of New-York, Medical Department, *Annual Announcement of Lectures, Session of 1841–42* (New York, 1841).

University of Pennsylvania, Medical Faculty Papers, General Archives, "Communication from the Medical Faculty to the Trustees on Introducing the Dissections into the Common Course of Study for Graduates in Medicine, 1824," in Simon Baatz, ed., "'A Very Diffused Disposition': Dissecting Schools in Philadelphia, 1823–1825," *Pennsylvania Magazine of History and Biography* 108 (1984): 203–17.

L. Valentine, *The Funny Little Darkies* (New York, n.d. [1875?]) [AAS].

Thaddeus Burr Wakeman, *In Memory of Edward Bliss Foote, M.D.: A "Beloved Physician," of the New, Scientific, Human, Social, "Agnostic" Faith. . . . The Funeral Address Delivered. . . .* (New York, 1907).

Horace Walpole, *Anecdotes of Painting in England; with Some Account of the Principal Artists; and Incidental Notes on Other Arts; Collected by the Late George Vertue* (1762; London, 1786).

Nehemiah Walter, *The Body of Death Anatomized: a brief essay concerning the sorrows and the desires of the regenerate, upon their sense of indwelling sin; delivered at the Lecture in Boston, 12 d. 7 m. 1706 by Nehemiah Walter, paster of the church in Roxbury* (2d ed., Boston, 1736) [MHS].

Edward Warren, *The Life of John Collins Warren, M.D., compiled chiefly from his autobiography and journals* (Boston, 1860), 2 vols.

James Webster, *Facts Concerning Anatomical Instruction in Philadelphia* (Philadelphia, 1832) [HS].

——— et al., *To the Medical Profession of the City of New-York* (New York, 1846) [CPP].

David Wechsler, "The New York Morgue," *Detroit Evening News* (2-3-1889).

Eleazar M.P. Wells, *Preparation for Death, delivered at Trinity Church, Boston, on the sixth Wednesday in Lent, A.D. MDCCCLII* (n.p., 1852) [MHS].

John Wesley, *Primitive Physic. . . .* [facs. 23 ed., London, 1797], ed. A. Wesley Hill (London: Epworth Press, 1960).

Andrew Dickson White, *The History of the Warfare of Science with Theology in Christendom* (New York, 1896), 2 vols.

Sophia White, *Dialogues, Essays, and Stories for the use of children* (Boston, 1859) [AAS].

Walt Whitman, *An 1855–56 Notebook Toward the Second Edition of Leaves of Grass*, intro. and annot. Harold Blodgett (Carbondale: Southern Illinois Press, 1959).

———, *Notebooks and Unpublished Prose Manuscripts*, ed. Edward F. Grier (New York: New York University Press, 1984).

Stephen Wickes, *Sepulture: Its History, Methods and Sanitary Requisites* (Philadelphia, 1884).

Mary Elizabeth Wieting, *Prominent Incidents in the Life of Dr. John M. Wieting. . . .* (New York-London, 1889).

Burt Green Wilder, *What Young People Should Know: The Reproductive Function in Man and the Lower Animals* (Boston, 1875).

Marcius Willson, *The Fourth Reader of the School and Family Series* (New York, 1861) [AAS].

Rev. A. B. Winfield, *Sermon at the Interment of the Bodies of John G. Van Nest, Mrs. Sarah Van Nest, Mrs. Sarah Van Nest, G.W. Van Nest, Their Son, and Mrs. Phebe Wykoff [mother in law], who were murdered March 12th inst., by a colored man named William Freeman, Preached in the R.D. Church, at Sand Beach, Owasco Lake, March 15th* (Auburn, NY, 1846) [NYHS].

Samuel B. Woodward, *Hints for the Young, in Relation to the Health of Body and Mind* (3d ed., Worcester, 1839) [AAS].

Jeffries Wyman, "Twelve Letters from Jeffries Wyman, M.D.: Hampden-Sydney Medical College, Richmond, Virginia, 1843–1848," ed. George Gifford, Jr., *Journal of the History of Medicine & Allied Sciences* 20 (1965): 309–33.

Lunsford P. Yandell, *History of the University of Louisville: An Introductory Lecture, delivered November 1st, 1852* (Louisville, 1852).

PERIODICALS

Albany Argus, 1851–54.

Albany Atlas, 1851–54.

Albany Evening Journal, 1851–54.

Alta Californian (San Francisco), 1867.

American Journal of Homeopathy, 1852.

American Journal of Medical Reform, 1851.

American Journal of the Medical Sciences, 1836–37, 1840.

American Lancet (New York), 1830–31.

Annals of Phrenology (Boston), 1835.

Baltimore Republic and Daily Argus, 1844.

Boston Courier, 1831.

Boston Daily Globe, 1885.

Boston Gazette, 1771.

Boston Guide to Health and Journal of Arts and Sciences, 1843.

Boston Medical Intelligencer, 1823; continues as *Boston Medical & Surgical Journal*.

Boston News Letter, 1773.

Boston Weekly Newsletter, 1825–26.

Boston Post-Boy, 1753.

Botanico-Medical Investigator and Journal of Health (Springfield, MA), 1843.

Brooklyn Daily Eagle, 1854.

Brookville Republican, 1915.

Buffalo Morning Express, 1854–67.

Chicago Inter-Ocean, 1878.

Cincinnati Evening Post, 1884.

Cleveland Plain Dealer, 1852.

Colored American (New York), 1837–40.

Detroit Evening News, 1889.

Dr. Foote's Health Monthly 1–20 (New York), 1876–1895.

Freedom's Journal (New York), 1827–30.

Freeman's Journal (New York), 1854.

Graham's Journal of Health and Longevity (Boston), 1836–39.

Greenleaf's New York Journal and Patriotic Register, 1792.

Harper's New Monthly Magazine (New York), 1854–82.

Hartford Daily Times, 1850.

The Homoeopathic Advocate and Guide to Health (Keene, NH), 1851 [AAS].

Indianapolis Recorder, 1902.

Journal of Medical Reform (New York), 1854.

Journal of the Assembly of the State of New-York, 1820–54.

Journal of the Senate of the State of New-York, 1820–54.

Juvenile Rambler; Designed for Families and Schools (Boston), 1832–33.

Library of Health 1 (Boston), 1837.

Maryland Gazette, 1762.

Medical Eclectic, 1876.

Medical Record (New York), 1874–90.

Medical Reformer, 1823.

Medico-Legal Journal, 1888.

Moore's Rural New-Yorker (Rochester, NY/New York City), 1874.

The Moral Reformer and Teacher of the Human Condition (Boston), 1835–36.

The National Era (Washington, DC), 1847–48.

New-England Weekly Journal (Boston), 1734.

New York City, Documents of the Board of Aldermen 12 (New York, 1846).

———, *Proceedings of the Board of Aldermen of the City of New York* 34 (1848).

———, *Proceedings and Documents of the Board of Assistant Aldermen* 31 (1848).

———, *Proceedings of the Board of Councilmen of the City of New York* 53 (1854).

[New York] Daily Advertiser, 1788.

The New-York Dissector: A Quarterly Journal of Medicine, Surgery, Magnetism, Mesmerism and the Collateral Sciences, with the mysteries and fallacies of the faculty, 1844–47 [ed. Henry Hall Sherwood] [CPP].

New York Evening Post, 1824

New York Gazette, 1763.

New York Herald, 1843–88.

New York Independent, 1874.

New York Medical Enquirer, 1830–31.

New York Mirror and Ladies Literary Gazette, 1824.

New York Morning Journal, 1888.

New York Times, 1854–88.

New York Tribune, 1851–88.

New York Star, 1888.

New York Sun, 1835, 1888.

New York World, 1874, 1887–88, 1896.

North American Review, 1831, 1861.

The North Star (Rochester, NY), 1847–49 [ed. Frederick Douglass].

Parley's Magazine (Boston), 1833–34.

Pennsylvania Chronicle, and Universal Advertiser, 1767.

Pennsylvania Gazette, 1765, 1770.

Pennsylvania Journal and Weekly Advertiser, 1771, 1786.

Pennsylvania Mercury, 1790.

The People's Medical Journal, and Home Doctor 1–2 (New York), 1853–54 [ed. Frederick C. Hollick] [FC].

Philadelphia Botanic Sentinel, 1843.

Potter's American Monthly, 1878.

Proceedings of the National Medical Conventions, Held in New York, May 1846, and in Philadelphia, May, 1847 (Philadelphia, 1847).

Providence Gazette, and Country Journal, 1773.

Providence Journal, 1830.

The Quaker City (Philadelphia), 1849.

Rhode Island Medical Reformer: A Family Journal for the Promotion of Health and Longevity (Providence), 1843.

Royal Gazette (New York), 1781.

The Scalpel (New York), 1846–58.

Southern Botanico-Medical Journal (Forsyth, GA), 1841.

Teacher of Health and Laws of the Human Constitution (Boston), 1843.

Thomsonian Manual (Boston), 1835–38 [continues as *Boston Thomsonian Manual and Lady's Companion*, 1938–39].

Thomsonian Recorder (Columbus, OH), 1832–35.

Thomson's Almanac for the Year 1844 (Boston), 1843.

University of New-York, Medical Department, Announcements of Lectures, 1841–85.

Vermont Journal, 1789.

Wayne County [NY] Sentinel, 1824.

Weekly Magazine of Original Essays (Philadelphia), 1798.

Westminster Review, 1824, 1829.

Secondary Works

Emily K. Abel, "Family Caregiving in the Nineteenth Century: Emily Hawly Gillespie and Sarah Gillespie, 1858–1888," *Bulletin of the History of Medicine* 68 (1994): 573–99.

Harold J. Abrahams, *Extinct Medical Schools of Nineteenth-Century Philadelphia* (Philadelphia: University of Pennsylvania Press, 1966).

Ruth J. Abram, ed., *"Send Us a Lady Physician": Woman Doctors in America, 1835–1920* (New York: Norton, 1985).

M. E. Abrams et al., *The Norton Anthology of English Literature* (New York: Norton, 1968).

Erwin Ackerknecht, *A Short History of Medicine* (Baltimore: Johns Hopkins University Press, 1955).

Bluford Adams, *E Pluribus Barnum: The Great Showman and the Making of U.S. Popular Culture* (Minneapolis: University of Minnesota Press, 1997).

George Worthington Adams, *Doctors in Blue: The Medical History of the Union Army in the Civil War* (New York: Henry Schuman, 1952).

Robert Allen, *Horrible Prettiness: Burlesque and American Culture* (Chapel Hill: University of North Carolina Press, 1993).

Frederick S. Allis, Jr., et al., *Medicine in Colonial Massachusetts, 1620–1820* (Boston: Colonial Society of Massachusetts, 1980).

Richard D. Altick, *The Shows of London* (Cambridge, MA and London: Belknap Press of Harvard University Press, 1978).

Toby A. Appel, "Physiology in American Women's Colleges: The Rise and Decline of a Female Subculture," *Isis* 85 (1994): 29.

Philippe Ariès, *Western Attitudes Toward Death: From the Middle Ages to the Present,* tr. Patricia M. Ranum (Baltimore: Johns Hopkins University Press, 1974).

———, *Hour of Our Death,* tr. Helen Weaver (Oxford University Press: Oxford, 1981).

Simon Baatz, "'A Very Diffused Disposition': Dissecting Schools in Philadelphia, 1823–1825," *Pennsylvania Magazine of History and Biography* 108 (1984): 203–17 [edited text of "Communication from the Medical Faculty to the Trustees on Introducing the Dissections into the Common Course of Study for Graduates in Medicine, 1824," in Medical Faculty Papers, General Archives, University of Pennsylvania].

William Bachop, "Minimizing Risks and Maximizing Benefits in the Gross Anatomy Laboratory," *Transactions of the Illinois Academy of Science* 79.3–4 (1986): 279–82.

———, "Educational Abuses in the Teaching of Anatomy," *Vox* 1.1 (1987): 27–31.

C. W. Bardeen, *Anatomy in America,* Bulletin of the University of Wisconsin 115, Science Series 3:4 (Madison: University of Wisconsin Press, 1905).

G. J. Barker-Benfield, *The Culture of Sensibility : Sex and Society in Eighteenth-Century Britain* (Chicago: University of Chicago Press, 1992).

William Barlow and David O. Powell, "A Dedicated Medical Student: Solomon Mordecai, 1819–1822," *Journal of the Early Republic* 7 (1987): 377–97.

Jonathan Barry, "The Making of the Middle Class?", *Past & Present* 145 (11–1994): 194–208.

Jesse F. Battan, "'The Word Made Flesh': Language, Authority, and Sexual Desire in Late 19th-Century America," *Journal of the History of Sexuality* 3 (1992): 223–44.

Edward L. Bell, "The Historical Archaeology of Mortuary Behavior: Coffin Hardward from Uxbridge, Massachusetts," *Historical Archaeology* 24 (1990): 54–78.

Whitfield J. Bell, Jr., "Doctors' Riot, New York, 1788" [letter of William Heth to Edmund Randolph, 4-16-1788], *Bulletin of the New York Academy of Medicine* 47 (1971): 1501–3.

———, "Nathan Smith Davis: An Autobiographical Letter, Previously Unpublished" [Binghamton, NY, 1840], *Journal of the American Medical Association* 224 (1973): 1014–16.

———, "Medicine in Boston and Philadelphia: Comparisons and Contrasts, 1750–1820," in *Medicine in Colonial Massachusetts, 1620–1820,* Publications of the Colonial Society of Massachusetts, 57 (Boston, 1980): 159–83.

Alex Berman, "Neo-Thomsonianism in the United States," *Journal of the History of Medicine* 11 (1956): 133–52.

W. T. Berry and H. E. Poole, *Annals of Printing* (Toronto: University of Toronto Press, 1966).

Catherine Birney, *Sarah and Angelina Grimké: The First Women Advocates of Abolition and Woman's Rights* [1885] (rpt. Westport, CT: Greenwood Press, 1969).

John B. Blake, "The Development of American Anatomy Acts," *Journal of Medical Education* (August 1955) 30: 431–39.

——, "Anatomy and the Congress," in L.G. Stevenson and R.P. Multhauf, eds., *Medicine, Science and Culture: Historical Essays in Honor of Owsei Temkin* (Baltimore: Johns Hopkins Press, 1968).

——, "Anatomy," in Ronald Numbers, ed., *The Education of American Physicians: Historical Essays* (Berkeley: University of California Press, 1980).

Robert L. Blakely and Judith M. Harrington, eds., *Bones in the Basement: Postmortem Racism in 19th-Century Medical Training* (Washington, DC: Smithsonian Institution Press, 1997).

Stuart Blumin, *The Emergence of the Middle Class: Social Experience in the American City, 1760–1900* (Cambridge: Cambridge University Press, 1989).

Pierre Bourdieu, *The Logic of Practice*, trans. Richard Nice (Cambridge: Polity Press, 1990).

James O. Breeden, "Body Snatchers and Anatomy Professors: Medical Education in Nineteenth-Century Virginia," *Virginia Magazine of History & Biography* 83 (1975): 321–45.

Amy Bridges, *A City in the Republic: Antebellum New York and the Origins of Machine Politics* (Ithaca: Cornell University Press, 1984).

David R. Brigham, *Public Culture in the Early Republic: Peale's Museum and its Audience* (Washington, DC: Smithsonian Institution Press, 1995).

Laurence Brockliss and Colin Jones, *The Medical World of Early Modern France* (Oxford: Clarendon Press, 1997).

Janet Farrell Brodie, *Contraception and Abortion in Nineteenth-Century America* (Ithaca: Cornell University Press, 1994).

Elisabeth Bronfen, *Over Her Dead Body: Death, Femininity, and the Aesthetic* (New York: Routledge, 1992).

Gillian Brown, *Domestic Individualism: Imagining Self in Nineteenth-Century America* (Berkeley: University of California Press, 1990).

Peter G. Buckley, "The Culture of 'Leg-Work': The Transformation of Burlesque after the Civil War," in James Gilbert et al., eds., *The Mythmaking Frame of Mind: Social Imagination and American Culture* (Belmont, CA: Wadsworth Publishing Company, 1993).

Stanley Buder, *Pullman: An Experiment in Industrial Order and Community Planning, 1880–1930* (New York: Oxford University Press, 1967).

Joan Burbick, *Healing the Republic: The Language of Health and the Culture of Nationalism in Nineteenth-Century America* (New York: Cambridge University Press, 1994).

Martin J. Burke, *The Conundrum of Class: Public Discourse on the Social Order in America* (Chicago: University of Chicago Press, 1995).

W. L. Burrage and H. A. Kelley, *Dictionary of American Medical Biography* (1928; rpt. Boston: Milford House, 1971).

Richard L. Bushman, *Joseph Smith and the Beginnings of Mormonism* (Urbana, IL: University of Illinois Press, 1984).

————, *The Refinement of America: Persons, Houses, Cities* (New York: Vintage, 1992).

Judith Butler, *Bodies That Matter: On the Discursive Limits of "Sex"* (New York: Routledge, 1993).

Richard Butsch, "Bowery B'hoys and Matinee Ladies: The Re-Gendering of Nineteenth-Century American Theater Audiences," *American Quarterly* 46 (1994): 374–405.

Caroline Walker Bynum, *Fragmentation and Redemption* (New York: Zone, 1992).

————, "Why All the Fuss about the Body? A Medievalist's Perspective," *Representations* 22.1 (1995): 1–33.

David Cannadine, "War and Death, Grief and Mourning in Modern Britain," in Joachim Whaley, ed., *Mirrors of Mortality: Studies in the Social History of Death* (New York: St. Martin's Press, 1981).

Harry J. Carman, *Social and Economic History of the United States, Vol. 2: The Rise of Industrialism, 1820–1875* (Boston: D. C. Heath, 1934).

Philip Cash, "The Professionalization of Boston Medicine," in Frederick S. Allis, Jr., et al., *Medicine in Colonial Massachusetts, 1620–1820* (Boston: Colonial Society of Massachusetts, 1980).

James H. Cassedy, *Medicine in America: A Short History* (Baltimore: Johns Hopkins University Press, 1991).

Vincent J. Cirillo, "Edward Foote's *Medical Common Sense*: An Early American Comment on Birth Control," *Journal of the History of Medicine* 25 (1970): 341–45.

————, "Edward Bliss Foote [1829–1906]: Pioneer American Advocate of Birth Control," *Bulletin of the History of Medicine* 47 (1973): 471–79.

Emily Jane Cohen, "Enlightenment and the Dirty Philosopher," *Configurations* 5 (1997): 369–424.

Charles Colbert, *A Measure of Perfection: Phrenology and the Fine Arts in America* (Chapel Hill and London: University of North Carolina Press, 1997).

F. J. Cole, *History of the Anatomical Museum* (London, 1914), rpt. from *A Miscellany: Presented to J.M. Mackay, L.L.D.*

Roger Cooter, *The Cultural Meaning of Popular Science: Phrenology and the Organization of Consent in Nineteenth-Century Britain* (Cambridge: Cambridge University Press, 1984).

———— and Stephen Pumfrey, "Separate Spheres and Public Places: Reflections on the History of Science Popularization and Science in Popular Culture," *History of Science* 32.3 (1994): 237–67.

Alain Corbin, *The Foul and the Fragrant: Odor and the French Social Imagination* [1982], trans. Miriam Kochan (Cambridge: Harvard University Press, 1986).

George W. Corner, *Anatomy* (New York: Paul B. Hoeber, 1930).

————, "The Role of Anatomy in Medical Education," *Journal of Medical Education* 33 (1958): 1–8.

————, *Two Centuries of Medicine: A History of the School of Medicine, University of Pennsylvania* (Philadelphia: J. B. Lippincott, 1965).

H.L. Coulter, *Divided Legacy: The Conflict between Homœopathy and the American Medical Association* (Richmond, CA: North Atlantic, 1973).

David Cressy, "Death and the Social Order: The Funerary Preferences of Elizabethan Gentlemen," *Continuity and Change* 5 (1989): 99–119.

Andrew Cunningham, *The Anatomical Renaissance: The Resurrection of the Anatomical Projects of the Ancients* (Hants, U.K. and Brookfield, VT: Scolar Press, 1997).

Julia Curtis, "Philadelphia in an Uproar: *The Monks of Monk Hall*, 1844," *Theatre History Studies* 5 (1985): 41–47.

Robert Darnton, *Mesmerism and the End of the Enlightenment in France* (Cambridge: Harvard University Press, 1968).

Lorraine Daston, rev., "The Factual Sensibility," *Isis* 79 (1988): 452–67.

———, and Katharine Park, *Wonders and the Order of Nature, 1150–1750* (New York: Zone, 1998).

Arnold I. Davidson, "How to Do the History of Psychiatry: A Reading of Freud's *Three Essays on the Theory of Sexuality*," *Critical Inquiry* 18 (1987): 266–67.

John Dunn Davies, *Phrenology, Fad and Science: A 19th-Century American Crusade* (New Haven: Yale University Press, 1955).

Michael Denning, *Mechanic Accents: Dime Novels and Working-Class Culture in America* (London-New York: Verso, 1987).

Mark Dery, "Anatomy Lesson: The Visceral Pleasures of Medical Museums," in Sara Diamond and Sylvere Lotringer, eds. *Flesh Eating Technologies* (New York: Semiotexte and the Banff Centre, 1999).

Adrian Desmond, *The Politics of Evolution: Morphology, Medicine and Reform in Radical London* (Chicago: University of Chicago Press, 1989).

Kenneth Allen de Ville, *Medical Malpractice in Nineteenth-Century America: Origins and Legacy* (New York: New York University Press, 1990).

R. Dingwall and P. Lewis, eds., *The Sociology of the Professions* (London: MacMillan, 1983).

T. Doby and G. Alker, *Origins and Development of Medical Imaging* (Carbondale: Southern Illinois University Press, 1997).

Jay P. Dolan, *The Immigrant Church: New York's Irish and German Catholics, 1815–1865* (Notre Dame: University of Notre Dame Press, 1975).

Ann Douglas, "Heaven Our Home: Consolation Literature in the Northern United States, 1830–1880," in Stannard et al., ed., *Death in America* (Philadelphia: University of Pennsylvania Press, 1975), 49–68.

———, *The Feminization of American Culture* (New York: Knopf, 1977).

Jacalyn Duffin, *Langstaff: A Nineteenth-Century Medical Life* (Toronto: University of Toronto Press, 1993).

———, *To See with a Better Eye: A Life of R. T. H. Laennec* (Princeton: Princeton University Press, 1998).

Ronald Dworkin, Thomas Nagel, Robert Nozick, John Rawls, Thomas Scanlon, and Judith Jarvis Thomson, "Assisted Suicide: The Philosophers' Brief [amicus curiae brief presented in the cases of *State of Washington et al.* v. *Glucksberg et al.* and *Vacco et al.* v. *Quill et al.*, argued before the U.S. Supreme Court, 1-8-1997], *New York Review of Books*, 1-27-1997: 41–47.

Terry Eagleton, *Ideology: An Introduction* (New York: Verso, 1991).

Myrl Ebert, "The Rise and Development of the American Medical Periodical, 1797–1850," *Bulletin of the Medical Library Association* 40 (1952): 243–76. [HS]

James Edmonson, "The Medical Period Room," *Caduceus* 3.4 (Winter 1987): 27–43.

J. Edwards and M. J. Edwards, *Medical Museum Technology* (London: Oxford University Press, 1959).

Linden F. Edwards, "Body Snatching in Ohio During the Nineteenth Century," *Ohio State Archaeological & Historical Quarterly* 59 (1950): 329–51.

———, "The Ohio Anatomy Law of 1881," *Ohio Medical Journal* 46 (1950): 1190–92; 47 (1951): 49–52, 143–46.

———, "Resurrection Riots During the Heroic Age of Anatomy in America," *Bulletin of the History of Medicine* 25 (1951): 178–84.

———, "Cinci's 'Old Cunny': A Notorious Purveyor of Human Flesh," *Ohio Medical Journal* 50 (1954): 466–69.

———, "The Famous Harrison Case and Its Repercussions," *Bulletin of the History of Medicine* 31 (1957): 162–71.

———, "Dr. Frederick C. Waite's Correspondence with Reference to Grave Robbery," *Ohio State Medical Journal* 54 (1958): 480–82, 600–2.

Mircea Eliade, *Shamanism: Archaic Techniques of Ecstasy* [1951], trans. Willard R. Trask (Princeton: Princeton University Press, 1964).

Norbert Elias, *The History of Manners: The Civilizing Process, Vol. 1* [1939], trans. Edmund Jephcott (New York: Pantheon, 1978).

John H. Ellis, *Medicine in Kentucky* (Lexington: University Press of Kentucky, 1977).

Frantz Fanon, *Black Skin, White Masks* [1952], trans. Charles Lam Markmann (New York: Grove Press, 1967).

James J. Farrell, *Inventing the American Way of Death, 1830–1920* (Philadelphia: Temple University Press, 1980).

Margaretta V. Faugeres, *The Ghost of John Young the Homicide. . . .* (New York, 1797).

Howard M. Feinstein, *Becoming William James* (Ithaca: Cornell University Press, 1984).

Anita Clair Fellman and Michael Fellman, *Making Sense of Self: Medical Advice Literature in Late Nineteenth-Century America* (Philadelphia: University of Pennsylvania, 1981).

H. W. Felter, "Pathfinders," *National Eclectic Medical Quarterly* 1.2 (12–1909): 81–96.

Paula Findlen, *Possessing Nature: Museums, Collecting and Scientific Culture in Early Modern Italy* (Berkeley: University of California Press, 1994).

David Hackett Fischer, *Albion's Seeds: Four British Folkways in America* (New York: Oxford University Press, 1989).

Steven Earl Forry, "The Hideous Progenies of Richard Brinsley Peake: *Frankenstein* on the Stage, 1823 to 1826," *Theatre Research International* 11 (1986): 13–31.

Michel Foucault, *The Order of Things: An Archaeology of the Human Sciences* (New York: Pantheon, 1971).

———, *The Birth of the Clinic: An Archaeology of Medical Perception*, trans. A.M. Sheridan Smith (New York: Pantheon, 1973).

———, *Discipline and Punish: The Birth of the Prison*, trans. A.M. Sheridan (New York: Vintage, 1979).

———, *The History of Sexuality, Volume I: An Introduction* [1976], trans. Robert Hurley (New York: Vintage, 1990).

George Fredrickson, *The Black Image in the White Mind: The Debate on Afro-American Character and Destiny, 1817–1914* (New York: Wesleyan University Press, 1971).

Robert C. Fuller, *Mesmerism and the American Cure of Souls* (Philadelphia: University of Pennsylvania Press, 1982).

W. Bruce Fye, *The Development of American Physiology: Scientific Medicine in the Nineteenth Century* (Baltimore: Johns Hopkins University Press, 1987).

Philip Gaskell, *A New Introduction to Bibliography* (New York and Oxford: Oxford University Press, 1972).

Gordon E. Geddes, *Welcome Joy: Death in Puritan New England* (Ann Arbor: UMI Research Press, 1981).

Clifford Geertz, *Interpretation of Cultures* (New York: Basic Books, 1973).

Patsy A. Gerstner, "A Note on Body Snatching in the United States," *Bulletin of the Cleveland Medical Library Association* 18 (July 1971): 64–65.

George Gifford, Jr., ed., "Twelve Letters from Jeffries Wyman, M.D.: Hampden-Sydney Medical College, Richmond, Virginia, 1843–1848," *Journal of the History of Medicine & Allied Sciences* 20 (1965): 309–33.

Paul A. Gilje, *The Road to Mobocracy: Popular Disorder in New York City, 1763–1834* (Chapel Hill: University of North Carolina Press, 1987).

Lori D. Ginzberg, "'The Hearts of Your Readers Will Shudder': Fanny Wright, Infidelity, and American Freethought," *American Quarterly* 46 (1994): 195–226.

Claire Gittings, *Death, Burial and the Individual in Early Modern England* [1984] (rpt., London: Routledge, 1988).

Donald F. Glut, *The Frankenstein Catalogue* (Jefferson, NC: MacFarland Publishers, 1984).

Barbara Goldsmith, *Other Powers: The Age of Suffrage, Spiritualism and the Scandalous Victoria Woodhull* (New York: Knopf, 1998).

Jan Golinski, *Science as Public Culture: Chemistry and Enlightenment in Britain, 1760–1820* (Cambridge: Cambridge University Press, 1992).

F. Gonzalez-Crussi, *The Day of the Dead and Other Mortal Reflections* (New York: Harcourt, Brace and Co. 1993)

W.H. Goodrich, *The History of the Medical Department of the University of Georgia* (Augusta, GA: University of Georgia Press, [1928]).

Linda Gordon, *Woman's Body, Woman's Right* (New York: Penguin, 1974).

Stephen Jay Gould, *The Mismeasure of Man* (Norton: New York, 1981).

———, "Boyle's Law and Darwin's Details," *Natural History* (8–1995): 9–11, 32–34.

Robert M. Green, "J. V. C. Smith," in W. L. Burrage and H. A. Kelley, eds., *Dictionary of American Medical Biography* (1928; rpt. Boston: Milford House, 1971), 1128–29.

Stephen Greenblatt, *Renaissance Self-Fashioning: From More to Shakespeare* (Chicago: University of Chicago Press, 1980).

James R. Griesemer and Susan Leigh Star, "Institutional Ecology, 'Translations,' and Boundary Objects: Amateurs and Professionals in Berkeley's Museum of Vertebrate Zoology, 1907–39," *Social Studies of Science* 19 (1989): 387–420.

Michael Gross, "The Lessened Locus of Feelings: A Transformation in French Physiology in the Early 19th Century," *Journal of the History of Biology* 12 (1979): 231–71.

Alan F. Guttmacher, "Bootlegging Bodies: A History of Body-Snatching," *Bulletin of the Society of Medical History of Chicago* 4 (1935): 353–402.

Frederic W. Hafferty, *Into the Valley: Death and the Socialization of Medical Students* (New Haven: Yale University Press, 1991).

David D. Hall, *Worlds of Wonder, Days of Judgment: Popular Religious Belief in Early New England* (Cambridge: Harvard University Press, 1990).

John S. Haller, Jr., *Medical Protestants: The Eclectics in American Medicine, 1825–1939* (Carbondale: Southern Illinois University Press, 1994).

Karen Halttunen, *Confidence Men and Painted Women: A Study of Middle-Class Culture in America, 1830–1870* (New Haven: Yale University Press, 1982).

Hannibal Hamlin, "The Dissection Riot of 1824 and the Connecticut Anatomical Law," *Yale Journal of Biology & Medicine* 7 (1934–35): 275–89.

David Harley, "Political Post-Mortems and Morbid Anatomy in Seventeenth-Century England," *Social History of Medicine* 7 (1994): 1–28.

Donna Harraway, "A Game of Cat's Cradle: Science Studies, Feminist Theory, Cultural Studies," *Configurations* 2.1 (1994): 71.

Rom Harré, *Physical Being: Theory for a Corporeal Psychology* (Oxford: Blackwell, 1991).

Thomas F. Harrington, *The Harvard Medical School: A History, Narrative, and Documentary* (New York: Lewis, 1905).

Neil Harris, *Humbug; the Art of P. T. Barnum* (Boston: Little, Brown, 1973).

Steven J. Harris, "Long-Distance Corporations, Big Sciences, and the Geography of Knowledge," *Configurations* 6 (1998): 269–304.

Nathan O. Hatch, *The Democratization of American Christianity* (New Haven: Yale University Press, 1989).

Claude Heaton, "Body Snatching in New York City," *New York State Journal of Medicine* 43 (1943): 1861–65.

William H. Helfand, "Advertising Health to the People," in *"Every Man His Own Doctor": Popular Medicine in Early America*, Exhibition Catalogue, Library Company of Philadelphia (Philadelphia, 1998).

Glenn Hendler, "Pandering in the Public Sphere: Masculinity and the Market in Horatio Alger," *American Quarterly* 48 (1996): 415–38.

Robert Hertz, "A Contribution to the Study of the Collective Representation of Death" [*Années Sociologique* 10 (1907)], in idem, *Death and the Right Hand*, trans. R. and C. Needham (Glencoe, IL: Free Press, 1960), 27–86.

Arthur E. Hertzler, *The Horse and Buggy Doctor* (New York: Knopf, 1938).

Norman E. Himes, *Medical History of Contraception* (New York: Gamut Press, 1970).

Dirk Hoerder, *Crowd Action in Revolutionary Massachusetts 1765–1780* (New York: Academic Press, 1977).

Frederick L. Hoffman, *History of the Prudential Insurance Company of America (Industrial Insurance), 1875–1900* (n.p.: Prudential Press, 1900).

———, *Pauper Burials and the Interment of the Dead in Large Cities* (Newark, NJ: Prudential Press, 1919).

Stewart H. Holbrook, *The Golden Age of Quackery* (New York: Macmillan Co., 1959).

Christian A. Hovde, "Cadavers: General Ethical Concerns," in Warren T. Reich, ed., *Encyclopedia of Bioethics* (New York: Free Press, 1978), 1:139–43.

David C. Humphrey, "Dissection and Discrimination: The Social Origins of Cadavers in America, 1760–1915," *Bulletin of the New York Academy of Medicine* 49.9 (1973): 819–27.

Lynn Hunt, ed., *The New Cultural History* (Berkeley: University of California Press, 1989).

Ivan Illich, *Medical Nemesis: The Expropriation of Health* (New York: Pantheon, 1976).

Kenneth Jackson and Camilo José Vergara, *Silent Cities: The Evolution of the American Cemetery* (Princeton: Princeton Architectural Press, 1989).

Ludmilla Jordanova, *Sexual Visions: Images of Science and Medicine Between the Eighteenth and Twentieth Centuries* (Madison: University of Wisconsin Press, 1989).

Robert J.T. Joy, "The Natural Bonesetters with Special Reference to the Sweet Family of Rhode Island," *Bulletin of the History of Medicine* 28 (1954): 416–39.

Amalie M. Kass, "The Obstetrical Casebook of Walter Channing, 1811–1822," *Bulletin of the History of Medicine* 67 (Fall 1993): 494–523.

John F. Kasson, *Rudeness and Civility: Manners in Nineteenth-Century Urban America* (New York: Hill & Wang, 1990).

Martin Kaufman, *Homeopathy in America: The Rise and Fall of a Medical Heresy* (Baltimore: Johns Hopkins University Press, 1971).

———, *American Medical Education: The Formative Years, 1765–1910* (Westport, CT: Greenwood Press, 1976).

———, "American Medical Education" in R. Numbers, ed., *The Education of American Physicians: Historical Essays* (Berkeley: University of California Press, 1980).

——— et al., *Dictionary of American Medical Biography* (Westport, CT: Greenwood Press, 1984).

——— and Leslie L. Hanawalt, "Body Snatching in the Midwest," *Michigan History* 55 (Spring 1970): 23–40.

Michael G. Kenny, *The Perfect Law of Liberty: Elias Smith and the Providential History of America* (Washington, DC: Smithsonian Institution Press, 1994).

Joseph F. Kett, *The Formation of the American Medical Profession: The Role of Institutions, 1780–1860* (New Haven: Yale University Press, 1968).

Jack Kevorkian, *The Story of Dissection* (New York: Philosophical Library, 1959).

Lester King, *Transformations in American Medicine* (Baltimore: Johns Hopkins University Press, 1991).

S. J. Kleinberg, "Death and the Working Class," *Journal of Popular Culture* 11.1 (1977): 193–209.

Sally Kohlstedt, "The 19th-Century Amateur Tradition: The Case of the Boston Society of Natural History," in G. Holton and W. Blanpied, eds., *Science and Its Public* (Dordrecht: D. Reidel, 1976), 173–90.

———, "Curiosities and Cabinets: Natural History Museums and Education on the Antebellum Campus," *Isis* 79 (1988): 405–26.

E. B. Krumbhaar, "The Early History of Anatomy in the United States," *Annals of Medical History* 4 (1922): 271–86.

———, "History of the Autopsy and Its Relation to the Development of Modern Medicine," *Hospitals* 12 (1938): 68–74.

Jules C. Ladenheim, "The Doctor's Mob," *Journal of the History of Medicine* 5 (1950): 23–53.

George Lakoff and Mark Johnson, *Metaphors We Live By* (Chicago: University of Chicago Press, 1980).

Thomas Laqueur, "Bodies, Death, and Pauper Funerals," *Representations* 1.1 (1983): 109–31.

————, *Making Sex: Body and Gender from the Greeks to Freud* (Cambridge: Harvard University Press, 1990).

A. M. Lassek, *Human Dissection: Its Drama and Struggle* (Springfield, IL: Charles C. Thomas, Publisher, 1958).

Susan Lawrence, "Beyond the Grave: The Use and Meaning of Human Body Parts: A Historical Introduction," in Robert F. Weir, ed., *Stored Tissue Samples: Ethical, Legal, and Public Policy Implications* (Iowa City: University of Iowa Press, 1998).

William Leach, *True Love and Perfect Union: The Feminist Reform of Sex and Society* (New York: Basic Books, 1980).

Judith Walzer Leavitt and Ronald L. Numbers, *Sickness and Health in America* (3d rev. ed., Madison: University of Wisconsin Press, 1997).

Drew Leder, "Medicine and Paradigms of Embodiment," *Journal of Medicine and Philosophy* 9 (1984): 29–43.

Timothy Lenoir, "Was the Last Turn the Right Turn?: The Semiotic Turn and A. J. Greimas," *Configurations* 2.1 (1994): 122.

Gerda Lerner, *The Grimké Sisters from South Carolina: Rebels Against Slavery* (Boston: Houghton Mifflin, 1967).

Herbert Leventhal, *In the Shadow of the Enlightenment: Occultism and Renaissance Science in 18th-Century America* (New York: New York University Press, 1976).

David Michael Levin and George F. Solomon, "The Discursive Formation of the Body in the History of Medicine," *Journal of Medicine and Philosophy* 15 (1990): 515–37.

R. M. Lewis, "William Andrus Alcott," in W. L. Burrage and H. A. Kelley, eds., *Dictionary of American Medical Biography* (1928; rpt. Boston: Milford House, 1971), 10–11.

Sidney E. Lind, "Poe and Mesmerism," *PMLA* 62.4 [pt. 1] (12–1947): 1077–94.

Peter Linebaugh, *The London Hanged: Crime and Civil Society in the Eighteenth Century* (London: Allen Lane-Penguin, 1991).

————, "The Tyburn Riot Against the Surgeons," in D. Hay et al., eds., *Albion's Fatal Tree: Crime and Society in 18th-Century England* (New York: Pantheon Books, 1977).

Uri Lloyd, "A Review of the Principal Events in American Medicine," *Eclectic Medical Journal* 86 (1926): 262–69.

Margaret Lock and Nancy Scheper-Hughes, "The Mindful Body: A Prolegemon to Future Work in Medical Anthropology," *Medical Anthropology* 1.1 (1987): 6–41.

Bette London, "Mary Shelley, *Frankenstein*, and the Spectacle of Masculinity," in *Publications of the Modern Language Association* 108.2 (March 1993): 253–67.

Eric Lott, *Love and Theft: Blackface Minstrelsy and the American Working Class* (New York: Oxford University Press, 1993).

Irvine Loudon, "The Making of Man-Midwifery" [rev. of A. Wilson, *The Making of Man-Midwifery*], *Bulletin of the History of Medicine* 70 (1996): 507–15

Kenneth M. Ludmerer, *Learning to Heal: The Development of American Medical Education* (New York: Basic Books, 1985).

T. O. Mabbot, *Collected Writings of E. A. Poe* (Boston: Belknap, 1975), 3: 1024–42.

George E. Macdonald, *Fifty Years of Freethought: The Story of the Truthseeker* (New York: Truthseeker, 1929).

Arien Mack, ed., *Death in American Experience* (New York: Schocken Books, 1973).

C. B. Macpherson, *The Political Theory of Possessive Individualism: From Hobbes to Locke* (New York: Oxford University Press, 1962).

H. L. Malchow, "Frankenstein's Monster and Images of Race in Nineteenth-Century Britain," *Past & Present* 139 (May 1993): 90–130.

Dumas Malone, ed. *Dictionary of American Biography* (New York: Scribners, 1935).

Tim Marshall, *Murdering to Dissect: Grave-robbing, Frankenstein and the Anatomy Literature* (Manchester: Manchester University Press, 1995).

Luther H. Martin, Huck Gutman, and Patrick H. Hutton, eds., *Technologies of the Self: A Seminar with Michel Foucault* (Amherst: University of Massachusetts Press, 1988).

Albert Matthews, "Notes on Early Autopsies and Anatomical Lectures," *Publications of the Colonial Society of Massachusetts* 19 (1916–1917): 273–90.

Russell C. Maulitz, *Morbid Appearances: The Anatomy of Pathology in the Early Nineteenth Century* (Cambridge: Cambridge University Press, 1987).

Pauline M. H. Mazumdar, "Anatomical Physiology and the Reform of Medical Education: London, 1825–1835," *Bulletin of the History of Medicine* 57 (1983): 230–46.

Grant McCracken, *Culture and Consumption* (Indiana University Press: Bloomington, IN, 1988).

Thomas M. McDade, ed., *The Annals of Murder: A Bibliography of Books and Pamphlets on American Murders from Colonial Times to 1900* (Norman, OK: University of Oklahoma Press, 1961).

Brooks McNamara, *Step Right Up* (rev. ed., Jackson, MI: University Press of Mississippi, 1995).

Martha McPartland, "The Bonesetter Sweets of South County, Rhode Island," *Yankee* (1–1968): 80–102.

Carolyn Merchant, *The Death of Nature: Women, Ecology, and the Scientific Revolution* (San Francisco: Harper & Row, 1983).

A. W. Meyer, "Anatomy Acts of California: A Survey of Former and Present Laws," *California & Western Medicine* 33 (1930): 703–7.

Jessica Mitford, *The American Way of Death* (New York: Simon and Schuster, 1963).

Mark Monmonier, *How to Lie with Maps* (Chicago: University of Chicago Press, 1991).

Horace Montgomery, "Prescholastic Anatomical Instruction as a Factor in Medical Professionalization in British North America" in K. Lanzinger, ed., *Americana-Austriaca* (rpt. Vienna: W. Braunmiller, [n.d.]).

——— "A Body Snatcher Sponsors Pennsylvania's Anatomy Act," *Journal of Medical History* 21 (1966): 374–93.

Regina Markell Morantz, "Nineteenth-Century Health Reform and Women: A Program of Self-Help," in Guenter B. Risse, Ronald L. Numbers, and Judith Walzer Leavitt, eds., *Medicine Without Doctors: Home Health Care in American History* (New York: Science History Publications, 1977), 73–94.

———, Cynthia Stodola Pomerleau, and Carol Hansen Fenichel, eds., *In Her Own Words: Oral Histories of Women Physicians* (New Haven: Yale University Press, 1982).

Regina Morantz-Sanchez, *Sympathy & Science: Women Physicians in American Medicine* (New York: Oxford University Press, 1985).

Jarvis Means Morse, *A Neglected Period in Connecticut's History, 1818–1850* (New Haven: Yale University Press, 1933).

Ornella Moscucci, *The Science of Woman: Gynæcology and Gender in England, 1800–1929* (Cambridge: Cambridge University Press, 1990).

Lamar Riley Murphy, *Enter the Physician: The Transformation of Domestic Medicine, 1760–1860* (Tuscaloosa: University of Alabama Press, 1991).

Stephen Nissenbaum, *Sex, Diet, and Debility in Jacksonian America* (Westport, CT: Greenwood Press, 1980).

Gregory Nobles, "Straight Lines and Stability: Mapping the Political Order of the Anglo-American Frontier," *Journal of American History* 80 (June 1993): 9–35.

Ronald Numbers, ed., *The Education of American Physicians: Historical Essays* (Berkeley: University of California Press, 1980).

———, "The Fall and Rise of the American Medical Profession," in Judith Walzer Leavitt and Ronald L. Numbers, eds., *Sickness and Health in America* (3d rev. ed., Madison: University of Wisconsin Press, 1997), 225–36.

David E. Nye, *Electrifying America: Social Meanings of a New Technology, 1800–1940* (Cambridge: MIT Press, 1990).

George C. D. Odell, *Annals of the New York Stage* (New York: Columbia University Press, 1931), 15 vols.

Richard Broxton Onians, *The Origins of European Thought about the Body, the Mind, the Soul, the World, Time, and Fate: New Interpretations of Greek, Roman and Kindred Evidence Also of Some Basic Jewish and Christian Beliefs* (Cambridge: Cambridge University Press, 1951).

Joel J. Orosz, *Curators and Culture: The Museum Movement in America, 1740–1870* (Tuscaloosa: University of Alabama Press, 1990).

Katharine Park, "The Criminal and the Saintly Body: Autopsy and Dissection in Renaissance Italy," *Renaissance Quarterly* 47 (1994): 1–33.

——— and Lorraine Daston, *Wonders and the Order of Nature, 1150–1750* (New York: Zone, 1998).

F. L. M. Pattison, *Granville Sharp Pattison: Anatomist and Antagonist, 1791–1851* (Tuscaloosa: University of Alabama Press, 1987).

Marcello Pera, *The Ambiguous Frog: The Galvani-Volta Controversy on Animal Electricity*, trans. Jonathan Mandelbaum (Princeton, NJ: Princeton University Press, 1992).

Martin S. Pernick, *A Calculus of Suffering: Pain, Professionalism and Anesthesia in Nineteenth-Century America* (New York: Columbia University Press, 1985).

———, "Back from the Grave: Recurring Controversies over Defining and Diagnosing Death in History," in Richard M. Zaner, ed., *Death: Beyond Whole-Brain Criteria* (Dordrecht: Kluwer Academic, 1988).

T. V. N. Persaud, *A History of Anatomy: The Post-Vesalian Era* (Springfield, IL: Charles C. Thomas, Publisher, 1997).

John V. Pickstone, "Museological Science? The Place of the Analytical/Comparative in 19th-Century Science, Technology and Medicine," *History of Science* 32.2 (1994): 111–38.

H. E. Poole and W. T. Berry, *Annals of Printing* (Toronto: University of Toronto Press, 1966).

Mary Poovey, *Uneven Developments: The Ideological Work of Gender in Mid-Victorian England* (Chicago: University of Chicago Press, 1988).

———, "Anatomical Realism and Social Investigation in Early 19th-Century Manchester," *Differences* 5.3 (1993): 1–30.

Charlotte M. Porter, "The Natural History Museum," in Michael S. Shapiro, ed., with Louise Ward Kemp, *The Museum: A Reference Guide* (New York: Greenwood Press, 1990).

Roy Porter, *Health for Sale: Quackery in England 1660–1850* (Manchester, U.K.: Manchester University Press, 1989).

———, *Doctor of Society: Thomas Beddoes and the Sick Trade in Late-Enlightenment England* (London: Routledge, 1992).

Anson Rabinbach, *The Human Motor: Energy, Fatigue, and the Origins of Modernity* (New York: Basic Books, 1990).

James Reed, *From Private Vice to Public Virtue: The Birth Control Movement and American Society Since 1830* (New York: Basic Books, 1978).

———, "Charles Knowlton," in John A. Garraty and Mark C. Carnes, eds., *American National Biography* (New York: Oxford University Press, 1999), 12: 829–30.

Stanley Joel Reiser, *Medicine and the Reign of Technology* (Cambridge: Cambridge University Press, 1978).

Benjamin Reiss, "P. T. Barnum, Joice Heth and Antebellum Spectacles of Race," *American Quarterly* 51 (1999): 78–107.

David S. Reynolds, *George Lippard* (Boston: Twayne Publishers, 1982).

———, ed., *George Lippard, Prophet of Protest: Writings of an American Radical* (New York: Peter Lang Publishers, 1983).

———, *Beneath the American Renaissance: The Subversive Imagination in the Age of Emerson and Melville* (New York: Knopf, 1988).

———, *Walt Whitman's America: A Cultural Biography* (New York: Knopf, 1995).

Evelleen Richards, "The 'Moral Anatomy' of Robert Knox: The Interplay between Biological and Social Thought in Victorian Scientific Naturalism," *Journal of the History of Biology* 22 (1989): 373–436.

———, "A Political Anatomy of Monsters, Hopeful and Otherwise: Teratogeny, Transcendentalism, and Evolutionary Theorizing," *Isis* 85 (1994): 377–411.

Ruth Richardson, *Death, Dissection and the Destitute* (London: Penguin, 1988).

——— and Brian Hurwitz, "Jeremy Bentham's Self Image: An Exemplary Bequest for Dissection," *British Medical Journal* 295 (7-18-1987): 195–98.

Felix Riesenberg, *East Side West Side* (New York: Harcourt, Brace and Company, 1927).

Karlem Riess, "The Rebel Physiologist: Bennet Dowler," *Journal of the History of Medicine & Allied Sciences* 16 (1961): 39–48.

Guenter B. Risse, Ronald L. Numbers, and Judith Walzer Leavitt, eds., *Medicine Without Doctors: Home Health Care in American History* (New York: Science History Publications, 1977).

David R. Roediger, *The Wages of Whiteness: Race and the Making of the American Working Class* (London–New York: Verso, 1991).

Naomi Rogers, "The Proper Place of Homeopathy: Hahnemann Medical College and Hospital in an Age of Scientific Medicine," *Pennsylvania Magazine of History and Biography* 108 (1984): 159–201.

Sidney Rosen, "The Origins of High School Biology," *School Science and Mathematics* 59 (1959): 473–84.

Charles E. Rosenberg, "Catechisms of Health: The Body in the Prebellum Class-room," *Bulletin of the History of Medicine* 69 (1995): 175–97.

———, "The Therapeutic Revolution: Medicine, Meaning, and Social Change in 19th-Century America," in Rosenberg, *Explaining Epidemics and Other Essays in the History of Medicine* (Cambridge: Cambridge University Press, 1992).

——— and Carroll-Smith Rosenberg, eds., *The Male-Midwife and the Female Doctor* (New York: Arno Press, 1974).

Dorothy Rosenthal and Rodger Bybee, "Emergence of the Biological Curriculum: A Science of Life or a Science for Living?", in T. S. Popkowitz, ed., *The Forma-tion of School Subjects* (New York: Falmer Press, 1987): 123–44.

Ira Rosenwaike, *Population History of New York City* (Syracuse: Syracuse University Press, 1972).

Dorothy Ross, *The Origins of American Social Science* (Cambridge: Cambridge Uni-versity Press, 1991).

Sydney Ross, *"Scientist:* The Story of a Word," *Annals of Science* 18 (1962): 65–84.

William G. Rothstein, *American Physicians in the Nineteenth Century: From Sects to Science* (Baltimore: Johns Hopkins University Press, 1972).

———, *American Medical Schools and the Practice of Medicine: A History* (Oxford: Oxford University Press, 1987).

Gayle Rubin, "The Traffic in Women: Notes on the 'Political Economy' of Sex," in Rayna R. Reiter, ed., *Toward an Anthropology of Women* (New York: Monthly Review Press, 1975).

Jay Ruby, *Secure the Shadow: Death and Photography in America* (Cambridge: MIT Press, 1995).

Cynthia Eagle Russett, *Sexual Science: The Victorian Construction of Womanhood* (Cam-bridge: Harvard University Press, 1989).

Mary Ryan, *Cradle of the Middle-Class: The Family in Oneida County, New York, 1790–1860* (Cambridge: Cambridge University Press, 1981).

Morris Harold Saffron, *Samuel Clossy, M.D. (1762–1786)* (New York: Haffner, 1967).

G. C. Sanchez, "John Collins Warren," in M. Kaufman et al., eds., *Dictionary of American Medical Biography* (Westport, CT: Greenwood Press, 1984) 2:779.

Karen Sánchez-Eppler, *Touching Liberty: Abolition, Feminism, and the Politics of the Body* (Berkeley: University of California Press, 1993).

Todd L. Savitt, "The Use of Blacks for Medical Experimentation in the Old South," *Journal of Southern History* 48 (1982): 331–48.

Jonathan Sawday, *The Body Emblazoned: Dissection and the Human Body in Renaissance Culture* (New York–London: Routledge, 1995).

A. H. Saxon, *P. T. Barnum: The Legend and the Man* (New York: Columbia University Press, 1989).

Alexander Saxton, *The Rise and Fall of the White Republic: Class Politics and Mass Culture in Nineteenth-Century America* (London–New York: Verso, 1990).

Londa Schiebinger, "Skeletons in the Closet: The First Illustrations of the Female Skeleton in 18th-Century Anatomy," *Representations* 14 (1986): 42–82.

———, *The Mind Has No Sex?: Women in the Origins of Modern Science* (Cambridge: Harvard University Press, 1989).

Esther Schor, *Bearing the Dead: The British Culture of Mourning from the Enlightenment to Victoria* (Princeton: Princeton University Press, 1994).

Hillel Schwartz, *The Culture of the Copy: Striking Likenesses, Unreasonable Facsimiles* (New York: Zone Books, 1996).

Donald A. Scott, "The Popular Lecture and the Creation of a Public in Mid-19th-Century America," *Journal of American History* 66 (1980): 791–809.

Hal D. Sears, *The Sex Radicals: Free Love in High Victorian America* (Lawrence: Regents Press of Kansas, 1977).

Eve Kosofsky Sedgwick, *Between Men: English Literature and Male Homosocial Desire* (New York, Columbia University Press, 1985).

Mark Seltzer, *Bodies and Machines* (New York: Routledge, 1992).

Susan Shifrin, "'The Worst Are Women Doctors': Nineteenth-Century Attitudes Toward the Appearance and Professionalism of Women Physicians," *Transactions & Studies of the College of Physicians of Philadelphia*, ser. 5, 16 (12–1994): 47–65.

Charles Shively, *A History of the Conception of Death in America, 1650–1860* (New York: Garland, 1988).

John Shrady, ed., *The College of Physicians and Surgeons, New York, and its Founders, Officers, Instructors, Benefactors and Alumni: A History* (New York-Chicago: Lewis, 1903).

Richard H. Shryock, *The Development of Modern Medicine: An Interpretation of the Social and Scientific Factors Involved* [1936] (Madison: University of Wisconsin Press, 1979).

——, *Medicine and Society in America, 1660–1860* (New York: New York University Press, 1960).

——, *Medicine in America: Historical Essays* (Baltimore: Johns Hopkins Press, 1966).

Suzanne M. Shultz, *Body Snatching: The Robbing of Graves for the Education of Physicians in Early Nineteenth Century America* (Jefferson, NC and London: MacFarland, 1992).

Richard A. Shweder and Edmund J. Bourne, "Does the Concept of the Person Vary Cross-Culturally?", in A. J. Marsella and G. M. White, eds., *Cultural Conceptions of Mental Health and Therapy* (Dordrecht: Reidel, 1982), 97–137.

Harry J. Sievers, *The Harrison Horror* (Fort Wayne, IN: Public Library of Fort Wayne and Allen County, 1956).

Nancy Siraisi, *Medieval and Early Renaissance Medicine: An Introduction to Knowledge and Practice* (Chicago: University of Chicago Press, 1990).

——, "Vesalius and the Reading of Galen's Teleology," *Renaissance Quarterly* 50 (1997): 1–37.

David Charles Sloane, *The Last Great Necessity: Cemeteries in American History* (Baltimore: Johns Hopkins University Press, 1991).

Philip Sohm, "Gendered Style in Italian Art Criticism from Michelangelo to Malvasia," *Renaissance Quarterly* 48 (1995): 759–808.

James Alfred Spalding, *Dr. Lyman Spalding: the Originator of the United States Pharmacopeia* (Boston: W.M. Leonard Publishers, 1916).

Barbara M. Stafford, *Body Criticism: Imaging the Unseen in Enlightenment Art and Medicine* (Cambridge: MIT Press, 1991).

David E. Stannard, "Death and Dying in Puritan New England," *American Historical Review* 78 (1973): 1305–30.

——, *The Puritan Way of Death: A Study in Religion, Culture, and Social Change* (New York: Oxford University Press, 1977).

————, ed., *Death in America* (Philadelphia: University of Pennsylvania Press, 1974).

Paul Starr, *The Social Transformation of American Medicine* (New York: Basic Books, 1982).

Gertrude Stein, *Three Lives* [1913] (New York: Penguin, 1990).

Nancy Stepan, *The Idea of Race in Science: Great Britain, 1800–1960* (London: Macmillan Press, 1982).

Madeleine B. Stern, *Heads & Headlines: The Phrenological Fowlers* (Norman: University of Oklahoma Press, 1971).

Taylor Stoehr, *Hawthorne's Mad Scientist: Pseudoscience and Social Science in Nineteenth-Century Life and Letters* (Hamden, CT: Archon Books, 1978).

————, ed., *Free Love in America: A Documentary History* (New York: AMS Press, 1979).

I. N. Stokes, *The Iconography of Manhattan Island* (New York, 1928).

Byron Stookey, "Samuel Clossy, A.B., M.D., F.R.C.P. of Ireland: First Professor of Anatomy, King's College (Columbia), New York," *Bulletin of the History of Medicine* 38 (1964): 153–67.

Bryan Strong, "Ideas of the Early Sex-Education Movement in America," 1890–1920," *History of Education Quarterly* 12 (1972): 129–61.

Charles W. Taylor, *Sources of the Self: The Making of Modern Identity* (Cambridge: Harvard University Press, 1989).

Graham Taylor, *Physiognomy in the European Novel: Faces and Fortunes* (Princeton: Princeton University Press, 1982).

John Tebbel, *The Media in America* (New York: Mentor, 1974).

James S. Terry, "Dissecting Room Portraits: Decoding an Underground Genre," *History of Photography* 7.2 (1983): 96–98.

Paul Theerman, "Dionysius Lardner's American Tour: A Case Study in Antebellum American Interest in Science, Technology, and Nature," in Theerman and K. Hunger Parshall, eds., *Experiencing Nature* (Amsterdam: Kluwer Academic, 1997), 211–36.

Kendall Thomas, "Beyond the Privacy Principle," *Columbia Law Review* 92 (1992).

Robert C. Toll, *Blacking Up: The Minstrel Show in Nineteenth-Century America* (New York: Oxford University Press, 1974).

Jonathan R. Topham, "Beyond the 'Common Context': The Production and Reading of the Bridgewater Treatises," *Isis* 89 (1998): 233–62.

Laurel Thatcher Ulrich, *A Midwife's Tale: The Life of Martha Ballard, Based on Her Diary, 1785–1812* (New York: Knopf, 1990).

U.S. Department of Commerce, *Historical Statistics of the United States* (Washington, DC: GPO, 1975).

Philip Van Ingen, *The New York Academy of Medicine: Its First Hundred Years* (New York: Columbia University Press, 1949).

Martha H. Verbrugge, "The Social Meaning of Personal Health: The Ladies' Physiological Institute of Boston and Vicinity in the Mid-19th Century," in Susan Reverby and David Rosner, eds., *Health Care in America: Essays in Social History* (Philadelphia: Temple University Press, 1979).

————, *Able-Bodied Womanhood: Personal Health and Social Change in 19th-Century Boston* (New York: Oxford University Press, 1988).

Camilo José Vergara and Kenneth Jackson, *Silent Cities: The Evolution of the American Cemetery* (Princeton: Princeton Architectural Press, 1989).

Ralph G. Victor, "An Indictment for Grave Robbing at the Time of the 'Doctors' Riot,' 1788," *Annals of Medical History*, 3d ser., 2 (1940): 366–70.

Maris Vinovkis, "Angels' Heads and Weeping Willows: Death in Early America," in T. Hareven, ed., *Themes in the History of the Family* (Worcester: American Antiquarian Society, 1978).

F. B. Wagner and J. W. Savacool, eds., *Thomas Jefferson University: A Chronological History and Alumni Directory* (Philadelphia: Thomas Jefferson University, 1992).

Frederick Clayton Waite, "The First Independent Proprietary Medical School in New England, at Castleton, Vermont, in 1818," *Annals of Medical History* n.s. 7 (May 1935): 242–52.

———, "The Second Medical School in Ohio, at Worthington, 1830–1840," *Ohio State Medical Journal* 33 (1937): 1334–35.

———, "An Episode in Massachusetts in 1818 Related to the Teaching of Anatomy," *New England Journal of Medicine* 220 (1939): 221–28.

———, "The Development of Anatomical Laws in the States of New England," *New England Journal of Medicine* 233 (1945): 716–26.

———, "Grave Robbing in New England," *Bulletin of the Medical Library Association* 33 (1945): 272–94.

T. B. Wakeman, *In Memory of Edward Bliss Foote, M.D.: A "Beloved Physician," of the New, Scientific, Human, Social, "Agnostic" Faith. . . . The Funeral Address Delivered. . . .* (New York: Edward Bond Foote, 1907).

Judith R. Walkowitz, *Prostitution and Victorian Society: Women, Class, and the State* (Cambridge: Cambridge University Press, 1980).

———, *City of Dreadful Delight: Narratives of Sexual Danger in Late-Victorian London* (Chicago: University of Chicago Press, 1992).

Ronald G. Walters, *The Antislavery Appeal: American Abolitionism after 1830* (Baltimore: Johns Hopkins University Press, 1976).

James J. Walsh, *History of Medicine in New York: Three Centuries of Medical Progress* (New York: National American Society, 1919) 5 vols.

Mary Walsh, *Doctors Wanted: No Women Need Apply: Sexual Barriers in the Medical Profession, 1835–1975* (New Haven: Yale University Press, 1977).

Walter I. Wardwell, *Chiropractic: History and Evolution of a New Profession* (St. Louis: Mosby Year Book, 1992).

John Harley Warner, "Physiology," in Ronald Numbers, ed., *The Education of American Physicians: Historical Essays* (Berkeley: University of California Press, 1980).

———, *The Therapeutic Perspective: Medical Practice, Knowledge, and Identity in America, 1820–1885* (Cambridge: Harvard University Press, 1986).

———, "Ideals of Science and Their Discontents in Late Nineteenth-Century American Medicine," *Isis* 82 (1991): 454–78.

———, "Remembering Paris: Memory and the American Disciples of French Medicine in the 19th Century," *Bulletin of the History of Medicine* 65 (1991): 301–25.

———, "Science, Healing, and the Physician's Identity: A Problem of Professional Character in 19th-Century America," *Clio Medica* 22 (1991): 65–88.

————, *Against the Spirit of System: The French Impulse in Nineteenth-Century American Medicine* (Princeton: Princeton University Press, 1998).

Patricia A. Watson, *The Angelical Conjunction: The Preacher-Physicians of Colonial New England* (Knoxville: University of Tennessee Press, 1991).

Susan Wells, *Out of the Dead House: Nineteenth-Century Women Physicians and the Practice of Medicine* (Madison: University of Wisconsin Press, 2000).

Joachim Whaley, ed., *Mirrors of Mortality: Studies in the Social History of Death* (New York: St. Martin's Press, 1981).

James C. Whorton, "'Christian Physiology': William Alcott's Prescription for the Millenium," *Bulletin of the History of Medicine* 49 (1975): 466–81.

————, "William Andrus Alcott," in M. Kaufman et al., eds., *Dictionary of American Medical Biography* (Westport, CT: Greenwood Press, 1984), 1: 10–11.

Alexander Wilder, "Eclectic Medicine in the Eastern States," *Transactions, National Eclectic Medical Association* 20 (1892–93): 475–81.

Sean Wilentz, *Chants Democratic: New York City and the Rise of the American Working Class, 1788–1850* (New York: Oxford University Press, 1984).

Steven Robert Wilf, "Anatomy and Punishment in Late Eighteenth-Century New York," *Journal of Social History* 22 (1989): 507–30.

Raymond Williams, *Keywords: A Vocabulary of Culture and Society* (rev. ed., New York: Oxford University Press, 1983).

Adrian Wilson, *The Making of Man-Midwifery: Childbirth in England, 1660–1770* (Cambridge: Harvard University Press, 1995).

Mary Winkler, "The Anatomical Theater," *Literature and Medicine* 12 (1993): 65–80.

Joel Peter Witkin and Stanley Burns, *Masterpieces of Medical Photography: Selections from the Burns Archive* (Pasadena, CA: Twelvetree Press, 1987).

Arthur Wrobel, "Orthodoxy and Respectability in Nineteenth-Century Phrenology," *Journal of Popular Culture* 9 (1975): 38–50

————, "Phrenology as Political Science," in A. Wrobel, ed., *Pseudo-Science and Society in Nineteenth-Century America* (Lexington, KY: University Press of Kentucky, 1987).

Walter S. Wurzburger, "Cadavers: Jewish Perspectives," in W. T. Reich, ed., *Encyclopedia of Bioethics* (New York: Free Press, 1978), I: 144–45.

Viviana A. Zelizer, "Human Values and the Market: The Case of Life Insurance and Death in 19th-Century America," *American Journal of Sociology* 84/3 (November 1978): 591–610.

————, *The Social Meaning of Money* (New York: Basic Books, 1994).

Dissertations, Conference Papers, and Other Unpublished Works

Harold M. Childs, "A History of the School Health Education Program in New York State" (Doc. Educ. diss., Syracuse University, 1961).

Otto Christy, "The Development of the Teaching of General Biology in the Secondary Schools" (Ph.D. diss., education, George Peabody College for Teachers, 1936).

Eric Engles, "Biology Education in the Public High Schools of the United States from the Progressive Era to the Second World War: A Discursive History" (Ph.D. diss., sociology, University of California, Santa Cruz, 1991).

Sara S. Gronim, "Ambiguous Empire: The Knowledge of the Natural World in British Colonial New York" (Ph.D. diss., history, Rutgers University, 1999).

Jonathan Harris, "The Rise of Medical Science in New York 1720–1820" (Ph.D. diss., history, New York University, 1971).

Susan E. Lederer, "Human Experimentation and Antivivisectionism in Turn-of-the-Century America" (Ph.D. diss., history, University of Wisconsin–Madison, 1987).

Catha Grace Rambusch, "Museums and Other Collections in New York City, 1790–1870" (M.A., American civilization, New York University, 1965).

Dale C. Smith, "The Emergence of Organized Clinical Instruction in the 19th-Century American Cities of Boston, New York, and Philadelphia" (Ph.D. diss., history, University of Minnesota, 1979).

Martin Cornelius Van Buren, "The Indispensable God of Health: A Study of Republican Hygiene and the Ideology of William Alcott" (Ph.D. diss., history, University of California, Los Angeles, 1977).

Philip Van Ingen, Notes on private teaching organizations in New York City [New York, ca. 1940; NYAM].

————, Notes on the origin and history of medical schools in New York and New England [New York, ca. 1945; NYAM].

Patricia A. Vertinsky, "Education for Sexual Morality: Moral Reform & the Regulation of American Sexual Behavior in the 19th Century" (Ed.D. diss., University of British Columbia, 1975).

Abernethy, John, 118, 144, 146
Agnew, D. H., 74, 314, 340, 381–82
Alcott, Bronson, 176, 361
Alcott, William Andrus, 34, 64, 146, 175–92, 195, 202–3, 206–7, 210, 249, 282, 291, 300, 333, 339, 361–63, 368, 375
alternative medicine and anatomy, 7–8, 12, 136–67, 241, 244, 304, 352, 354, 359, 370–71, 379–80
American Medical Association, 69, 98, 339
American Museum of Natural History, 295
American Social Science Association, 323–24, 345
anatomical body, 1, 7–8, 12, 143, 151, 155, 160–61, 306–7, 315, 353; and alternative medicine, 143, 166, 353; and bourgeois identity, 166, 177, 182, 209, 238, 241; and Christianity, 187; as commodity, 320–21; and death, 179–80, 259–60; and electromagnetism, 155–60; compared to house, 178, 180–83; and illustration in print, 175–76, 185, 291; and pathology, 91–92, 154, 185, 227, 280, 283, 291, 207, 299–300, 304; and popular culture, 213; and radical cultural politics, 201, 207, 240–41; and race, 89, 254; and self, 8, 12, 182, 238, 241, 271, 273, 325–27; and sex, 85, 262–63, 280, 323; as spectacle, 192, 201, 209, 304
anatomical representation, 175
anatomist, fear of, 12, 74, 96, 235
anatomy: and bioethics, 98–135; and butchery, 4, 6, 31, 37, 137, 141–42, 270–71, 319; stance vs. cadaver, 5, 74–88, 95, 217, 231, 256, 258, 303; and class, 1–2, 4–7, 9, 321–23; criticism of, 7, 58, 79, 87–88, 95, 113, 138, 140, 145, 179; and cultural authority, 9, 12, 16, 19, 39, 41–43, 48, 52, 55, 59, 61, 64–65, 68, 71, 75–76, 95–100, 140, 143–45, 150–52, 154, 156, 161–62, 169, 172, 189, 193, 215, 225, 227, 236, 259–60, 266, 272–73, 280, 282, 292, 306–7, 316, 324, 326, 344, 368; decline of,

239, 313–14, 319; enthusiasm for, 6, 48–49, 53–60, 74–75, 105, 111–12, 138, 140, 197, 201, 278, 329; compared to geography, 6, 46, 78, 179, 182, 200–201, 249, 268, 282, 340, 361; history of, 2, 47–53, 77–78, 84, 96; and the law, 99–114, 117–24, 127–35; and medical education. *See* medical education; as the foundation of medicine, 69, 76, 79, 140, 143, 151, 227, 259; impact on physic and surgery, 53–57; as professional and public performance, 90–95; as photographic subject, 82–83, 89; and religion, 79, 149, 172, 187–89; and race, 1, 22, 45, 87, 89, 169, 184–85, 210, 241, 243, 246–48, 253, 255–59, 263, 265, 268, 272–73, 277, 306, 329, 335, 362, 365, 373; and school curriculum, 190, 249; as a science, 2, 4, 7, 17, 45, 47, 49, 53–58, 62, 65–66, 68, 75, 90, 95, 98, 100, 109, 123, 128, 130–31, 133, 140–41, 144–45, 147–48, 151, 156, 169, 172–74, 184, 219, 225, 227, 231, 236–37, 254, 276, 313–14, 323, 340, 347; and women, 1, 3, 6–7, 19, 49, 61–62, 81, 87–90, 148, 168–70, 173, 192–95, 201, 203–4, 206, 213, 216, 218, 239, 241, 247, 255, 263–66, 268, 270, 273–74, 292–93, 307, 322–24, 338–39, 343, 364
anatomy acts, 4–5, 12, 117–22, 125, 127–35, 173–74, 238, 316, 318, 321, 323, 350, 376; British (1832), 121–23; Connecticut (1833), 323; Massachusetts (1831), 121, 123; New York (1854), 105, 123, 126–35, 236–37
Anderson, James, 84
Andral, Gabriel, 52
animism, 16, 23, 77, 187, 256, 261
antivaccinationism, 245, 273
antivivisectionism, 19, 245, 273–74, 327, 376
Ariès, Philippe, 329
Army Medical Museum, 305
atheism, 42, 79, 149, 172, 189
auto-icon, 119, 129, 322, 349
autopsy, 42, 51–52, 57, 61, 71, 92–93, 103, 152, 154, 156, 247, 323–24, 329, 346

Bacon, Francis, and Baconian science, 55–56, 149, 164, 340

bacteriological revolution, 57, 314

Ballard, Martha, 61, 338

Bard, John, 346

Barnum, P. T., 92–93, 201, 292, 295, 307, 344, 377, 379–80

Baskette, Dr., Museum of Anatomy, 92,

Bayley, Richard, 105, 111

Beach, Wooster, 143, 161, 165, 278, 283, 290, 292–93, 308, 354, 359, 379

Beddoes, Thomas, 170, 359

Beecher, Catharine, 161, 193–95, 291, 364, 375

Beecher, Henry Ward, 198, 267, 371, 374

Bennett, D. M., 243, 370, 383

Bennett, Stella Kneeland, 187, 363

Bentham, Jeremy, 34, 118–19, 129, 322, 349

Bentley, William, 277–78, 307, 378

Bichat, Xavier, 52–53, 77, 162, 189

Bird, Lucy, 30, 332

blackness and death, 85, 256–58

Blackwell, Elizabeth, 26–27, 89, 195, 332, 343, 350

Boardman, Andrew, 350

body snatching, 3–5, 12–13, 35–38, 76, 84, 106, 108, 112–20, 125, 131, 134, 215, 236, 303, 316–17, 320–21, 325, 335, 343, 345–47, 348, 352, 376, 382; and class, 4, 87, 113, 120, 131, 215, 218–19, 223, 316, 321, 348; economics of, 113, 320; fear of, 13–14, 19, 113; Ipswich scandal (1818), 13, 18; and the law, 98–103, 109–113, 121–22, 134; as rape, 5, 87, 216, 220; and race, 87; in sensationalist fiction, 216–20, 222–24, 230, 366; as student ritual, 80–87, 95–96, 125, 343

Bone Bill. *See* anatomy acts, New York

bonesetting, 144, 163–67, 172, 358–59

Boston Physiological Society, 189

botanical medicine, 6, 98, 138–49, 165, 190, 242, 353–54, 363

Boyle, Robert, 56, 359

Bowery, the, 12, 274, 283, 294, 299, 298, 300, 304, 306–9, 381

Braman, Rev. Milton, 42

Bridgewater Treatises, 359

Brigham, Amariah, 174, 359

Broussais, François, 52, 162, 189

Buchner, Ludwig, 259

burial, 4, 18, 29, 33–34, 42, 110, 124, 134, 326, 347, 350; and class identity, 30–31, 35–38, 101, 104, 107, 115, 121, 131–35, 273, 322, 352; after dissection, 121; premature, 28, 223; and race, 107; societies, 130, 135; reform of, 37, 72, 243, 326, 334, 350, 352

Burke and Hare case, 118, 318–19

burking, in America, 236, 318–19

Bushman, Richard, 181, 332, 339, 348, 362

Butler, Benjamin, 318, 382

Butler, Judith, 11, 329

cabinet of curiosities, 276

cadaver: competition between schools for, 99, 114, 116, 119, 122, 124–27; defense against body snatching, 14, 18; material culture, 29; empathy with, 28; and gender, 85–90; power of, 4, 7, 14–18, 34, 47, 62, 77–78, 96, 119, 129–30, 163, 187, 227, 232, 251, 256, 258–59, 274, 277, 322, 324; provision for medical schools, 4, 6, 47, 99, 102, 105, 110–17, 120–29, 134, 138, 162, 172, 314, 316, 320, 348, 350, 353, 368; role in medical education, 74–80; and self, 20–24, 27–29; trade in, 117, 122, 317–20; uses of, 34, 117–21, 184, 341, 349

Carroll, Hermanus, 346

Cathell, D. W., 94, 344

Calvinism, 16, 22–24, 41, 244, 332,

cemeteries, 12, 29–30, 35, 42, 134, 168, 256, 316, 322, 332, 334, 352

Carroll, Lewis, 249

Channing, Walter, 338

Channing, William Ellery, 210

Child, Lydia Maria, 202, 206

chiropractic, 153, 167, 358, Chovet, Abraham, 277, 307

chrono-thermalism, 151, 351

Civil War, American, 238–39, 368, 372, 379

class, 10–12, 14–15, 18–19, 24–27, 30, 34–39, 51, 61–63, 66–67, 83, 87–88, 100, 116, 120–21, 128–29, 131–35, 139, 142, 149–50, 158–61, 163, 168–215, 219–20, 222, 236, 243, 245–46, 253–55, 264–65, 268, 270–74, 277–78, 280, 294–95, 298, 303, 306–8, 315–16, 318, 320–24, 332–34, 338, 349, 352–53, 359, 365, 367, 372–73, 383

Cleveland anatomy riot, 106, 136–37

Clinton, George, 108
Clirehugh, Vair, 151
Clossy, Samuel, 102–03, 105, 346
Coffin, John Gorham, 99
College of Physicians and Surgeons, Fairfield, 67
College of Physicians and Surgeons, New York (P&S), 68, 91, 111–12, 114, 116–17, 121–22, 343, 347, 370, 379
Collyer, Robert, 153, 174
Columbia College, 105–07, 111; King's College, 102–03, 105
Combe, George, 174–75, 186
comparative anatomy, 50–51, 140, 289, 313
Comstock, Anthony, 207, 241, 244, 248, 266–68, 273–74, 299–302, 305–7, 309–10, 358, 374–75, 380–81
Comstock laws, 244
Conkling, F. A., 129, 351,
Coventry, C. B., 169, 359,
Crowell, Rev. Robert, 13, 18, 38, 329–31, 334
cultural poetics, 2, 8, 76, 96, 136, 150, 220, 340
Cunningham, William, 236, 317
Cutter, Calvin, 157, 187–88, 192, 364, 375

Dartmouth , 101
Darwinism, 239, 373
Davis, Andrew Jackson, 152, 154, 156, 158, 357–58
Davis, Nathan S., 68–69, 339
Dawson, Peter, 130
death and the body, 1, 3–4, 13–43, 96, 217, 259–60, 329–34, 337; authority over, 41–43, 51, 97, 217, 327, 344; beautiful death, 5, 31, 35, 39, 41, 234; and capitalism, 133; Christian beliefs about, 22–23, 39; and the female body, 215–16, 220, 227, 233–35, 237, 366, 368; folk beliefs about, 14, 16–17, 34, 163; and funerary practice, 16, 18, 29–30, 39, 334; as conclusion of life narrative, 22, 30–35, 39, 41–43, 333; material culture of, 28–30, 33, 35–37, 334; medical authority over, 39–42, 51–53, 61, 80, 84; and photoportraiture, 39–41; and social identity, 4, 7, 13, 16, 34–39, 210, 219–20; stages of, 140, 217; and working people, 4, 16, 18, 34–38, 118, 130, 132, 134–35, 333
Descartes, René, 183

Dickson, Samuel, 151, 210, 356, 366
Dimanche, Madame, 289,
diplomas, medical, 47, 59, 62, 67, 70–71, 76, 92, 105, 120, 138–39 151 370
dissection: of criminals, 3, 45, 91, 94, 100–4; fear of, 104, 113, 118, 135, 273; as punishment, 131
dissecting room: efforts to clean up, 319; as liminal space, 217, 219, 235; pranks and jokery, 81, 84–85, 319
Dixon, E. H., 66–68, 79, 116–17, 339
Doctors' Mob, 105–9
Drake, Daniel, 73, 339–40
Draper, John William, 73, 128, 329, 350, 374, 381,
Ducachet, Henry William, 53–54, 336
Dunglison, Robley, 14, 16, 337, 340–41, 361

eclecticism, 137–38, 143–44, 152, 241, 244, 292, 304, 354, 359, 370–71, 379–80
Edgerly, Samuel, 168, 209–10, 359, 366
Edinburgh, as center of anatomical study, 49, 51, 53, 59, 118, 151, 313, 318
electrotherapy, 150, 152–62
Elias, Norbert, 332
Eliot, George, 78, 341
Eliot, John, 187
Elliot, Rev. Samuel Hayes, 31–32, 38, 132, 133, 333–34, 352
Ely, Ezra Stiles, 187, 363
Emerson, Ralph Waldo, 325, 383
entrepreneurship, anatomical, 6, 8, 64, 150, 152, 161, 204, 240–41, 244, 271, 307–8
eugenics, 144, 241, 243, 245, 248, 251, 262, 264–66, 273, 327
evolutionary theory, 239, 243, 251, 253, 262, 264, 354, 370, 374

Faraday, Michael, 153
Fernandez, Manuel, 95
Finch, Marianne, 208–9, 366
Fishbough, William, 154
Fisher, John D., 349
Fisher, Margaret, 103
Flint, Austin, 197
Foote, Edward Bliss, 8, 239–73, 324, 368–76; arrest by Comstock, 268; biography and social origins, 241–48
Foote, Edward Bond, 370
Forty Years in the Wilderness of Pills and Powders, 176–77, 333, 339, 361, 363

Foucault, Michel, 19, 21–22, 208, 211, 225, 331, 336, 340, 366–67
Fowler, Lydia, 148, 193
Fowler, Orson, 153
Fowlers & Wells, 154, 175, 360
Francis, Samuel Wakefield, 84
Frankenstein, 94, 308, 349, 367
funerals, 16, 29–30, 34–37, 42, 110, 120–21, 132, 330

Galen, 66,
Gall, Franz, 174, 361
Galvani, Luigi, 94, 153
galvanic experiments, 28, 32, 57, 93–95, 153–54, 159, 345, 365
Geneva Medical , 122, 125–26 162, 169, 342, 350, 359
gentility, 10–11, 20, 25–27, 29, 51, 61, 64–65, 99–100, 105, 141
Germania Society, 130
Gibbs, Charles, 279, 290, 344, 377
The Gilded Age, 88–89
Godman, John Davidson, 64–65, 77, 84, 114–15, 340, 348,
Goodrich, S. G., 161, 359
Gordon, Linda, 243, 369–70
Gove, Mary, 157, 179, 193, 195, 364, 375
Graham, Sylvester, 146, 177, 189–90, 193, 363
grave robbery. See body snatching
Grimké, Angelina, 23, 331–32

Hahnemann, Samuel, 138, 148–50, 355
Hamilton, Frank H., 14, 58, 77, 162–63, 330, 340, 358
Hammond, William A., 305, 381
Harper's Monthly, 12, 37, 83, 95, 133, 213–14, 308
Harré, Rom, 1,
Harrison bodysnatching scandal, 316–318, 382
Harvard Medical , 42, 49, 53, 60, 74, 81, 114, 125, 172, 193, 216, 307, 336, 338, 345, 348–50, 353, 366
Harvey, William, 21, 49, 55–56, 66, 272, 331
Helmholtz, Heinrich von, 313
Hering, Constantine, 149
Hersey, Thomas, 144–46
Hertzler, Arthur, 81, 83, 319, 342–43, 382
Heth, Joice, 93, 344, 379

Hippocrates, 66
Hosack, David, 346
Hoffman, Frederick, 334, 352
Hollick, Frederick C., 167, 195–96, 198–211, 213, 249, 291, 344, 359, 365–66, 375, 379
Holmes, E. W., 314, 382
Holmes, Oliver Wendell, 70, 85, 272, 292, 343
homeopathy, 138, 148–50, 152, 162, 317, 352, 355–56
homosociality, 80–84, 88, 90, 203, 217–20, 224, 324, 342
Hooker, Worthington, 355
Hopkinson, Francis, 44–47
Horner, W. E., 75, 112–15, 124–25, 348–49
House I Live In, The, 8, 175, 177–87, 189, 193, 291, 359, 361–64
Hubbardton raid, 343
Hughes, Archbishop John, 131, 351
Hunt, Harriot K., 32–34, 193, 333
Hunter, John, 49, 51, 66, 105, 337
Hunter, William, 47–49
Hunterian anatomy, 48–53, 55, 313
Hunterian Oration, 118
Huntington, Jedediah Vincent, 219, 367
Huxley, Thomas, 260, 372
Hygieia, 170, 359

iconography: anatomical 76, 92, 151, 185, 315, 319; of death, 35
Illich, Ivan, 333
insurance, 36, 135, 352
interracial love, 247, 265, 268
introductory lectures, 14, 126, 162, 313,
Irish Emigrant Society, 130
irregular medicine. See alternative medicine and anatomy

Jay, John, 108, 110
Jefferson, Thomas, 44, 54, 336, 347
Jefferson Medical , 14, 60, 116, 278
Judd, G. R., 187
Jordan, Henry, 283, 290, 308–9, 378–79
Jordan, Louis J., 283, 308–9, 378
juvenile fiction, 241, 249, 255, 371
Juvenile Rambler, The, 176–77, 361

Kahn, Louis J., 275, 283, 300, 304–10, 377–78, 380–81
Keckley, Elizabeth, 39, 334

Keagy, John M., 186–87, 189, 363, 368
Keen, W. W., 77, 340
Kelly, H. A., 321, 323, 382
King, Dan, 149, 339, 355
King's College. *See* Columbia College

Ladies Physiological Society, 193, 208–09
Laënnec, R.T.H., 52, 336
Lambert, T. S., 161, 190, 249, 323, 364, 371, 374–75
lectures, anatomical, 1, 6, 8, 51–52, 68, 76–77, 102–04, 106, 111–12, 114, 140, 144, 147, 165–66, 168–73, 189–90, 193, 197–98, 201–03, 206, 209, 230, 240–41, 246–47, 258, 265, 270, 308, 315, 317, 342, 360, 364–65, 378; introductory, 14, 162, 313, 336, 338–40, 342–43, 345, 349–59, 354, 358, 377, 383; popular, 6–8, 12, 152, 163, 167–73, 189–93, 196–98, 201–02, 206, 208–210, 213, 239–41, 246–47, 256, 258, 265–66, 270, 278, 291–92, 307–08, 310, 315, 323, 358, 360, 352, 364–65, 373, 375, 381; valedictory, 329–30, 335
Leidy, Joseph, 53, 303–04, 326, 380, 383
Lippard, George, 215, 221–37, 344, 366–67
Lott, Eric, 253–54, 258, 372–73

M'Clintock, James, 55, 330, 336
McDowell, Ephraim, 58
McKnight, W. J., 70, 87, 339, 343
Magoon, Nathan S., 146–47
man-midwifery, 51, 60–63
manikins, anatomical, 197–98, 201–2, 208–9, 280, 362–63, 376
Marietta, 215–20, 225, 235, 366–67
Martineau, Harriet, 29, 35, 332–33, 357
Marvell, Andrew, 25, 332
Masonic conspiracy, 33, 96
Massachusetts anatomy act of 1831, 4, 74, 105, 121–23, 125, 128, 169, 173, 337
Massachusetts Medical Society, 70, 173, 337, 339
Mather, Cotton, 22–23, 331–32
medical education, 2, 4, 47–48, 51, 54–55, 59–60, 62, 64, 67, 74, 76, 89, 103, 105–7, 111–18, 122, 124–26, 128, 136–39, 142–44, 147–50, 167, 171–72, 210, 213, 270, 277, 303, 316, 319, 337, 341, 355–56, 359, 368, 376
medical electricity, 93, 144, 152–56, 162, 167, 198, 219, 259, 344

Medical Reformer, The, 140, 353
medical identity and anatomy, 44–97
medicine: advances in, 14, 19, 47–53, 56–59, 74, 77, 79, 90, 96, 132, 140, 276, 323, 327, 337, 357, 363; as anatomical cult, 44–97; as a bourgeois profession, 63–70; cultural authority of, 4, 12, 19, 39, 48, 55, 59, 61, 64–65, 68–73; vs. midwifery, 61–63; as a fusion of physic and surgery, 53–55; and religion, 40–42, 79; and science, 53–59
memento mori. *See* skeleton
mesmerism, 144, 154, 156, 224, 235, 303, 357, 360
Metropolitan Life Insurance Company, 135, 352
microscopic anatomy, 71, 239, 313
Middleton, Peter, 346
midwives vs. physicians, 60–63, 324, 335–36, 338–39, 353
Millet & Brown, 125
mind/body dichotomy, 2, 4, 8, 15, 19, 22–26, 32–33, 53, 76–77, 80–81, 88, 129, 133, 137, 142, 148, 150, 159, 180, 182–84, 217, 220, 226, 229, 232, 251, 258–61, 291, 299, 303, 325, 331, 373
minstrelsy, 8, 168, 215, 241, 253–58, 292, 315, 372–73
missionaries and anatomy, 184, 187–89
Monro dynasty, 49, 51, 360
Morgan, John, 51, 76, 336, 340,
Morrow, T. V., 143,
Morse, Samuel F. B., 153
Morton, Dr. Charles O., 317
Mott, Valentine, 58, 84, 276, 329, 343, 377, 383
museums and exhibitions, anatomical, 1, 6, 8, 12–13, 35, 71, 91, 136, 138, 144, 168, 193, 201, 210, 212–13, 215, 227, 235, 271, 274–309, 315, 322, 326, 330, 344–45, 349, 377–81

natural bonesetting. *See* bonesetting
natural theology, 6, 77, 170, 177–78, 189, 209, 354, 359; *Natural Theology,* 170, 178, 354, 359
Negro Burying Ground, 45, 107, 347
neo-Thomsonianism, 137, 147, 152, 354
nervous debility and neurasthenia, 265, 299, 299, 305, 378, 380–81

New England's Chattels, 31–32, 38, 132, 133, 333–34, 352
New York Academy of Medicine, 84, 322
New York anatomy act. *See* bone bill
New York City police, 274–75, 290, 300–7, 309
New York Colored Orphan Asylum, 32, 333
New-York Dissector, 154, 357
New York Medico-Legal Society, 305, 380–81
New York Society for the Suppression of Vice, 207, 274–75, 381
Newton, Isaac, 56, 186
novels and anatomy, 3, 8, 12, 88, 94, 212–237, 239, 249, 294, 299, 315, 366–67

An Oration, Which Might Have Been Delivered to the Students in Anatomy, 44–47, 100, 335–36, 341
osteopathy, 167

Paine, Martyn, 128
Paley, William, 144, 146, 170, 178, 354, 359, 361
Papillon, Fernand, 259–60
Parisian anatomy, 52–53, 59, 69–70, 111, 114, 118–19, 140, 152, 162, 278, 336
Parker, Willard, 128
Parkman, Samuel, 125, 192–93, 350
Parley's Magazine, 176, 178, 359
Parsons, Usher, 163, 171–72, 358, 360
pathological anatomy, 52–53, 58, 68, 71, 78, 91, 114, 140, 147, 149, 156, 162, 239, 276–77, 314, 336, 355, 357
Pattison, Granville Sharp, 117, 171–72, 349, 360
paupers' burials. *See* Potter's Field
Peale, Charles Wilson, 275, 295, 307, 308, 377, 380
periodicals, antebellum, 146
Philadelphia almshouse, 18
Philadelphia School of Anatomy, 60, 340
phrenology, 91, 144, 152–54, 174–75, 186, 189, 243–44, 259, 276, 286, 288, 290, 292, 308, 359–61, 370–71, 375, 379
physic, relation to surgery, 51–53
physiology: as a field of knowledge and sub-discipline, 52, 57–58, 68, 70–71, 147, 162, 247, 260, 327, 336, 356; and popular anatomy, 169, 173–74, 189–203, 206–08, 213, 239, 245, 267–73, 296, 315, 359,

361–62; and self-making, 6, 8, 34, 158–59, 170, 175, 178–89, 203–06, 208–13, 239–41, 248–49, 261, 268, 270–71, 291, 296, 35; as a subdiscipline, 239, 313–14, 368, 381
Pierce, Albertus, 321
Poe, Edgar Allan, 26, 215, 221, 332, 357,
popular anatomical museums, 158, 274–309
popular anatomy, 6, 8, 12, 144, 158, 160–61, 168–211, 213, 239–251, 270–309, 314, 323, 365, 380; Alcott, William, as pioneer, 175–78; and anatomy acts, 173–74; and bourgeois self-making, 158, 160–61, 169–70, 176, 178–89, 191–93, 206–7, 209–211; and the Civil War, 239; and domestic ideology, 178–83; and entrepreneurs, 195–207; and evangelical Christianity, 178–79, 184–89; origins of, 169–84, 359–60; and phrenology, 174–75, 360–61; and radicalism, 204–07; resistance and criticism of, 213; and sexuality, 172–73, 177, 181, 184–86, 189, 195, 201, 203–9, 365; and universal human subject, 184–86; and women, 193–95, 202–4, 206
postmortem dissection. *See* autopsy
potter's field, 4, 35–36, 45, 84, 107, 110, 114–15, 117, 124, 135, 138, 322, 350, 352
Powell, William Byrd, 259, 292
Poyen, Charles, 153
preparations. *See* anatomical objects
Prudential Insurance Company, 135, 352
Pullman, George, 322, 382
puritan theology, 22, 25–26, 331–32

Quaker City, The, 215, 220–37, 344, 366–67

Ramsay, Alexander, 53, 112, 170–73, 360
resurrectionism. *See* body snatching
Revere, John, 115, 348
Revere, Paul, 94, 115, 348
Rex v. Lynn (1788), 101
Richardson, Ruth, 16, 18, 23, 330–31, 349, 376
Richardson, James H., 60
riots, anatomy, 4, 19, 44–45, 69, 84, 99, 104, 117–18, 122, 128, 130, 142–43, 163, 176, 323; Cleveland anatomy riot (1852), 106, 136–37, 141–42, 352; Doctor's Mob (New York, 1788), 105–10, 346–47
Robinson, John Hovey, 215–17, 366
Rogers, David L., 91–93, 95

Rolph, John, 60,
Roman Catholicism, 16, 24, 37, 134, 138, 333; Protestant critique of, 16, 24, 138–39, 206, 236
Rosemary, or Life and Death, 219, 367
Rush, Benjamin, 313, 381
Rutgers Medical College, 114–16, 122

Sailors' Mob, 45, 106
Sammy Tubbs the Boy Doctor, 8, 239–41, 245–73, 368, 371–76
Sandwich Islands (Hawaiian islands), 187, 363
Sanford, John F., 77, 338
Sarti, Madame, 208
Scalpel, The, 66, 68, 339, 357
Sears, Hal D., 244, 369–70, 374
Sedgwick, Eve Kosofsky, 342
self making, 8, 12, 26, 38, 158, 174–75, 210, 238–39, 247, 258, 266, 273, 275, 280, 294–95, 325–27, 373, 376
sensationalism, 8, 209, 212–37, 271, 280, 290, 298–99, 315, 366–67
Sewall, Thomas, 13, 330
sex education, 243, 247, 267, 327
Sherwood, Henry Hall, 152–62, 356–58
Shippen, William, Jr., 45, 51, 90, 104, 346
Simons, J. C., 69
Sizer, Nelson, 174, 360–61
skeleton: as anatomical icon, 46, 50, 185; as anatomical object and teaching tool, 176, 193, 198, 201, 290, 300, 349; as death figure, 34, 179, 223, 228, 373; as effigy in riots, 137; as frame of the embodied self, 179, 185, 257; in physicians' offices, 66, 91–93, 151, 235, 256, 303; as prop in student photographs, 83, 89
Smith, Adam, 27, 120, 134, 332
Smith, Ashbel, 69
Smith, Rev. Elias, 353
Smith, Rev. Gibson, 154, 357
Smith, Jerome Van Crowninshield, 74, 175, 193, 339, 359, 361, 363–64
Smith, Joseph, 113, 348
Smith, Thomas Southwood, 119–21, 129, 341, 347–49
social performance, 8–12, 25–27, 30, 36–37, 39, 42, 51, 59, 63, 76, 87, 90, 92–93, 95–96, 132, 137, 141, 149, 151, 207, 211, 215, 217, 219, 225, 232, 235, 238, 240, 254,

258–59, 262, 268–69, 276, 278, 306, 321–25,
Soresi, George, 322–23
spirit/matter dichotomy. *See* mind/body dichotomy
spiritualism, 144, 152, 369–70
Spurzheim, Johann Gaspar, 174
Stephens, Alexander H., 63, 339
Stephens, H. L., 240, 245, 249, 263, 368, 375
Stewart, Frank, 212–13
Stout, Hannah, 1, 3–14
student pranks, 81–85, 319,
Sumner, William Graham, 324, 383
superstition, 4, 7–8, 14–17, 34, 47, 62, 77, 96, 119, 129–30, 163, 187, 232, 251, 256, 258–59, 322, 324
surgery, relation to physic and anatomy, 48–49, 51–54, 56–59, 69, 71, 74
Sweet family, 163, 167, 358
Sweet, Waterman, 162–67, 172, 187, 358–59
Sweeting, Whiting, 103–4, 346

Taylor, Jane, 195–96, 364
Taylor, Charles W., 31, 211, 333, 366
telegraphic body, 153, 158–59, 249, 260, 262, 358
Tewksbury Almshouse scandal, 318, 382
Theory of Moral Sentiment, 27–28, 118, 134, 332
therapeutic nihilism, 149
Thomson, Samuel, 65, 138–40, 142–44, 146–47, 149, 164, 166, 187
Thomson, Wilson, 144–47
Thomsonianism, 138–42, 152, 162, 164, 169, 190, 353–55, 370; adoption of anatomy, 144–48; anatomist's critique of, 142–44
Treatise on Domestic Economy, 193–95, 291, 364, 375
Turkel, Spencer, 346
Turner, William, 351, 356

Ulrich, Laurel Thatcher, 61, 338
universalism, 11–12, 184–85, 210, 241, 256, 258, 273, 291, 362, 372
University of New York (UNY), 73, 124–26, 128
University of Pennsylvania Medical School, 44, 59–60, 74, 111, 113, 116–17, 125, 314, 325, 335–36, 338, 340, 349–50

Ure, Andrew, 94–95, 344
Use of the Dead to the Living, 34, 117, 119–21,
     341, 349
utilitarianism, 5, 34, 118–19, 133, 247, 260,
     349, 373

venereal disease, 204–5, 208, 218, 262, 271,
     288, 296–97, 300, 302–3, 365
Vesalius, Andreas, 21–22, 49, 55–56, 77–78,
     185
von Hagens, Gunther, 327
von Steuben, Baron, 108

Wakeman, Theodore Burr, 242, 250, 270–
     71, 370–72
Walpole, Horace, 90, 343
Warren, John, 49, 60, 81, 93, 338, 342, 345,
     348
Warren, John Collins, 42, 48–49, 52, 72, 74,
     114–15, 125, 172, 193, 307, 322, 334–35,
     337, 339, 348–50, 360, 364
waxes. *See* anatomical objects
Webster, Daniel, 330

Webster, James, 349–50
Weeks, Cyrus, 125, 350
Wesley, John, 354
Whitman, Walt, 154, 170, 357, 359
Wiesenthal, Charles F., 45, 106
Wieting, John M., 195–98, 201, 213, 337,
     365
Wilder, Burt Green, 375
Wilf, Steven Robert, 19, 107, 329, 331, 346–
     47
Williams, H., 278, 378
Williams, Raymond, 9
Willis, Thomas, 49
Wines, Frederick, 324, 383
Woods, James R., 128
Worthington Reformed Medical College,
     106, 143
Wyman, Jeffries, 360

Yale Medical College, 101–2, 106, 117, 123,
     176
Yeldall, Dr. Anthony, 277, 307, 377
Young, John, 105, 347